Critical Reviews in Psychiatry
Second Edition

WITHDRAWN 19/06/24.

Critical Reviews in Psychiatry
Second Edition

Edited by
Tom Brown &
Greg Wilkinson

GASKELL

First edition ©1998 The Royal College of Psychiatrists
©2000 The Royal College of Psychiatrists

British Library Cataloguing-in-Publication Data
A catalogue record for this book is available from the British Library.
ISBN 1-901242-41-2

Distributed in North America by American Psychiatry Press, Inc.

The views presented in this book do not necessarily reflect
those of the Royal College of Psychiatrists, and the publishers
are not responsible for any error or omission of fact. College
seminars are produced by the Publications Department of
the College; they should in no way be construed as providing
a syllabus or other material for any College Examination.

Gaskell is an imprint of the Royal College of Psychiatrists,
17 Belgrave Square, London SW1X 8PG.

The Royal College of Psychiatrists is a registered charity (no. 228636).

Typeset by Dobbie Typesetting Limited, Tavistock, Devon
Printed in Great Britain by Bell & Bain Limited, Thornliebank, Glasgow

Contents

Critical reviews

Contributors

Dr Tom Brown, Consultant Psychiatrist, St John's Hospital at Howden, Livingston, EH4 6PP

Dr John Cookson, Consultant Psychiatrist and Honorary Senior Lecturer, Tower Hamlets Healthcare NHS Trust, The Royal London Hospital (St Clements), 2A Bow Road, London E3 4LL

Dr J. Eagles, Consultant Psychiatrist, Clerkeat Building, Royal Cornhill Hospital, Cornhill Road, Aberdeen AB25 2ZF

Professor Anne E. Farmer, Social, Genetic and Developmental Psychiatry Research Centre, Institute of Psychiatry, 111 Denmark Hill, London SE5 8AF

Dr John Geddes, Senior Clinical Research Fellow and Honorary Consultant Psychiatrist, Department of Psychiatry, Warneford Hospital, Oxford OX3 7JX

Dr Stephen M. Lawrie, Senior Clinical Research Fellow, Department of Psychiatry, Royal Edinburgh Hospital, Edinburgh EH10 5FT

Professor Glyn Lewis, Professor of Community and Epidemiological Psychiatry, University of Wales College of Medicine, Department of Psychological Medicine, Heath Park, Cardiff CF4 4NX

Dr Andrew McIntosh, Lecturer in Psychiatry, Kennedy Tower, Royal Edinburgh Hospital, Morningside Park, Edinburgh EH10 5HF

Dr Angus Mackay, Physician Superintendent and Clinical Director, Argyll and Bute Hospital, Lochgilphead, Argyll PA31 8LD

Dr Max Marshall, Senior Lecturer and Honorary Consultant Psychiatrist, University of Manchester, Department of Community Psychiatry, Guild Academic Centre, Royal Preston Hospital, Sharoe Green Lane North, Fulwood, Preston PR2 9HT

Dr David Owens, Senior Lecturer in Psychiatry, University of Leeds, Academic Unit of Psychiatry, 15 Hyde Terrace, Leeds LS2 9LT

Dr Michael Sharpe, Senior Lecturer, University Department of Psychiatry, Kennedy Tower, Royal Edinburgh Hospital, Edinburgh EH10 5HF

Professor S. C. Wessely, Department of Psychological Medicine, King's College School of Medicine, 103 Denmark Hill, London SE5 9RS

Professor Greg Wilkinson, Department of Psychiatry, University of Liverpool, Liverpool L69 3GA

Acknowledgements

The initiative and preliminary proposal for *Critical Reviews in Psychiatry* arose from discussions among the editors and colleagues at Neurolink. Neurolink is an independent multi-disciplinary advisory board that produces educational materials relating to the management of depressive illness, and is sponsored by Wyeth.

The members of the Neurolink Board are:

> Professor Greg Wilkinson (Chairman), Dr Tom Brown, Dr Phil Cowen, Mr Martin Davies, Dr Chris Freeman, Professor Hugh Freeman, Dr Linda Gask, Dr Graham Jackson, Dr George Kassianos, Dr Amanda Kirby, Dr Siân Koppel, Professor David Nutt, Dr Peter Shaw, Dr Andre Tylee and Ms Kathie Walker.

A detailed proposal was prepared and submitted by the editors, Tom Brown and Greg Wilkinson, to Gaskell Publications. Production costs of *Critical Reviews in Psychiatry* were met in full by Gaskell Publications.

Dr Stephen Tyrer, Chief Examiner, and Tom Sensky, Chairman of the Critical Review Paper Panel of the Examinations Sub-Committee, were informed about the production of *Critical Reviews in Psychiatry* and kindly gave permission for us to reprint the Critical Review Paper Information Pack and the new Critical Review Papers from the Spring 1999 examination onwards. We would also like to thank the *Journal of the American Medical Association* and the *British Medical Journal* for permission to reprint the articles on which the papers were based. The Chief Examiner and colleagues on the Examinations Sub-Committee involved in the preparation of the MRCPsych Part II Examination played no other part in the preparation or production of this book. John Geddes is a member of the Critical Review Working Party and received permission from the Chairman of the Working Party to contribute to this book.

The most challenging task was met by our 'specimen candidates' and to them must go our gratitude and appreciation — we have spared them the embarrassment of awarding marks!

We thank the authors of the original papers for supporting our use of their work for this purpose.

Reference list of papers subject to critical review

Duffett, R. & Lelliott, P. (1998) Auditing electroconvulsive therapy. *British Journal of Psychiatry*, **172**, 401–405.

Hawton, K., Fagg, J., Simkin, S., *et al* (1997) Trends in deliberate self-harm in Oxford, 1985–1995. *British Journal of Psychiatry*, **171**, 556–560.

Hickie, I., Lloyd, A., Wakefield, D., *et al* (1990) The psychiatric status of patients with the chronic fatigue syndrome. *British Journal of Psychiatry*, **156**, 534–540.

Hotopf, M., Hardy, R. & Lewis, G. (1997) Discontinuation rates of SSRIs and bicyclic antidepressants: a meta-analysis and investigation of heterogeneity. *British Journal of Psychiatry*, **170**, 120–127.

Kuipers, E., Garety, P., Fowler, D., *et al* (1997) London–East Anglia randomised controlled trial of cognitive–behavioural therapy for psychosis. *British Journal of Psychiatry*, **171**, 319–327.

Lindsay, M., Crino, R. & Andrews, G. (1997) Controlled trial of exposure and response prevention in obsessive–compulsive disorder. *British Journal of Psychiatry*, **171**, 135–139.

Mason, P., Harrison, G., Croudace, T., *et al* (1997) The predictive validity of a diagnosis of schizophrenia. *British Journal of Psychiatry*, **170**, 321–327.

Oehrberg, S., Christiansen, P. E., Behnke, K., *et al* (1995) Paroxetine in the treatment of panic disorder. A randomised, double-blind, placebo-controlled study. *British Journal of Psychiatry*, **167**, 374–379.

Vollmer-Conna, U., Wakefield, D., Lloyd, A., *et al* (1997) Cognitive deficits in patients suffering from chronic fatigue syndrome, acute infective illness or depression. *British Journal of Psychiatry*, **171**, 377–381.

Wing, J. K., Beevor, A. S., Curtis, R. H., *et al* (1998) Health of the Nation Outcome Scales (HoNOS). *British Journal of Psychiatry*, **172**, 11–18.

Papers used in examinations

Fleming, M. F., Lawton Barry, K., Baier Manwell, L., *et al* (1997) Brief physician advice for problem alcohol drinkers. A randomised controlled trial in community-based primary care practices. *Journal of the American Medical Association*, **277**, 1039–1045.

Kessler, D., Lloyd, K., Lewis, G., *et al* (1999) Cross sectional study of symptom attribution and recognition of depression and anxiety in primary care. *British Medical Journal*, **318**, 436–440.

Mason, P., Harrison, G., Glazebrook, C., *et al* (1995) Characteristics of outcome in schizophrenia at 13 years. *British Journal of Psychiatry*, **167**, 596–603.

Sadowski, H., Ugarte, B., Kolvin, I., *et al* (1999) Early life family disadvantages and major depression in adulthood. *British Journal of Psychiatry*, **174**, 112–120.

Introduction

This book is aimed at psychiatrists in training who are taking the MRCPsych Part II Examination, which introduced a Critical Review Paper in 1999. We are pleased to include the first three MRCPsych Critical Review Papers in this second edition (Appendix 1).

Critical Review Paper

Psychiatrists should be able to evaluate published literature both in terms of its scientific validity and its clinical relevance. In the Information Pack (Appendix 2) issued by the College in relation to the introduction of the Critical Review Paper the College highlights the fact that good clinical practice is based on a combination of clinical judgement and sound application of research-based evidence. It is noted that pscyhiatrists will need to acquire new skills and confidence in critical appraisal of research and its application to their clinical work.

In preparation for the introduction of the Critical Review Paper the College conducted two pilot examinations and took cognisance of comments from both examiners and the candidates who sat them. The Information Pack for candidates contains two pilot papers and a reading list. The stated intention of the paper is to test candidates in the principles and methodology of evidence-based medicine (EBM).

Aims of the Critical Review Paper

These are clearly stated in the Information Pack (in Appendix 2). They include.

- (a) Understanding research design and methodology.
- (b) Understanding sources of problems and bias in different kinds of research methodology.
- (c) Understanding basic statistics.
- (d) Definitions and meanings of measures important in critical appraisal, for example: sensitivity, specificity, odds ratio.
- (e) Knowledge of methodology of systematic reviews and meta-analysis.
- (f) How to determine reliability and validity of results.
- (g) (Clinical relevance of) results in scientific papers.
- (h) How to detect errors in research methodology and design.
- (i) Understanding the process and results of critical appraisal of a scientific paper.
- (j) Ability to suggest further experiments which would confirm or increase understanding in the field under investigation.
- (k) Placing important results of scientific papers in their clinical context and seeing how they might alter clinical practice.

Critical Reviews in Psychiatry

At the time we decided to produce the first edition of this book, as far as we were aware, there was no other book on the psychiatric aspects of critical review. We therefore wanted to produce a book which would be useful reading for all psychiatric trainees taking the MRCPsych Examination. We ourselves only had access to information from the College which was in the public domain and had seen no more than the two pilot papers produced by the College. Given the aims of the Critical Review Paper we decided it was more important when selecting our papers to include those representative of different types of research methodology, for example, randomised controlled trials, cohort studies, case–controlled studies, qualitative studies and meta-analyses. This, in our view, took precedence over any attempt to cover different areas of psychiatry.

We asked all of our contributors to assess the papers we sent them under exam conditions. Each was sent an edited version of a paper and a specimen examination paper with the instruction to take 60 minutes to complete the task. We felt this would bring an important realism and credibility to the material contained in this book. Just as there is no such thing as the perfect study, there is no such thing as the perfect answer. Also bear in mind that the edited version contains less information than the original paper. Some of the questions would have been answered differently if the full article had been made available. Our reviewers all have considerable research expertise and we are sure you will find their illustrative answers informative. However, it is only fair to confess that although some followed our instructions, others admitted to taking longer. Dr Eagles, for example, advised us: "to emphasise . . . that when authors are providing specimen answers, they are pretty keen for them to be good specimen answers which leads to cheating. Naturally, today's trainees might be much sharper than I am, but if they are not then we risk demoralising them if they think an ordinary psychiatrist could write such a lengthy answer in an hour."

Please note the Critical Review Paper is now allotted 90 minutes not 60 minutes, as for the pilot papers!

How to use this book

Begin by familiarising yourself with the College Information Pack in Appendix 2 and by reading Lawrie's introductory chapter on EBM. In addition, we would particularly recommend the book by Sackett et al (1996, 1999) as a concise introductory text on evidence-based medicine. We also draw attention to Dr McIntosh's 'Trainee's Viewpoint' (pp. 11–12).

Critical Reviews in Psychiatry is structured as follows. Following the introductory material, there are 10 critical reviews comprising:

(a) A specimen article for critical review.

(b) An examination-style question paper.

(c) Illustrative answers.

(d) The full published article for reference and close reading (in Appendix 3).

Finally, there are the first three MRCPsych Critical Review Papers. We invite you to attempt each paper under 'exam conditions'.

Some tips

To make your task easier when you attempt these critical reviews – and the real thing – remember these tips:

(a) Read the question paper before reading the article for critical review.

(b) Prepare your thoughts using rough notes before answering the question paper and make sure you understand, in particular, the type of study and the subject of the investigation.

(c) Re-read each question carefully and make sure you tackle each component of it.

(d) Choose an order in which you wish to answer the questions posed, beginning with questions you can answer fully and at once leaving until later those that may require more consideration.

(e) Look at the number of marks allotted to each question and allocate your time for each answer in the same proportion. For example, a question with 10 marks may have five components each with two marks or *vice versa*.

(f) Answer only the question that is being asked.

(g) Pay attention to the wording of the questions and structure your answers appropriately. If you are asked to 'list' – use words or short phrases. If you are asked to 'discuss' – use sentences and short paragraphs. If you are asked to 'compare and contrast' remember to do both.

(h) Attempt an answer for each question.

(i) Write clearly and make your answer for each component of a question clear (using the appropriate numbers or headings) so that the examiner can properly evaluate your answer.

(j) Refer to established work (author, date) if you are confident it is relevant to your answer.

We hope you find *Critical Reviews in Psychiatry* interesting, useful and enjoyable. We would welcome receipt of all constructive criticism and comments directed at making improvements to future editions.

Tom M. Brown
Greg Wilkinson

References

Sackett, D., Richardson, W., Rosenburg, W., *et al* (eds) (1996) *Evidence-Based Medicine: How to Practice and Teach EBM*. London: Churchill Livingstone.

—— , Straus, S. E., Richardson, W. S., *et al* (eds) (1999) *Evidence-Based Medicine: How to Practice and Teach EBM* (2nd edn). London: Churchill Livingstone.

Making sense of the numbers in evidence-based medicine
Stephen M. Lawrie

As doctors, we diagnose, treat and make prognoses about our patients. These decisions are guided by our training and clinical experience, but must be informed by important new research findings. Relevant studies must first be located, which is probably most effectively done by reading secondary publication sources such as the journal *Evidence-Based Mental Health*. Identified studies must then be 'critically appraised' in terms of scientific merit and clinical importance. Statistically significant results, even from rigorously conducted clinical research, are not necessarily clinically significant. For example, large treatment trials may report statistical differences, which might only benefit a small number of patients in clinical practice. The development of reliable and useful indices of clinical importance has been a central concern of the pioneers of the evidence-based medicine movement (Sackett *et al*, 1996, 1999). This brief review aims to explain these indices to a psychiatric audience.

Let's imagine that you have been asked by local general practitioners to provide useful information about the diagnosis, treatment and prognosis of depression in primary care. In particular, they want to know about a potential simple screening test, the efficacy of new antidepressants and how many patients will recover within one year. It just so happens that you are able to locate three relevant articles that look promising, and you set about devising clinically useful summary information.

Diagnosis

The hypothetical diagnosis paper evaluated the performance of a number of questions in identifying depressive illness as compared with the 'gold standard', that is, a structured psychiatric interview and diagnostic criteria. Crucially, all eligible subjects received both assessments from interviewers who were blind to the results of the other test. Let's say that many of the screening questions performed adequately, but the best balance of sensitivity and specificity was obtained with the simple question "Have you felt depressed for the past two weeks?" The performance of the screening and standard tests are shown in Table 1.

The screening question found 25 of the 30 patients identified as being depressed by the gold standard, and 60 of the 70 patients identified by the gold standard as not being depressed. These comparative

Table 1. Diagnosis. Gold standard diagnostic interview

	Depressed	Not depressed	Total
Screening question			
Depressed	25 (a)	10 (b)	35 (a+b)
Not depressed	5 (c)	60 (d)	65 (c+d)
Total	30 (a+c)	70 (b+d)	100 (N)

rates are the 'sensitivity' and 'specificity' of the screening question respectively, that is, the ability of the test to detect true positives and true negatives as judged by the gold standard. These can be expressed algebraically.

Equation 1

Sensitivity=a/(a+c), which in this example is 25/30=0.83, that is, 83% of people with the disease will test positive on the screening test.

Equation 2

Specificity=d/(b+d), which in this example is 60/70=0.86, that is, 86% of people without the disease will test negative on the test.

Sensitivity and specificity are properties of the test, whereas clinicians are interested in patients' results – of those patients who score as cases, how many actually have the disease and of those patients who score as non-cases, how many do not actually have the disease. These are the positive predictive values (PPVs) and negative predictive values (NPVs) respectively, which quantify the predictive power of particular test results.

Equation 3

PPV=a/(a+b), which in this example is 25/35=0.71, that is, 71% of those scoring positive on the test will actually have the disease.

Equation 4

NPV=d/(c+d), which in this example is 60/65=0.92, that is, 92% of those scoring negative on the test will actually not have the disease.

Unfortunately, the PPV and NPV are dependent on the prevalence of the disease. For example, if the prevalence of depression was only 10%, with similar sensitivity and specificity (as they are usually constant), the cell values in Table 1 would change (to approximately a=8, b=15, c=2 and d=75), the PPV would drop substantially (to about 8/23) and the NPV would increase (to about 75/77). Conversely, if the prevalence was higher, the PPV would increase and the NPV would fall. Few tests work well if the prevalence is less than 10% or more than 90%.

A useful way of summarising the performance of a diagnostic test regardless of prevalence is to calculate a likelihood ratio, as this can be done from the sensitivity and specificity. The likelihood ratio of a positive test result (LR+) is the likelihood that a positive test result comes from a person with the disease rather than one without; while the likelihood ratio of a negative result (LR−) is the likelihood that a negative test result comes from a person with the disease rather than one without.

Note that we are dealing with the 'odds' or relative probabilities of results in one group compared with another. It may help you to know that the probability of an event includes the observation in the numerator and denominator of the equation, whereas the odds of two events are represented separately in the numerator and denominator. For example, the probability of throwing any number with a die is one in six whereas the odds are one to five. Probabilities (P) and odds (O) are clearly related, such that P=O/(1+O) and O=P/(1−P).

Equation 5

LR+=[a/(a+c)]/[d/(b+d)], or sensitivity/(1−specificity), which in this example is 0.83/1−0.86=5.93, that is, a positive result is 5.93 times more likely to be found in a patient with the disease rather than one without.

Equation 6

LR−=[c/(a+c)]/[d/(b+d)], or (1−sensitivity)/specificity, which in this example is 1−0.83/0.86=0.20, that is, a negative result is 0.2 times more likely − or five times less likely − to be found in a patient with the disease than without.

The likelihood ratio, as a relative measure, is multiplied by the pre-test odds of having the disorder to generate the post-test odds. Probabilities are easier to interpret than odds, so the post-test odds are converted back into a post-test probability, that is, the probability that a person scoring positive (or negative) on the test actually has the disorder.

Equation 7

Pre-test odds=pre-test probability/(1−pre-test probability), which in this example is 0.3/(1−0.3)=0.43, that is, any patient is about a half as likely to have the disease as not. (It is worth noting that the pre-test probability is the same as the prevalence rate and that the pre-test odds are simply the rates in those with, relative to those without, the disease − 0.3 to 0.7.)

Equation 8

Post-test odds (of a positive result)=pre-test odds × LR+, which in this example is 0.43 × 5.93=2.55, that is, a patient scoring positive on the test is 2.55 times more likely to have the disease than not.

Equation 9

Post-test probability (of a positive result)=post-test odds/(1+post-test odds), which in this example is 2.55/(1+2.55)=0.72, that is, 72% of patients scoring positive on the test will actually have the disease.

The same, rather laborious, calculations can be conducted for a negative test − prevalence is 0.3, pre-test odds 0.43, LR−0.20, post-test odds 0.086, post-test probability=0.079 (i.e. 7.9% of those scoring negative on the test will actually have the disease). Fortunately, nomograms are available to avoid the need for these calculations − as long as we know the LR+ and LR−, the pre-test probabilities are simply converted to post-test probabilities.

Returning to our hypothetical situation, you are now in a position to tell general practitioners that simply asking their patients if they have felt depressed for the past two weeks will mean that 72% of those responding positively will actually be depressed and that only 7.9% of those responding negatively will be falsely regarded as not depressed. Whether general practitioners regard this simple strategy as worthwhile might depend on their psychiatric experience, average consultation times and if there is a simple and safe therapeutic intervention for the identified cases.

Treatment

Any new treatment should ideally be evaluated in a randomised placebo-controlled double-blind trial, in which the outcomes of interest are measured in all subjects who enter the trial. Suppose that such a

Table 2. Treatment

	New antidepressant	Placebo	Total
Outcome			
Not depressed	40	20	60
Depressed	10	30	40
Total	50	50	100

trial compared the rates of treatment success, as measured by an arbitrary, but reliable 50% reduction in symptom levels, with a new antidepressant and a placebo in 100 patients with depression in a primary care setting. The hypothetical results are shown in Table 2.

Thus, 40 (80%) out of 50 patients treated with the new antidepressant responded as compared with 20 (40%) out of 50 patients treated with placebo. These are the experimental event rate (EER) and the control event rate (CER), respectively. The difference between them is likely to be statistically significant, but is it clinically important? The traditional measure of this is the proportional or relative risk reduction (RRR).

Equation 10

RRR=(EER−CER)/CER, which in this example is (80−40)/40=1 (or 100%), that is, antidepressants increase the relative response by 100%. (Note that, strictly speaking, this is a relative benefit increase (RBI) as a desirable event is being considered.)

The problem with the RRR (or RBI) is that it cannot distinguish large treatment effects from trivial effects. The RRR in this example would still be 1 if the EER and CER were 100% and 50% respectively and even if they were 2% and 1%. This is because the RRR does not consider the underlying chances of events (such as spontaneous recovery) in patients entering trials. In contrast, the simple difference between experimental and control event rates − the absolute risk reduction (ARR) − does allow for baseline risks.

Equation 11

ARR=EER−CER, which in this example is 80−40=40%, that is, antidepressants increase the absolute response rate by 40%. (Note that, strictly speaking, this is an absolute benefit increase (ABI) as a desirable event is being considered.)

Some readers will almost intuitively realise that if the average benefit is 40% then 2.5 (100/40) people will need to be treated to obtain recovery in one. This is the number needed to treat (NNT) and is simply calculated as the reciprocal of the ARR (or ARI).

Equation 12

NNT=1/ARR, which in this example is 1/0.4=2.5 (which is rounded up to 3.0 'whole' people).

This is the best estimate of the magnitude of the treatment effect from this hypothetical study, but when dealing with different patients from various populations we need to know the likely range of results. This is best expressed as a 95% confidence interval (95% CI), that is, the range of results within which we can be 95% confident or sure that the true value lies. There are a number of ways of calculating (usually approximate) confidence intervals, which also depend on the measure of interest, and one could not be expected to memorise them all. Interested readers are referred to Sackett *et al* (1997) for some of the more commonly used methods. It is, however, worth knowing that the confidence intervals on the NNT are simply the reciprocals of the confidence intervals on the ARR.

Equation 13

The 95% CI of the NNT is 1/higher confidence interval of the ARR to 1/lower confidence interval of the RR, which in this example is (using arbitrary values) 1/0.5 to 1/0.3=2 to 3.3 (rounded up to 4.0).

Provided an NNT is reasonably low, and the 95% CI around it is not too wide, one can be confident that a given intervention will work, in similar patients, in routine clinical practice. Whether a particular treatment was used will, however, also depend on likely adverse effects (and cost). Adverse effects can also be quantified, as a number needed to harm (NNH), in an analogous way to the NNT, that is, the NNH equals the reciprocal of the absolute difference in the rates of adverse events in the experimental and control groups.

Finally, as clinicians, we deal with individual patients rather than populations. Some of our patients are similar to those in randomised controlled trials but many are not. The NNT can be adapted for individual patients in a number of ways – with reference to our clinical experience, to the results of clinical audit or from figures in a prognosis paper on similar patients. The former technique is the easiest as it simply requires one to make an estimate of a patient's likely susceptibility to an outcome as compared to the average control patients in the reported trial. This estimate should be expressed as a decimal fraction (F) and divided into the NNT to produce an 'adjusted NNT'.

Equation 14

Adjusted NNT=NNT/F, which in this example if (say) a patient was judged to be half as likely to respond to antidepressants is 2.5/0.5=5.

The other techniques are likely to be more accurate, but are more difficult and time-consuming and are best used when considering whether a treatment reduces the rates of an undesirable event rather than increases the chance of a desirable one (see Sackett *et al*, 1996, 1999).

Returning to our general practitioners, you could inform them that they would need to treat three typical patients (confidence interval two to four patients) with the antidepressant to get one recovery that would have not occurred without treatment over the time scale of the trial.

Prognosis

Reliable data on prognosis is best obtained from (a meta-analysis of) cohort studies, where a group of patients at similar stages of their illness are prospectively followed-up for an adequate length of time to monitor the rates of outcomes of interest – such as recovery, relapse and death.

Suppose that such a study reported recovery rates from depression, in primary care, of 80% at one year. This is also the probability or chances of recovery. Note, however, that the confidence intervals around this estimate would need to be relatively narrow (say 70–90%) for this information to be clinically useful. Confidence intervals are actually quite simply calculated on probabilities (P) or proportions, such that it is worth running through the calculation of a 95% CI for this example.

Equation 15

The 95% CI of a proportion=P±(1.96 × the standard error). The standard error of a proportion is the square root of [P × (1−P)/N]. In this example, the 95% CI is therefore $0.8 \pm (1.96 \times \sqrt{[0.8 \times (1-0.8)/100]}) = 0.8 \pm (1.96 \times \sqrt{[0.16/100]}) = 0.8 \pm (1.96 \times 0.04) = 0.8 \pm 0.08 = 0.72$ to 0.88 (or 72% to 88%).

Note that the standard error is heavily influenced by the size (*n*) of any study. If the same P was found in a study of 1000 subjects, the standard error would be about 0.01 and 95% CI would be approximately 70% to 82%. In other words, the larger a study is, the more confident one can be that the result is accurate.

Conclusions

At first glance, some of these concepts and calculations may seem a bit complicated. Relatively little practice, preferably in real-life clinical situations, will however, quickly accustom you to their use. In time, you will probably find them very useful, even essential, in guiding clinical decisions and communicating with your colleagues and your patients. They will certainly help you pass the membership exam and should facilitate your continuing professional development.

Acknowledgements

I thank Andrew McIntosh and Sanjay Rao for reading through a draft of this review.

References

Sackett, D. L., Richardson, S., Rosenberg, W., et al (eds) (1996) Evidence-Based Medicine: How to Practice and Teach EBM. London: Churchill Livingstone.
—— , Straus, S. E., Richardson, W. S., et al (eds) (1999) Evidence-Based Medicine: How to Practice and Teach EBM (2nd edn). London: Churchill Livingstone.

Further reading

Lawrie, S. M. & Geddes, J. R. (1998) Evidence-based medicine and psychiatry. In Edinburgh Companion to Psychiatric Studies (eds E. C. Johnstone, C. P. Freeman & A. Zealley). Pp. 865–877. Churchill Livingstone: Edinburgh.
Streiner, D. & Geddes, J. (1998) Some useful concepts and terms in articles about diagnosis. Evidence-Based Mental Health, 1, 6–7 (erratum in press).
Szatmari, P. (1998) Some useful concepts and terms used in articles about treatment. Evidence-Based Mental Health, 1, 39–40.

How to approach the MRCPsych Critical Review Paper. A trainee's viewpoint

Andrew McIntosh

What follows is based on my experience of sitting (and passing) the first Critical Review Paper. I found the experience enjoyable, useful and I've continued to use the methods since. The new paper tests the skills of the clinician of appraising published literature and then applying the evidence of their own practice. If you are sitting the exam you should be confident that it is not just a paper exercise, but a useful addition to your clinical skills that will help you decide whether the books and papers you read are valid, important and whether they can be used in caring for your patients. You should not be worried if you actually enjoy the experience!

The Critical Review Paper covers the use of articles on diagnosis, treatment, meta-analysis and systematic reviews, prognosis, economics, audit and clinical practice guidelines. Although the subject matter is familiar, some of the terms (such as NNT, likelihood ratios, confidence intervals) will not be familiar and some will seem daunting. Therefore, each area will need to be read and re-read many times before the concepts are finally grasped. Many people will read one or two of the books in the area (Brown & Wilkinson, 1998; Sackett *et al*, 1999), although arguably this is one of the hardest ways of establishing confidence in the subject matter if it is done without any of the other methods mentioned below.

The most effective means of passing the exam is to begin to practise evidence-based medicine in your everyday work and to see the benefits and questions this raises about your own clinical practice. The following five-step plan is perhaps the ideal way to maximise your chances.

(a) Read one of the many texts. Don't worry about any of the mathematical terms you don't understand initially, these will become intuitive eventually with repeated practice. You will find that there is a great deal that you already understand or that is common sense.

(b) Join an evidence-based journal club. Ask yourself questions about the evidence for the interventions you make in your working day. Then find and appraise the evidence at the journal club. Using the journal club to learn from other people's clinical problems and appraisal of the literature will make this an efficient use of your time.

(c) Subscribe to, or read, the journal *Evidence-Based Mental Health* or other secondary publications such as *Clinical Evidence*. The journals publish critically appraised papers regularly, selecting only the most methodologically sound material. *Evidence-Based Mental Health* also includes a glossary and two brief pieces of an aspect of evidence-based psychiatry.

(d) Visit the many websites on evidence-based mental health (www.cebmh.com) or evidence-based medicine (cebm.jr2.ox.ac.uk, hiru.mcmaster.ca). The websites are useful reference guides and also include critically appraised topics (CATS) that are similar to the critical appraisal of published material that takes place at an evidence-based journal club.

(e) At least three months before the examination, start trying the sample questions included in this book. Save some questions to complete under exam conditions with others in your postgraduate class or study group. Get others to set questions under exam conditions: hopefully there will be teachers at your centre who will do this for you.

Finally, perhaps the most helpful means of passing the exam is to approach it with the right attitude. Those who see the 'evidence-based' approach as helpful and relevant will be more likely to enjoy the subject, pass the exam and continue using the methods in their own clinical practice afterwards. Your patients will also benefit from your efforts, therefore any time spent studying will not be wasted.

References

Brown, T. & Wilkinson, G. (1998) *Critical Reviews in Psychiatry* (1st edn). London: Gaskell.

Sackett, D. L., Strauss, S. E., Richardson, W. S. *et al* (eds) (1999) *Evidence-Based Medicine. How to Practice and Teach EBM* (2nd edn). Edinburgh: Churchill Livingstone.

A CRITICAL REVIEW PAPER

Questionnaire development and validation
Model answers by John Eagles

Health of the Nation Outcome Scales (HoNOS)

Research and development

J. K. WING, A. S. BEEVOR, R. H. CURTIS, S. B. G. PARK, S. HADDEN and A. BURNS

The Government White Paper *Health of the Nation* (Department of Health, 1992, 1993) identified five key areas, one of which was mental health, where priority should be given to the development of local strategies for reducing mortality and morbidity. One of the mental health targets was "to improve significantly the health and social functioning of mentally ill people". In order to set a quantified target and to measure how far it was being met, a dedicated instrument would be needed that could be used routinely, within the context of other necessary information, in the National Health Service.

PLAN OF DEVELOPMENT

To be useful to clinicians, the instrument would need to be brief enough for routine use by keyworkers, cover common clinical problems and social functioning, be sensitive to change or lack of it and have known reliability and relationship to more established scales.

TWO PILOT PHASES

HoNOS-1 was a 20-item instrument, drafted with the help of consultants and covering four key areas of functioning: behaviour, impairment, symptoms and social functioning. Item 20 was a global (0–100) disability score. This version was tested during a first pilot study (*n*=152) to discover how it performed in terms of clinical acceptability, simple structure and sensitivity to change. The results were satisfactory. In the light of comments from users it was shortened to 12 items, each rated on a 0–4 scale of severity. HoNOS-2 was then tested again (*n*=100) with results closely similar to those of the first pilot. HoNOS-3, used in the main field trials, reflected the lessons learned.

FIELD TRIALS – HoNOS-3

Large-scale trials were needed in order thoroughly to test feasibility and clinical acceptability and establish a substantial base of data from ratings made by clinicians as part of their everyday work.

The task in each area was routinely to collect HoNOS data on a consecutive series of up to 200 patients (Time 1), and to follow as many as possible for at least three months or to the end of the episode of contact.

Sensitivity to change

Table 1 shows the means for sub-scores A–D, the total score derived from items 1–11 (0–44) and the global item 12 (0–100), at Time 1 and Time 2 (first and second ratings).

Test–retest reliability

The intraclass correlation coefficients for items, the total score (sum of items 1–11) and the global score were all between 0.74 and 0.88, except for aggression (0.61).

Rating styles

Nearly all raters were nurses (*n*=399) or doctors (*n*=60) and the statistical analysis is heavily weighted by their data.

RELIABILITY AND RELATIONSHIP TO OTHER SCALES

Studies in Nottingham and Manchester

The fourth phase consisted of tests to show whether the final form of the instrument remained acceptable to clinicians, had comparable characteristics to its predecessor, performed well when subjected to independent tests of reliability, and had reasonable compatibility with larger instruments with a long track record. The studies were carried out in academic departments in Nottingham and Manchester, in consultation with the Royal College of Psychiatrists Research Unit team.

Comparisons

An update of the earlier search, and reference to a similar survey by Andrews & Morris-Yates (1994), found no instrument of reasonable length that covered both the clinical and the social items in HoNOS. Two sets of scales, the 24-item Brief Psychiatric Rating Scale (BPRS-24) (Overall & Gorham, 1962; Ventura *et al*, 1993) and the Role Functioning Scale (RFS; Goodman *et al*, 1993), were selected because of a long track record and because, between them, they cover most of the content of the final HoNOS. However, both instruments have a much wider range and the BPRS is intended to be completed at an interview with the patient, which is only an option for HoNOS.

In Nottingham, the trainer completed the comparison instruments for 33 of the patients in the reliability study. The product–moment correlation between the total HoNOS and total RFS scores was 0.65. That between the four social HoNOS items

Table I HoNOS-3 sub-scores and summary scores at Time I (TI) and Time 2 (T2): by type of rater pairs

Type of score	Same raters[1] (*n*=871)		Different raters[1] (*n*=798)	
	TI	T2	TI	T2
A (0–12) Behaviour	1.97	1.08	2.62	1.35
B (0–8) Impairment	1.03	0.83	1.22	0.85
C (0–12) Symptoms	3.92	2.41	4.13	2.23
D (0–12) Social	2.91	2.43	3.04	2.45
Total (0–44)	9.77	6.67	10.96	6.86
Global (0–100)	43.37	33.65	44.37	34.10

1. Numbers vary because of missing data.
All TI–T2 differences are significant (*P* < 0.001). Difference between same-rater pairs and different-rater pairs: A *P* < 0.001; total *P* < 0.001; Interaction: A *P* < 0.001; B *P* < 0.013; C *P* < 0.002; total *P* < 0.001.

(9–12) and RFS 1–4 was 0.75. The correlation between total HoNOS and total BPRS scores was 0.84 and that between the clinical items HoNOS 1–8 and BPRS 1–15 (omitting the behavioural items 16–24) was 0.85.

The exercise in Manchester was more complicated and less appropriate for comparisons, since nine consultants rated a total of 97 patients. Five contributed too few BPRS and RFS forms for separate analysis; a total of 20. The other four between them provided a total of 77 score sheets. Of these, 37 (22 with a diagnosis of dementia) were contributed by one rater. The correlations between total HoNOS and total RFS scores, in order of magnitude, were 0.52, 0.64, 0.67 and 0.73. The equivalents for total HoNOS and total BPRS scores were 0.49, 0.57, 0.71 and 0.71.

REFERENCES

Andrews G. & Morris-Yates, A. (1994) Ethical implications of the electronic storage of medical records. In *Computers in Mental Health*, Vol. 1 (eds G. Andrews, T. B. Ustun, H. Dilling, *et al*), pp. 129–135. St Andrews: Churchill Livingstone/WHO.

Department of Health (1992) *Health of the Nation*. White Paper. London: HMSO.

— **(1993)** *Key Area Handbook. Mental Health*. London: Department of Health.

Goodman, S. H., Sewell, D. R., Cooley, E. L., et al (1993) Assessing levels of adaptive functioning: the Role Functioning Scale. *Community Mental Health Journal*, **29**, 119–131.

Overall, J. E. & Gorham, D. R. (1962) The Brief Psychiatric Rating Scale. *Psychological Reports*, **10**, 799–812.

Ventura, J., Green, M. F., Shaner, A., et al (1993) Training and quality assurance with the BPRS. 'The drift busters'. *International Journal of Methods in Psychiatric Research*, **3**, 221–244.

WING *ET AL*

Please write your answers to questions I to IV in the spaces provided.

I.   Background

A.   Discuss the concept of mental health, giving three general definitions.   [6 marks]

....
....
....
....
....
....

B.   List six strategies for reducing mortality (3) and morbidity (3) related to mental health.
                                                                                                                      [6 marks]

....
....
....
....
....
....

C.   List six targets that could be measured, so as to indicate significant change in the health (3)
      and social functioning (3) of people with mental illnesses.   [6 marks]

....
....
....
....
....
....

D.   List three types of instrument that could be used in a study of this topic to set and measure
      'a quantified target'. Discuss the pros and cons of each.   [6 marks]

....
....
....
....
....
....

II. Method

A. Define reliability in relation to questionnaires. List types of reliability examined by the authors. Also list any other forms of reliability not addressed by the authors. [8 marks]

....
....
....
....
....
....

B. List statistical measures of reliability used in this study, and two others you know of. How have these authors measured sensitivity to change? Suggest logical additions to the methodology shown. [8 marks]

....
....
....
....
....
....

C. Criticise the pros and cons of what the authors did to enhance reliable rating when using the instrument in different settings? How would you assess the effect of different rating styles by nurses and doctors in this study? [8 marks]

....
....
....
....
....
....

D. Compare and contrast the terms 'feasibility study, pilot study and field trial'. Which two groups (other than nurses, psychiatrists and psychologists) would you have involved in the drafting of HoNOS-1? Give your reasons. [8 marks]

....
....
....
....
....
....

III. Results

A. What are the main findings shown in Table 1? What does the term 'interaction' signify?

[8 marks]

....
....
....
....
....
....

B. In what ways might the results be biased because raters were used in ward and non-ward settings? Give a possible reason why the means from different-rater pairs were all higher at Time 1 than those from same-rater pairs?

[8 marks]

....
....
....
....
....
....

C. Give reasons why the intraclass correlation coefficient (ICC) was lowest for aggression. What steps would you take to improve the ICC for aggression?

[4 marks]

....
....
....
....
....
....

D. How did the authors assess the validity of HoNOS? What are the key results? How would you interpret the differences in different centres? Define the validity in this context giving example(s) of different ways in which the validity of HoNOS could be assessed, suggesting statistical measures, as appropriate. What is the importance of the global HoNOS score in this context?

[12 marks]

....
....
....
....
....
....

....
....
....
....
....
....

IV. Summary

A. What are the main conclusions of this study? What are the main clinical implications of this work? [6 marks]

....
....
....
....
....
....

B. Identify the limitations of the development of HoNOS, indicating how each could be addressed in future work. [6 marks]

....
....
....
....
....
....

I. Background

A. Discuss the concept of mental health, giving three general definitions.

Mental health is notoriously difficult to define. It can mean the absence of serious mental disorder (such as a categorical distinction as to whether a person is or is not psychotic), but when one looks at dimensional variables (such as degree of mood fluctuations or obsessional personality traits) there are no clear 'cut-off points' between mental health and mental ill health. The other use of the term 'health' is to denote 'positive mental well-being' rather than just an absence of significant psychopathology or impaired social functioning. Three possible definitions would be as follows:

(a) An absence of significant psychopathology.
(b) The attainment of positive mental well-being.
(c) A level of psychological functioning which permits full enjoyment of life and mutually satisfactory interpersonal relationships.

B. List six strategies for reducing mortality (3) and morbidity (3) related to mental health.

Strategies to reduce mortality generally address the rates of suicide among people with mental illnesses. While it should be noted that there is no evidence of the effectiveness of any suicide prevention strategy, approaches would include:

(a) Reducing the availability of the means of suicide (e.g. catalytic converters on motor cars).
(b) More widespread long-term use of lithium and/or antidepressants for patients with recurrent depressive disorders.
(c) Alleviating unemployment among young men, a group whose suicide rate has increased significantly over recent years.

Strategies which may improve mental health morbidity include:

(a) Better recognition and treatment of depressive disorders (as through the Defeat Depression Campaign).
(b) Attempting to ameliorate the stigma which relates to mental illness.
(c) Earlier detection and treatment (e.g. of alcohol problems identified in the workplace).

C. List six targets that could be measured, so as to indicate significant change in the health (3) and social functioning (3) of people with mental illnesses.

Measurable targets which would indicate a significant change in the health of mentally ill people would include:

(a) Days per annum spent as a hospital in-patient.
(b) Rates of out of hours/emergency contacts with services.
(c) Suicide rates (although this may well relate in part to social functioning).

Measurable targets which would indicate a significant change in the social functioning of mentally ill people would include:

(a) Whether the patient returns to or acquires full-time employment.
(b) The number of occasions per week on which a patient goes out of the house.
(c) The number of different people seen socially during a given period.

D. List three types of instrument that could be used in a study of this topic to set and measure 'a quantified target'. Discuss the pros and cons of each.

Observer ratings of psychopathology such as the Brief Psychiatric Rating Scale (BPRS) which purports to cover a wide range of symptomatology. An advantage is the use of one instrument for all patients, the corresponding disadvantage being that it may be insufficiently specific to cover the broad range of psychiatric illnesses and symptomatology. Instruments specific to particular conditions (schizophrenia, depression, eating disorders, etc.) may give more meaningful information about outcomes. Observers usually need to be trained to use these scales and observer-rated instruments may be contaminated by 'observer bias' especially when the observer is a professional who is treating a patient and is thus keen for the patient to make progress.

Self-rated instruments of psychopathology such as the General Health Questionnaire (GHQ) which is also designed to cover a wide range of conditions and again has the advantage of allowing comparisons between conditions. Again it is rather non-specific and condition specific self-rating scales (such as the Hospital Anxiety and Depression Scale (HADS)) that may be preferable. Patients may be too disturbed to complete self-rating scales accurately and even when patients are less acutely ill, compliance with scale completion may be unsatisfactorily low.

Ratings of social functioning in relation to health, such as the Medical Outcomes Study Short Form–36 (SF–36) which is a self-rated scale (see disadvantages of self-rated scales above) of social functioning which includes the concept of 'quality of life'. This has the advantage of being a broad and generalisable outcome. Again, it may suffer from being insufficiently specific to particular patient groups, for example, a patient with schizophrenia may not see his or her quality of life as being enhanced by going out to a restaurant.

II. Method

A. Define reliability in relation to questionnaires. List types of reliability examined by the authors. Also list any other forms of reliability not addressed by the authors.

The reliability of a questionnaire is essentially the degree to which it will produce the same result when administered repeatedly to an individual, given that the person's well-being does not change between administrations.

The types of reliability examined by the authors were:

(a) Test–re-test reliability.
(b) Alternate measures of reliability (i.e. comparison with other scales, also partly a measure of validity).

A form of reliability not addressed: internal consistency (e.g. split half coefficients, item-total correlations). Inter-rater reliability is not mentioned in the précis shown, but the authors did investigate inter-rater reliability at another point in the paper.

B. List statistical measures of reliability used in this study and two others you know of. How have the authors measured sensitivity to change? Suggest logical additions to the methodology shown.

The main statistical measure of reliability used in the study was intraclass correlation coefficients for test–re-test reliability, inter-rater reliability and alternate measures of reliability.

Reliability can also be calculated by Pearson's r, by Kappa (which takes account of ratings agreeing by chance), Spearman's r (which looks at the ranking of ratings rather than their absolute values) or by Cronbach's alpha (which is a measure of internal consistency).

The authors have compared the mean scores on sub-scales and mean total scores at Time 1 and Time 2 indicating that analysis of variance was used, although this is not stated. There was no apparent attempt at external validation of the change, that is, ensuring that patients who are found to have changed (i.e. improved) on the scale actually had improved when other forms of assessment were used. Better methodology would compare the ratings of groups of patients who were shown to have changed (as judged by other criteria) with those who have not changed. A satisfactorily high proportion of patients who have changed should show improvement on HoNOS (sensitivity) and a satisfactorily low number of patients who have not changed should show improvement on HoNOS (specificity).

C. Criticise the pros and cons of what the authors did to enhance reliable rating when using the instrument in different settings? How would you assess the effect of different rating styles by nurses and doctors in this study?

The studies of reliability were carried out in "academic departments in Nottingham and Manchester". It is an advantage that two centres were used, but arguably this is too few. Since HoNOS is an instrument which should be equally applicable in hospital and non-hospital settings, it should have been used in a variety of settings (it was in fact tested in ward and non-ward settings – see Question IIIB – but this is not stipulated in the summary).

To assess possible nurse–doctor differences, one could investigate whether the inter-rater reliability of nurse–nurse ratings and of doctor–doctor ratings differed from those of nurse–doctor ratings. To assess whether nurses or doctors tended to rate consistently lower or higher, the mean totals could be compared for patients assessed in particular settings. If this did occur, it would be of interest to determine on which sub-scale(s) nurse–doctor differences were most prominent.

D. Compare and contrast the terms 'feasibility study, pilot study and field trial'. Which two groups (other than nurses, psychiatrists and psychologists) would you have involved in the drafting of HoNOS-1? Give your reasons.

Feasibility study – this looks at whether a proposed course of action or intervention is practicable, possible and desirable.

Pilot study – this is a small scale trial of a study protocol which seeks to identify unforeseen problems within the protocol.

Field trial – this tests out an instrument or intervention 'in the real world' to establish whether one can generalise from research findings to more ordinary clinical circumstances.

Two other groups who might have been involved in drafting HoNOS-1 are:

(a) Patients, since they have first hand knowledge and experience of symptoms and often valid views about what constitutes a good or a bad outcome.

(b) Carers, since they see patients at close quarters from a 'non-medical perspective' and again often have valid views about what constitutes a good or a bad outcome.

III. Results

A. What are the main findings shown in Table 1? What does the term 'interaction' signify?

Table 1 shows the means of the four sub-scales, the means of the total scores and the means of the global ratings at the times of the first ratings and the times of the second ratings of patients. The data are subdivided into the means of 871 ratings by the same rater at Time 1 and Time 2 and 798 ratings by different raters at Times 1 and 2. The means show a statistically significant fall (i.e. an improvement) at a level of $P<0.001$, whether they are derived from same-rater or different-rater pairs. The changes on sub-scale A (behaviour) and on the total score were significantly greater for different-rater pairs than for same-rater pairs ($P<0.001$).

The term interaction signifies that there was an apparent influence of the type of rater pair (different-rater versus same-rater) upon the scores allocated by the raters.

B. In what ways might the results be biased because raters were used in ward and non-ward settings? Give a possible reason why the means from different-rater pairs were all higher at Time 1 than those from same-rater pairs?

In non-ward settings, it is perhaps more likely that the same rater (for example a community psychiatric nurse) would rate the patient at both Time 1 and Time 2, while in ward settings different raters (nurses working shifts) would be more likely to rate the patient.

If different-rater pairs were more likely in acute ward settings than in non-ward settings, the patients rated by different-rater pairs would be more severely ill and would score more highly on HoNOS.

C. Give reasons why the interclass correlation coefficient (ICC) was lowest for aggression. What steps would you take to improve the ICC for aggression?

It is likely that ratings of aggression are more subjective than 'harder' symptoms (e.g. psychosis) and that aggression will show significant fluctuations across time compared with more enduring symptoms (e.g. cognitive problems), giving rise to greater fluctuations in ratings and reduced reliability.

To improve the ICC for aggression one could attempt to tighten the definition, to engage in further training of raters and to encourage raters to 'average out' their ratings of aggression across several meetings with the patient.

D. How did the authors assess the validity of HoNOS? What are the key results? How would you interpret the differences in different centres? Define the validity in this context giving example(s) of different ways in which the validity of HoNOS could be

assessed, suggesting statistical measures, as appropriate. What is the importance of the global HoNOS score in this context?

The validity of HoNOS was assessed through five raters (one in Nottingham, four in Manchester) who rated patients on the HoNOS, the BPRS and the Role Functioning Scale (RFS). Scores were correlated (Pearson's r) between HoNOS total scores plus relevant sub-scale scores and BPRS and RFS total scores.

(a) HoNOS total/BPRS total correlations ranged from 0.49–0.84.
(b) HoNOS total/RFS total correlations ranged from 0.52–0.73.

With regard to differences between centres, one rater assessed 33 patients in Nottingham and three of the raters in Manchester rated only 40 patients between them, while the majority of the patients rated by the fourth Manchester rater had dementia. Differing 'diagnostic mixes' of patients, differences in numbers of patients rated and differences in rating style could give rise to the differences between centres.

Validity relates to whether a measure does indeed measure what it purports to measure and HoNOS purports to measure the 'health and social functioning of mentally ill people' across all diagnostic categories. Ideally, validity of HoNOS would be measured against so called 'gold standards'. Gold standards can be other established measures (e.g. Hamilton Depression Rating Scale (HDRS)) or even more ideally, objective measures of pathology (e.g. correlating ratings of cognitive problems against brain morphology). It would be instructive to determine the validity of each individual item (e.g. ratings of depression against HDRS scores). Given the (perhaps unrealistically) optimistic aim of using the HoNOS in people with all types of mental illness, it would be desirable to establish its validity among homogeneous groups of diagnosed patients, again comparing HoNOS scores and subscores against gold standards of severity for that particular condition. Relevant statistical tests are correlation coefficients either Pearson's r or Spearman's r (when data are not normally distributed).

The 'global HoNOS' gives an overall rating of disability by an experienced clinician. As such, it is a rating which could be used as a gold standard of impairment. However, gold standards in the assessment of validity are more credible if they derive from an independent rating by a different observer. A global score is likely to be contaminated by the ratings made concurrently on the HoNOS, thus exaggerating the validity of the scale when HoNOS is correlated with global scores.

IV. Summary

A. What are the main conclusions of this study? What are the main clinical implications of this work?

The authors appeared to conclude that they have produced a brief observer rated instrument which will be useful, reliable and valid in assessing the health and social functioning (and changes therein) among people with mental illnesses. Some of the points raised above may indicate that these conclusions may not be entirely justified.

The clinical implications depend upon the debatable conclusions. Clinicians who are happy with HoNOS may well wish to use it routinely to assess the progress of patients and the success of treatment interventions across the whole range of patients whom they see, thus perhaps providing an overview of the efficacy of service provision. Clinicians who are less happy with the instrument may wish to postpone the routine use of HoNOS until further data become available as has been suggested by the authors themselves.

B. Identify the limitations of the development of HoNOS, indicating how each could be addressed in future work.

Several limitations in the development of HoNOS are mentioned in the previous answers. Four such limitations are as follows.

(a) As in Answer IID, widespread multi-disciplinary consultation, including patients and carers might have been of help during the drafting of the first HoNOS and it would have been preferable to have consulted other professionals as well as patients and carers.
(b) The issue of nurse–doctor differences in ratings is described in the Answer IIC. Since the scale is designed to be used widely by different professional groups and purports to have inter-rater reliability between different professional groups, it would be instructive to conduct further tests of inter-rater reliability (as described in the Answer IIC) more widely with larger numbers of raters from differing professional groups.
(c) Validity was assessed by looking at the scores on observer-rated scales conducted by the same raters. It would be instructive to compare the scores of different raters on different observer-rated scales. Furthermore,

it would be of interest to know how closely observer ratings, and observer ratings of change, correlated with patients' self-ratings of symptomatology and of changes in symptomatology.

(d) Given the intention that HoNOS will rate patients in all diagnostic groups, it would be important to know if the instrument is equally reliable and valid in patients within each major diagnostic category and comparisons could be made with rating scales designed specifically for patients within each of these diagnostic categories.

A CRITICAL REVIEW PAPER

Clinical audit
Model answers by Angus Mackay

Auditing electroconvulsive therapy

The third cycle

RICHARD DUFFETT and PAUL LELLIOTT

PREVIOUS AUDITS OF ELECTROCONVULSIVE THERAPY IN BRITAIN

The College first set standards for the administration of electroconvulsive therapy (ECT) in 1977 (Royal College of Psychiatrists, 1977). Pippard & Ellam (1981) subsequently conducted a review of practice by visiting 180 ECT clinics in the UK – about one-half of the total number. The audit revealed that some centres were using obsolete machines and that training of junior doctors in the administration of ECT was generally poor. In response to these findings the College produced its first ECT handbook in 1989 (Royal College of Psychiatrists, 1989).

In a second audit, Pippard (1992) evaluated the administration of ECT against standards contained in the 1989 handbook during visits to 35 National Health Service (NHS) and five private ECT clinics in the old North East Thames and East Anglia Regions. Although he reported an improvement since 1981 in the standard of ECT facilities and some aspects of practice, many clinics were still failing to meet the 1989 recommendations, particularly with regard to the training of junior doctors and the use of modern machines.

After his second evaluation, Pippard (1992) made a number of further recommendations. These focused on the role of the College and its members in ensuring that ECT clinics meet certain standards. These included the allocation of consultant sessions to administer and supervise ECT, accreditation of consultants in charge of ECT clinics, external inspection visits and better training of junior doctors.

The College established a working group to consider Pippard's suggestions and recent research findings. The revised College recommendations related both to structures (including the quality of ECT suites and equipment for administering ECT and monitoring seizures) and to processes (the administration of the electrical current, management of anaesthesia and recovery, the training and supervision of personnel). These revised guidelines were disseminated in the 2nd ECT handbook (Royal College of Psychiatrists, 1995), a video for psychiatrists involved in administering ECT (400 had been sold by the autumn of 1996), two articles in a journal supporting continuing medical education of psychiatrists (Lock, 1994; Robertson & Fergusson, 1996) and a series of training courses organised by the College.

THE THIRD AUDIT

Method

Two hundred and fifteen ECT clinics, and the consultant responsible for ECT, were identified by telephoning all NHS mental health trusts in England and Wales. Private clinics in North Thames and East Anglia were also identified. There were two components to the audit.

Component 1: visits to ECT clinics

All 33 NHS clinics in the North East Thames and East Anglia regions and 17 in Wales were visited by R.D. between September 1995 and July 1996. In addition, visits were made to the two private clinics in the North East Thames and East Anglia regions and to three private clinics in north-west London. Whenever possible, visits were made on a day when ECT was due to be given. Clinics were rated using a schedule of standards derived from the 1995 ECT handbook. Some standards, such as presence of adequate equipment, could be rated simply as present or absent. The standards of rooms, personnel and training were given a summary rating of poor, average or good and each clinic was also assigned a global rating using a similar scale. Each of these ratings took account of a number of factors (see Results). Similar methods were used to those employed by Pippard, who was consulted both on the design of the rating methods and on assigning ratings to individual clinics.

A total of 130 ECT treatments were observed in 40 (80%) of the NHS clinics and five treatments in three of the private clinics. During the sessions, observations were made about the testing of equipment, preparation of the patient, nursing care, stimulus used and the adequacy of medical records.

Component 2: the postal questionnaire

An eight-page postal questionnaire was sent to the consultant responsible for the 165 ECT clinics in England which were not visited as part of Component 1. The questionnaires were posted at the end of 1995 with a second mailing made to non-responders in spring 1996. The questionnaire was also completed by 10 of the consultants whose units were visited.

RESULTS

Returns were received from 129 of the 165 clinics in Component 2. Thus, data were available from 184 of the 220 clinics identified (response rate of 84%). Comparison of information from the 10 clinics which completed both the postal questionnaire and received a visit suggested that the two approaches yielded results which were sufficiently similar for the data from both methods to be combined; this is done in the Results, where possible. The relevant standards (derived from Royal College of Psychiatrists (1995)) are displayed at the beginning of each Results sub-section.

The ECT suite

> ECT suites should consist of separate waiting room, treatment room and recovery room, and be warm, clean and of an adequate size. Clinics should provide a separate office for staff and a further recovery area for patients when they no longer need to be on the treatment trolley

An overview of the results is presented in Table 1.

Equipment

> ECT machines should be capable of a wide range of current settings (machines from four manufacturers are recommended in the 1995 handbook).

By 1996, 108 clinics (59%) had installed these 'state of the art' machines (see Table 2). About one-third of clinics were using the Ectron 5 which can deliver a less than three-fold range of current and so limits

Table 1 Standards of rooms in the electroconvulsive therapy suite

	Visited sites (%) $n=55$	Rest of England (%) $n=129$	Total (%) $n=184$
Good	14 (25)	47 (36)	61 (33)
Deficient in some areas	27 (49)	73 (57)	100 (54)
Poor	14 (25)	9 (7)	23 (13)

Table 2 Electroconvulsive therapy (ECT) machines in use

ECT machines in use	Visited sites (%) $n=55$	Rest of England (%) $n=129$	Total (%) $n=184$
Thymatron[1]	9 (16)	24 (18)	33 (18)
Mecta[1]	3 (5)	18 (12)	21 (11)
Neurotronics[1]	1 (2)	8 (6)	9 (5)
Ectron 5 a/b[1]	12 (22)	33 (24)	45 (24)
Ectron 5	27 (49)	37 (26)	64 (34)
Older Ectrons	3 (5)	9 (7)	12 (7)

1. Currently recommended by the Royal College of Psychiatrists.

the ability to titrate the current delivered. Twelve clinics (7%) were still using machines that were no longer recommended in the 1989 handbook.

> Anaesthetic equipment should include tilt trolleys, suction facilities, a supply of oxygen in the recovery and treatment rooms, electrocardiograms, pulse oximeters and capnographs.

Only two services visited provided capnographs and nine did not have tilt trolleys, otherwise these standards were generally well met; 21 clinics (41%) had pulse oximiters in both the treatment and recovery room.

Personnel, supervision and training

> The consultant psychiatrist responsible for ECT should attend the clinic regularly and be acquainted with College recommendations on ECT practice.

In all services a named consultant psychiatrist was identified as being responsible for the ECT clinic. Of the clinics visited only three consultants (6%) had sessional time allocated specifically for ECT. For the remainder, the times at which ECT was given often conflicted with other fixed commitments such as ward rounds and outpatient clinics. Twenty (36%) had read the 1995 ECT handbook and 23 consultants in the clinics visited (42%) had personally attended the ECT training course run by the College. In five (9%) of the clinics visited the consultants never attended ECT sessions; in 18 (33%) the consultant attended

on average every 2–6 months; in 23 (42%) once a month and in nine (16%) once a week. The respondents to the postal survey reported spending on average three hours a month devoted to ECT (range 0–20). Sixty-six per cent of respondents to the postal questionnaire ($n=85$) claimed to have read the College handbook.

> Junior doctors should observe ECT being given before they administer it themselves and should be supervised for the first few treatments they administer by a psychiatrist who has passed the Membership examination.

In brief, junior psychiatrists usually give ECT; all but four of the 184 clinics included senior house officers and registrars in psychiatry on the roster to give ECT and 140 (76%) included general practice vocational trainees. The College does not encourage the latter practice.

> Anaesthetists should be sufficiently trained and experienced to manage any complication likely to arise during ECT administration (particularly if ECT is given at a site without an anaesthetic department). Rosters should include a consultant anaesthetist and be arranged to provide some continuity of care for patients over their course of treatment.

Standards relating to anaesthetic practice were derived from the College's ECT handbook and measures agreed with a Council representative from the Royal College of Anaesthetists. In only four services visited (7%) was anaesthetic input rated as poor, either due to the inexperience of staff or to a failure to provide regular cover. Eight

clinics (15%), however, reported experiencing difficulty in obtaining anaesthetic cover at least once a month resulting in cancelled clinics or the need to transport patients between hospitals.

> Nursing staff should be familiar with ECT procedures and trained in recovery techniques. There should be at least one senior nurse with special responsibility for ECT who is supported during the clinic by additional appropriately trained staff.

The quality of nursing input to the clinic varied greatly. When staff had sessional time allocated for ECT, nurses were keen to ensure high standards and in some services routinely met patients prior to them starting a course of ECT. In 23 clinics visited (42%) the senior nurse was dual trained (Registered Mental Nurse and State Registered Nurse).

Policies and procedures

> There must be policies giving guidance on what settings to use to stimulate patients, what to do in the absence of a seizure and when to terminate a prolonged seizure.

ECT is a relatively simple and circumscribed medical procedure, and is a good subject for locally developed structured protocols for its administration. Despite this, 36 of the clinics visited (67%) lacked any clear written stimulation policy, 35 (65%) gave no written guidance on re-stimulating patients with short seizures and 48 (89%) gave no guidance on terminating prolonged seizures. Of the clinics visited, 13 (24%) had ECT recording forms which were judged to be inadequate.

Overall performance of clinics

Table 3 shows summary ratings of the quality of aspects of facilities and staffing. The global rating took account of facilities,

Table 3 Summary ratings of the 55 clinics visited

	Poor (%)	Average (%)	Good (%)
ECT suite	14 (25.5)	27 (49)	14 (25.5)
ECT/anaesthetic equipment	5 (9)	31 (56)	19 (34)
Psychiatric staff	10 (18)	34 (62)	11 (20)
Anaesthetic staff	4 (7)	30 (56)	20 (37)
Nursing staff	11 (20)	23 (42)	21 (38)
Global rating	12 (22)	27 (49)	16 (29)

ECT, electroconvulsive therapy.

personnel and how smoothly the clinic ran and were influenced by the level of patient care and the effectiveness of the observed ECT session. It was therefore a better rating of the quality of clinics where treatment was actually observed. R.D.'s view was that, had he required it, he would have been reluctant to receive ECT in 13 of the clinics visited (24%).

Impact of the College initiative

Consultants responsible for 147 (80%) of all clinics surveyed reported that they had seen the College video. In the clinics visited, 17 of the 23 consultants (74%) who had attended the one-day training course run by the College had also read the 1995 handbook compared with only three (9%) in the 32 clinics where the consultant had not attended the course ($\chi^2=24$, $P<0.001$). The overall performance of clinics whose consultants had attended the course was rated better than those where the consultant had not and none of the former received a poor rating; this association was statistically significant ($P<0.05$).

Although some of its recommendations related to nursing practice, in only 21 of the clinics visited (38%) had any nursing staff heard of the handbook.

DISCUSSION

Changes since the previous audit

There has been improvement between 1991 and 1996 in some aspects of ECT administration. ECT machines are no longer wheeled from patient to patient (evident in three clinics in the 1991 audit), operating department assistants have been introduced and further recovery areas made available for patients prior to them returning to their ward. ECT machines pre-dating the Ectron 5 (used by 46% of clinics in 1991) have been largely phased out. Fewer of the consultants responsible for ECT had never visited the clinic during its operation (9% v. 40% in 1991) and the number of services where anaesthetic practice was rated as poor has fallen from 28% to 7%.

Problems of implementation of ECT guidelines

The extent to which the slow improvement in ECT practice can be attributed to the College's actions could only have been gauged by a prospective, controlled study which, even if methodologically possible, would have been prohibitively expensive. There is, however, circumstantial evidence that the activities of the College over the years have had some impact. Consultants who had attended the College course had better clinics (although consultants keen to raise standards are probably also more likely to attend the College course). Also, staff in good clinics often attributed their high standards to following the College recommendations and reported using the results of the 1991 audit to argue for resources to improve facilities.

Although the 1996 audit was conducted only a few months after the publication of the ECT handbook, it is disappointing that only one-third of the consultants in the clinics visited had actually read it, most of whom had also attended the College course. Dissemination of the College recommendations across professional boundaries was also poor, with two-thirds of senior nurses in ECT clinics not even aware of the handbook's existence (despite liaison with the Royal College of Nursing at the time the standards were set). The College video had been more widely circulated, having been seen by more than one-half of junior doctors administering ECT (Duffett & Lelliott, 1997) and about 80% of consultants.

It is known that even after well-planned dissemination, guidelines frequently reach only a small proportion of their target audience (Grol, 1992; Lomas, 1993). The College ECT initiative is consistent with what is known about effective dissemination of guidelines in that it included presentation through a variety of media (video, workshops, a handbook, papers in peer review journals and journals of continuing professional development), interventions targeted at the key audience (the ECT course for responsible consultants) and the involvement

of respected colleagues (in teaching and promoting good practice; Lomas, 1993).

CURRENT STANDARDS IN ECT

Many aspects of the organisation and administration of ECT improved between 1991 and 1996. Very old ECT machines have largely been replaced, senior psychiatrists are more actively involved and anaesthetic input is better. However, two-thirds of ECT clinics fall short of the most recent College standards, particularly in relation to the frequency of consultant attendance and the training of junior doctors. These problems have not been fully resolved by 20 years of audit and College activity. There should be a continuing debate as to what further interventions might be considered.

REFERENCES

Duffett, R. & Lelliott, P. (1997) Junior doctors training in the theory and practice of electroconvulsive therapy. *Psychiatric Bulletin,* **21,** 563–565.

Grol, R. (1992) Implementing guidelines in general practice care. *Quality Health,* **1,** 184–191.

Lock, T. (1994) Advances in the practice of electroconvulsive therapy. *Advances in Psychiatric Treatment,* **1,** 47–56.

Lomas, J. (1993) Diffusion, dissemination, and implementation; who should do what? *Annals of New York Academy of Science,* **703,** 226–235.

Pippard, J. (1992) Audit of electroconvulsive treatment in two national health service regions. *British Journal of Psychiatry,* **160,** 621–637.

___ **& Ellam, L. (1981)** Electroconvulsive treatment in Great Britain: a report to the college. *British Journal of Psychiatry,* **139,** 563–568.

Robertson, C. & Fergusson, G. (1996) Electroconvulsive therapy machines. *Advances in Psychiatric Treatment,* **2,** 24–31.

Royal College of Psychiatrists (1977) The Royal College of Psychiatrists' memorandum on the use of electroconvulsive therapy. *British Journal of Psychiatry,* **131,** 261–272.

___ **(1989)** *The Practical Administration of Electroconvulsive Therapy.* London: Gaskell.

___ **(1995)** *The ECT Handbook: The 2nd Report of the Royal College of Psychiatrists' Special Committee on ECT.* Council Report CR39. London: Royal College of Psychiatrists.

DUFFETT & LELLIOT

Please write your answers to questions I to IV in the spaces provided.

I.   Background

A.(i) List the key components of the audit cycle.   [10 marks]

....
....
....
....
....
....
....
....

(ii)   Illustrate how these have been met in this audit.   [5 marks]

....
....
....
....

B.(i) List potential problems in the way the revised guidelines were disseminated.   [5 marks]

....
....
....
....
....
....
....
....

(ii)   Can you suggest other ways in which the guidelines could have been
         disseminated?   [10 marks]

....
....
....
....
....
....
....
....

C.   Was a new guideline justified by the results of previous audits? Discuss the issues, including new evidence and the public interest.   [15 marks]

....
....
....
....
....
....
....
....
....
....
....

II.   Method

A.   What is problematic about the way the ratings at each clinic visited were carried out?
                                                                                               [10 marks]

....
....
....
....
....
....
....
....

III.   Results

A.(i) How do the authors justify combining data from Component 1 and Component 2?
                                                                                               [5 marks]

....
....
....
....

(ii)   What are the pitfalls in this approach?   [10 marks]

....
....
....
....
....
....
....
....
....

(iii)   What aspects of ECT practice had improved most since the previous audit?   [10 marks]

....
....
....
....
....

IV.   Summary

A.   List five major clinical implications of this audit.   [10 marks]

....
....
....
....
....
....

B.   What barriers are there to implementing these guidelines?   [5 marks]

....
....
....

C.   Identify any general limitations or shortcomings in this audit.   [5 marks]

....
....
....

I.   Background

A.(i) List the key components of the audit cycle.

Choose a topic of importance and/or controversy in which performance is theoretically modifiable. Define a set of standards. Evaluate current practice against these standards. Suggest/implement change. Re-evaluate practice and redefine standards if necessary.

(ii)   Illustrate how these have been met in this audit.

ECT is of wide public interest and is clinically important. Previous audits had revealed widely variable standards throughout the UK. A new set of standards (Handbook II) was issued in 1995 and the current audit evaluated practice against these. This is the third round of this particular audit cycle.

B.(i) List potential problems in the way the revised guidelines were disseminated.

By several modalities: a bulky handbook, a training video, training courses, and published articles. All might be perceived as 'top down', some were time consuming, none had local involvement at a formative stage and none was a shared experience between psychiatrists and nurses. Perhaps crucially, commissioners of mental health care were not directly involved.

(ii)   Can you suggest other ways in which the guidelines could have been disseminated?

A handbook and executive summary might have been sent, free of charge, to the clinical director and senior nurse manager of every psychiatric clinic providing ECT, and executive summaries and a statement of minimal contract standards sent (with a firm recommendation) to chief executives of relevant trusts and to the officer responsible for commissioning at the relevant health authority. The directive might have recommended the immediate establishment of local multi-disciplinary ECT committees, to be responsible for operationalising the guideline in the local context, with particular attention to the joint involvement of psychiatric (senior and junior), nursing and anaesthetic staff.

C.   Was a new guideline justified by the results of previous audits? Discuss the issues, including new evidence and the public interest.

Previous audits revealed continuing wide variation between clinics and several serious shortcomings – particularly in the delivery of ECT (the use of obsolete machines and poor or absent protocols for stimulus delivery), poor training and inadequate consultant supervision. However, evidence of improvement had emerged from the earlier audit cycle which followed publication of the first guideline. Since the last audit by Pippard in 1992 new evidence had emerged clarifying the need for ECT machines with a wide range of current deliveries, and for more careful matching of the stimulus to the patient. Critical public interest had reawakened, provoked by dramatic and ill-informed media and press descriptions. The 'one flew over' image was as intense as ever, and something had to be seen to be done.

II.   Method

A.   What is problematic about the way the ratings at each clinic visited were carried out?

These were a mixture of hard and soft observations – the objective assessment of the ECT equipment and the subjective ratings of general amenity and atmosphere in the clinic environment. Global ratings took account of several factors including the facilities, the personnel, how 'smoothly' the clinic ran, and the 'effectiveness' of the session observed. What constituted effectiveness is not specified. The observer must, to some extent, have influenced the atmosphere and the single observer's assessment, although likely to have been reproducible between clinics, might have been reproducibly idiosyncratic (despite the involvement, by proxy, of Pippard). These were 'snapshots' and by definition may have been non-representative of the clinics' usual operation. A more structured and detailed series of ratings carried out by a pair of observers (with measures of inter-rater agreement) and a test–re-test assessment would have been preferable.

III. Results

A.(i) How do the authors justify combining data from Component I and Component 2?

In 10 clinics double data were obtained – from both visit and questionnaire. The results were felt to be 'sufficiently similar' to warrant combination of data from both sources in the final data analysis.

(iii) What are the pitfalls in this approach?

Combining data was justified because results were sufficiently similar from a small subsample, but it is not clear what is meant by sufficiently similar. It is not clear how these 10 clinics were selected – was it randomly? If not, systematic bias could operate. Even if random, 10 clinics represents only 5% of the total, a dangerously small sample in a situation where the between-clinic variation is wide. Also the choice of clinics to be visited in Component 1 was not random; it was prompted partly in order to reproduce Pippard's second audit, and the addition of Wales was presumably convenient. Thus, ample room exists for selection bias. Like is not being combined with like; mixing data from Components 1 and 2 is equivalent to performing a faulty meta-analysis in which data derived from disparate methodologies are combined; one was an observer-rated snapshot, the other a self-report which allowed the respondents to give an overall description of their clinic and one in which there would be a strong tendency to underrate the negative and overrate the positive. Thus the validity of the conclusions might have been seriously compromised.

(iii) What aspects of ECT practice had most improved since the previous audit?

ECT machines no longer were wheeled from bed to bed, operating department assistants had appeared in some and recovery areas created. Obsolete machines were much less in evidence, consultants were more directly involved in clinic operation and anaesthetic services had improved.

IV. Summary

A. List five major clinical implications of this audit.

    (a) Consultant time must be specifically and rigidly dedicated to supervision.
    (b) Junior doctors must have more structured training and supervision.
    (c) Local clinical guidelines should be derived which are enforceable, auditable, and yet faithful to the national handbook.
    (d) Production and implementation of local protocols should emerge from inter-professional discussion between, and involvement of, psychiatric, nursing and anaesthetic staff.
    (e) Structured local audit and protocol modification should become a regular ongoing practice, carried out by a multi-disciplinary group.

B. What barriers are there to implementing these guidelines?

Lack of a feeling of local involvement, lack of specific time allowance in job plans, lack of nursing involvement, the Handbook is not 'handy' (needs a separate executive summary) and the importance has not been emphasised to commissioners in terms of contract specifications.

C. Identify any general limitations or shortcomings in this audit.

This was an audit of structure and process. The question of outcome was not addressed, although curiously the authors included effectiveness in their global clinical rating. The recipients of ECT and/or their families/informal carers were not included and so even outcome in terms of patient satisfaction, let alone symptom improvement, was not measured.

A CRITICAL REVIEW PAPER

Case register study
Model answers by David Owens

Trends in deliberate self-harm in Oxford, 1985–1995

Implications for clinical services and the prevention of suicide

KEITH HAWTON, JOAN FAGG, SUE SIMKIN, ELIZABETH BALE
and ALISON BOND

Rates of deliberate self-harm (DSH) (self-poisoning and self-injury) in the UK escalated during the late 1960s and early 1970s to such an extent that it became a major health problem (Bancroft *et al*, 1975; Holding *et al*, 1977). This problem was particularly marked in adolescents and young adults (Kreitman & Schreiber, 1979; Hawton & Goldacre, 1982). Following a decline in rates during the late 1970s and early 1980s, notably in older teenage girls (Platt *et al*, 1988; Sellar *et al*, 1990*a*), we subsequently reported that rates in Oxford had begun to rise again in the late 1980s (Hawton & Fagg, 1992*a*), especially in older adolescent females (Hawton & Fagg, 1992*b*). Subsequently, it became clear that the rates of DSH in the UK are among the highest in Europe (Schmidtke *et al*, 1996). Because of the size of the problem of DSH and its associated significant risk of suicide (Hawton & Fagg, 1988), any changes in its prevalence can have important clinical implications both for general medical and psychiatric services and for suicide prevention. The aims of this study were to review trends in DSH which are relevant to the prevention of self-harm and service provision for this population. In this paper we have utilised data collected through the Oxford Monitoring System for Attempted Suicide (Hawton & Fagg, 1992*a*) to review trends in DSH in Oxford during the 11 years 1985 to 1995.

METHOD

The study population consisted of all persons referred to the general hospital in Oxford between 1985 and 1995 following self-poisoning or self-injury. The general hospital receives all hospital-referred cases from Oxford City and the surrounding area. Patients referred to the hospital following self-poisoning or self-injury are identified by the Monitoring System maintained by the University Department of Psychiatry (Hawton & Fagg,

1992*a*). Most attempted suicide patients are routinely referred to the emergency psychiatric service in the hospital. All patients referred to the service receive a detailed psychosocial assessment by a specially trained psychiatrist, psychiatric nurse, or social worker. Most assessments are discussed in detail with a senior psychiatrist. A range of patient characteristics and clinical items are recorded by the assessors on data sheets which are then coded and the data entered into a computerised data file. Through scrutiny of the records of the accident and emergency department a limited amount of information is also available on patients presenting to the hospital but not seen by the psychiatric service. We have previously demonstrated the reliability of our method of data collection (Sellar *et al*, 1990*b*).

Self-poisoning is defined as the intentional self-administration of more than the prescribed dose of any drug whether or not there is evidence that the act was intended to cause self-harm. This category also includes overdoses of 'drugs for kicks' and poisoning by non-ingestible substances and gas, provided the hospital staff consider that these are cases of deliberate self-harm. Alcohol intoxication is not included unless accompanied by other types of self-poisoning or self-injury. Self-injury is defined as any injury recognised by hospital staff as having been deliberately self-inflicted.

Calculation of rates

In the calculation of annual rates and examination of trends in rates, each individual could only contribute to the data once in any one year. However, they were included in the calculations of rates for other years if they made further attempts in those years. Where findings for the whole study period are averaged this is either on the basis of persons, in which case each individual could only contribute to the data once (i.e. 'true' persons), or episodes.

Clinical variables

Findings with regard to demographic variables, methods of self-harm, and repetition of attempts, are based on the total population of patients referred to the hospital. Most of the other clinical information was only available for patients assessed by the clinical service. We have reported on the problems patients referred in 1995 were facing, these problems being indicated by the clinical assessors on a standard check-list. A problem was defined as 'a factor which was causing current distress for the patient and/or contributed to the attempt'.

Repetition of attempts has been studied according to (a) previous attempts leading to hospital referral before the first referral during the study period, and (b) repeat attempts resulting in re-referral to the general hospital in Oxford during the year following the first referral in any one year (1985–1994 only).

Suicide rates

Data on annual suicide rates for England and Wales were obtained from the Office for National Statistics. Rates of suicide in the category 'suicide' (E950–E959) and 'undetermined cause' (E980–E989) were combined to provide a more valid estimate of the overall rates of suicide (Charlton *et al*, 1992).

Statistical analysis

The data were analysed with the SPSSX statistical package (SPSS, 1993) using χ^2 and Spearman's rho (two-tailed) tests where appropriate. In testing for trends the χ^2 test for trend was used where trends were approximately linear and χ^2 for proportions in grouped years where the trends were clearly non-linear.

RESULTS

Referrals to the general hospital

During the 11 years 1985 to 1995, 7437 persons presented to the hospital following 10 631 episodes of DSH. There was an increase in both the annual number of persons (mean annual increase +4.6% per year) and episodes (+7.2% per year) during the study period. This was more marked for males (persons +5.8% per year; episodes +7.9% per year) than females (persons +3.8% per year; episodes +5.6% per year). The gender ratio for episodes steadily declined, from

1.43 (F:M) in 1985 to 1.35 in 1990 and 1.23 in 1995.

Rate of DSH

Person-based rates for Oxford City reflected these changes (Fig. 1). The overall rate rose between 1985 and 1995 by 50.9% (χ^2 for trend=26.18, 1 d.f., $P<0.0001$), the rates in males by 62.1% (χ^2 for trend=19.59, 1 d.f. $P<0.0001$) and the rate in females by 42.2% (χ^2 for trend=8.42, 1 d.f., $P<0.01$). The gender ratio for rates decreased from 1.40 (F:M) in 1985 to 1.33 in 1990 and 1.23 in 1995.

When the trends were examined according to gender and age groups it was apparent that the increase in male rates (Fig. 2) was especially marked in 15–24-year-olds. The annual rates per 100 000 in 15–24-year-old males increased from 162.2 in 1985 to 477.1 in 1995, an increase of 194.1% (χ^2 for trend based on raw data=27.72, 1 d.f., $P<0.0001$). Rates also increased in females aged 25–34 years, with a 35.6% increase during the study period (χ^2 for trend=3.98, 1 d.f., $P<0.05$), and 35–54 years, with a 67.7% increase during the study period (χ^2 for trend=4.56, 1 d.f., $P<0.05$). Rates in other age groups did not change significantly.

Associations with rates of suicide

In males aged 15–24 years, annual rates of DSH in Oxford correlated positively with the combined annual rates of suicide (ICD codes E950–E959) and undetermined cause of death (E980–E989) in England and Wales between 1985 and 1995 (Spearman's rho=0.60, $P=0.053$). When the association was examined in 15–24-year-old females, it was also close to statistical significance (rho=0.58, $P=0.06$). The correlations in other age groups for both males and females were much smaller, although all were posi-

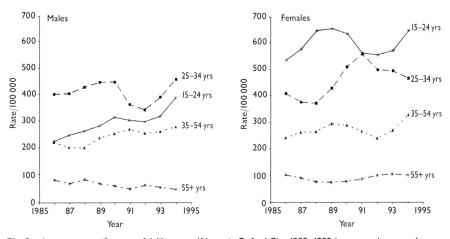

Fig. 2 Age group specific rates of deliberate self-harm in Oxford City, 1985–1995 (rates are shown as three-year moving averages).

tive apart from those for females aged 35–54 years and 55 years and over.

Repetition of DSH

Repetition of DSH also increased, as reflected in an increase in the episodes: persons ratio from an annual average of 1.15 in 1985–1990 to 1.24 in 1991–1995. The repetition rate within a year of an episode in each calendar year also increased, averaging 13.1% in 1985–1989 and 16.1% in 1990–1994 (χ^2=13.81, $P<0.001$). While the repetition rate within a year of a first episode in each year was generally higher in males (mean=15.8%) than females (mean=14.0%), the increase in annual repetition rates was more marked in females (11.9% in 1985–1989 to 15.8% in 1990–1994; χ^2=15.05, $P<0.01$) than males (15.0% to 16.5%, NS).

There was some indication of a diminution in the percentage of individuals (who received a psychiatric assessment) carrying out their first episodes of DSH (hospital referred or otherwise) during the study period. This proportion declined from 58.7% in 1985–1990 to 51.3% in 1991–1995. However, the mean annual numbers of 'first-timers' were very similar in the two time periods, being 353 in 1985–1990 and 350 in 1991–1995.

Methods used

During the period of the study, 87.9% (n=9345) of episodes of DSH involved self-poisoning, 8.3% (n=887) involved self-injury, and 3.8% (n=399) both self-poisoning and self-injury. There were major changes in the substances used for self-

poisoning. There was a steady increase in the use of non-opiate analgesics (χ^2 for trend=38.14, $P<0.0001$), this increase being entirely accounted for by the massive increase in the use of paracetamol (including paracetamol-containing compounds). Thus whereas in 1985 31.3% of overdoses involved paracetamol, by 1995 this figure had risen to 49.6% (χ^2 for trend=98.14, $P<0.0001$). This increase was most marked in females, in whom paracetamol overdoses increased from 29.6% in 1985 to 52.6% in 1995. The comparable increase in males was from 34.1 to 45.9%.

There was also an increase in antidepressant overdoses, from 11.6% in 1985 to 18.2% in 1995 (χ^2 for trend=55.46, $P<0.0001$). This increase was somewhat more marked in males (from 8.0% in 1985 to 18.1% in 1995) than in females (from 13.9% in 1985 to 18.3% in 1995). Of those who took antidepressant overdoses in 1995, 58.9% used tricyclics and 29.5% used selective serotonin reuptake inhibitors (SSRIs). The previously noted decline in overdoses of minor tranquillisers and sedatives continued between 1985 and 1995, with a drop from 25.5 to 15.6% (χ^2 for trend=49.19, $P<0.0001$).

Problems preceding self-harm

The most frequent problems identified as being present at the time of self-harm in the patients who presented in 1995 and were assessed by a member of the hospital psychiatric service showed some marked gender differences. Problems concerning a partner, employment or studies, alcohol, drugs and finances were all more common in the males and problems with family members other

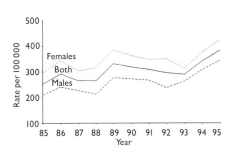

Fig. 1 Rates of deliberate self-harm in Oxford City in persons aged 15 years and over, by gender, 1985–1995.

than a partner were more common in the females.

In terms of living circumstances, an annual mean of 3.2% of individuals (6.4% of males and 1.0% of females) were of no fixed abode. This figure increased between 1985–1990 and 1991–1995, from 2.4 to 3.9% ($\chi^2=16.61$, $P<0.001$).

Admissions to the general hospital, psychiatric assessment and in-patient psychiatric admission

In spite of the considerable increase in the numbers of patients presenting to the general hospital following DSH the proportion admitted to an in-patient bed varied little during the study period, averaging 86.5% per year.

An average of 10.2% of all patients each year were admitted to in-patient psychiatric care from the general hospital, approximately half of whom were already in current psychiatric care and a third were current in-patients. This proportion increased from a mean of 7.9% in 1985–1987 to 12.5% in 1993–1995 ($\chi^2=30.78$, $P<0.001$). This change was more marked in females (from 7.7 to 13.5%; $\chi^2=27.82$, $P<0.001$) than males (from 8.2 to 11.2%; $\chi^2=5.33$, $P<0.05$).

DISCUSSION

Increased rates of DSH and implications for suicide prevention

The rising trends in DSH identified in Oxford appear to reflect what is happening elsewhere in the UK. We previously estimated on the basis of Oxford rates that the mean annual number of people presenting to hospitals following DSH in 1989 and 1990 in England and Wales would have been 120 000 (Hawton & Fagg, 1992a). On the basis of the 1995 rate the figure would be 142 000, a substantially increased proportion of whom are males.

The increase in DSH has been most marked in young males. This trend has clearly paralleled the recent trend in deaths from suicide and probable suicide.

One factor contributing to the recent rise in DSH appears to have been an increase in frequency of repetition, particularly in females. The reasons for this are unclear.

Implications for clinical services

The great increase in male DSH patients presents considerable problems for service provision. Not only do males, as we have shown, take their own discharge from hospital more often than females, a recent review of outcome of treatment studies following DSH has shown that they are less easy to engage in treatment and that currently available methods of treatment appear to be less efficacious in males (Hawton, 1997).

Changes in substances used in overdoses

The increasing rise in the use of paracetamol for self-poisoning and the concomitant rise in paracetamol-related deaths (Gunnell et al, 1997) clearly necessitates urgent preventive strategies. The rise in antidepressant overdoses in recent years presumably reflects more widespread prescribing, including greater use of SSRIs and other less toxic preparations in patients thought to be at risk of overdose.

Problems preceding DSH

The pattern of problems facing DSH patients showed an interesting change from that found in earlier studies in that whereas problems with partners used to be far more common in female DSH patients (e.g. Bancroft et al, 1977), the reverse was true in our study.

REFERENCES

Bancroft, J., Skrimshire, A., Reynolds, F., et al (1975) Self-poisoning and self-injury in the Oxford area: epidemiological aspects 1969–1973. British Journal of Preventive and Social Medicine, 29, 170–177.

__ , __ , Casson, J., et al (1977) People who deliberately poison or injure themselves: their problems and their contacts with helping agencies. Psychological Medicine, 7, 289–303.

Charlton, J., Kelly, S., Dunnell, K., et al (1992) Trends in suicide deaths in England and Wales. Population Trends, 69, 10–16.

Gunnell, D., Hawton, K., Murray, V., et al (1997) Use of paracetamol for suicide and non-fatal poisoning in the UK and France: Are restrictions on availability justified? Journal of Epidemiology and Community Health, 51, 175–179.

Hawton, K. (1997) Attempted suicide. In Science and Practice of Cognitive Behaviour Therapy (eds D. M. Clark & C. G. Fairburn), pp. 285–312. Oxford: Oxford University Press.

__ & Goldacre, M. (1982) Hospital admissions for adverse effects of medicinal agents (mainly self-poisoning) among adolescents in the Oxford Region. British Journal of Psychiatry, 141, 166–170.

__ & Fagg, J. (1988) Suicide, and other causes of death, following attempted suicide. British Journal of Psychiatry, 152, 359–366.

__ & __ (1992a) Trends in deliberate self-poisoning and self-injury in Oxford, 1976–90. British Medical Journal, 304, 1409–1411.

__ & __ (1992b) Deliberate self-poisoning and self-injury in adolescents: a study of characteristics and trends in Oxford, 1976–89. British Journal of Psychiatry, 161, 816–823.

Holding, T., Buglass, D., Duffy, J. C., et al (1977) Parasuicide in Edinburgh – a seven year review 1968–74. British Journal of Psychiatry, 130, 534–543.

Kreitman, N. & Schreiber, M. (1979) Parasuicide in young Edinburgh women, 1968–75. Psychological Medicine, 141, 37–44.

Platt, S., Hawton, K., Kreitman, N., et al (1988) Recent clinical and epidemiological trends in parasuicide in Edinburgh and Oxford: a tale of two cities. Psychological Medicine, 18, 405–418.

Schmidtke, A., Bille-Brahe, U., Deleo, D., et al (1996) Attempted suicide in Europe: rates, trends, and sociodemographic characteristics of suicide attempters during the period 1989–1992. Results of the WHO/EURO Multicentre Study on Parasuicide. Acta Psychiatrica Scandinavica, 93, 327–338.

Sellar, C., Hawton, K. & Goldacre, M. J. (1990a) Self-poisoning in adolescents: hospital admissions and deaths in the Oxford Region 1980–1985. British Journal of Psychiatry, 56, 866–870.

__ , Goldacre, M. J. & Hawton, K. (1990b) Reliability of routine hospital data on poisoning as measures of deliberate self-poisoning in adolescents. Journal of Epidemiology and Community Health, 44, 313–315.

SPSS (1993) SPSSX for Unix: Base System User's Guide, Release 5.0. Chicago, IL: SPSS Inc.

HAWTON *ET AL*

Please write your answers to questions I to IV in the spaces provided.

I.   Background

A.   Why are changes in incidence of deliberate self-harm so important?   [10 marks]

....
....
....
....
....
....
....
....

II.   Method

A.   What are the limitations of the data collection?   [15 marks]

....
....
....
....
....
....
....
....
....

B.   What is the basis of the authors' claim that combining the category 'suicide' and the category 'undermined cause' provides a more valid estimate of suicide rates?   [10 marks]

....
....
....
....
....
....
....
....
....

C. (i) What is a χ^2 test? [5marks]

....
....
....
....

(ii) What is a Spearman's rho test? [5 marks]

....
....
....
....

III. Results

A. List three reasons why there may have been a change in substances used for self-poisoning during the period of the study. [15 marks]

....
....
....
....
....
....
....
....

IV. Discussion

A. What are the main implications of this study for medical and psychiatric services? [15 marks]

....
....
....
....
....
....
....
....
....
....
....

B. What are the main implications of this study with regard to suicide prevention?   [15marks]

....
....
....
....
....
....
....
....
....
....

C. What are the limitations of the findings regarding repetition rates?   [5 marks]

....
....
....
....

D. In what way does the study provide evidence against effective primary prevention of
    deliberate self-harm?   [5 marks]

....
....
....
....

I. Background

A. Why are changes in incidence of deliberate self-harm so important?

Upward or downward trends in deliberate self-harm incidence affect physical care in accident and emergency and upon in-patient wards in the general hospital. In both these settings, change in incidence also results in altered need for psychosocial assessment. Alterations in the age- and gender-specific rates may influence need for particular types of service: for example, compared with older people, young people take different substances and have different psychosocial problems and characteristics.

A strong link has long been established between non-fatal self-harm and suicide. Any rise or fall in deliberate self-harm might be expected to influence subsequent suicide rates.

II. Method

A. What are the limitations of the data collection?

Although the paper tackles deliberate self-harm in Oxford, not all self-harm episodes in Oxford are represented. Some people take an overdose and do not contact health services; others will be dealt with by their general practitioner only. Some Oxford residents may attend another hospital (although we are told that the general hospital can expect to receive all the cases from the city and surrounding areas). The basic data include cases seen only in accident and emergency, but some will be missed because the 'diagnosis' of self-harm is not made or not recorded correctly.

Only limited data were collected on patients who attended hospital but were not referred to the specialist psychosocial assessment service; for example, the results concerning problems faced by the 1995 patients are based on only 72% (738/1020) of cases. Missing cases do not bring about random error: they are likely to include an excess of those who were uncooperative, those whose self-harm was thought to be trivial, those thought to have got over their problems and so on.

B. What is the basis of the authors' claim that combining the category 'suicide' and the category 'undetermined cause' provides a more valid estimate of suicide rates?

Coroners vary greatly in their willingness to assign a verdict of suicide – and there are time trends in coroners' practice. Where there is no suicide note, and no statement of intent to another person, then coroners are particularly likely to assign another verdict – some are described as accidents, others of undetermined cause. Clinical research involving close scrutiny of deaths supports the notion that many deaths of 'undetermined cause' and some by 'accidental poisoning' are really suicides. Regarding verdicts of suicide and undetermined cause as suicides is a widely used research procedure.

C. (i) What is a χ^2 test?

The χ^2 test is a significance test which has the effect of comparing two or more independent proportions (although the mathematics are carried out using raw numbers, not proportions). The null hypothesis is that the variables under scrutiny are evenly balanced between groups. The calculations involve examining the differences between the actual proportions found and those which might be expected if the null hypothesis were true.

(ii) What is a Spearman's rho test?

Spearman's rho is the result obtained from calculating a Spearman's rank correlation coefficient. By using the rank order of a variable rather than its actual values it is typical of distribution-free (or non-parametric) tests. The more commonly used Pearson's correlation coefficient should not be used unless one of the variables is reasonably normally distributed at given values of the other. In addition, some argue that distribution-free tests should usually be used when data are ordinal rather than continuous or ratio.

III. Results

A. List three reasons why there may have been a change in substances used for self-poisoning during the period of the study.

(a) There has been a decrease in use of tranquillisers and sedatives in self-poisoning episodes, in line with a decrease in the prescribing of these drugs.

(b) There has been an increase in use of antidepressants in self-poisoning episodes, accompanied by an increase in prescribing of antidepressants in recent years – especially since the introduction of newer anti-depressants whose side-effects and safety are alleged to be more favourable than those of older drugs.

(c) There has been a huge increase in use of paracetamol-containing drugs in deliberate self-poisoning. Reasons are not clear but may include increased availability in retail outlets and the home.

IV. Discussion

A. What are the main implications of this study for medical and psychiatric services?

Oxford rates of deliberate self-harm have been rising again since 1985, after steadying and then declining in the late 1970s and early 1980s. Oxford rates are borne out by other studies (although only Oxford has a comprehensive long-term monitoring system) and point to a national rise in numbers and rates.

More people attend accident and emergency where there is thereby more need for physical and psychosocial assessment and care. Similarly, in-patient general hospital (non-psychiatric) wards may be dealing with more cases. However, because there is an increase around the UK in discharge of deliberate self-harm patients from accident and emergency, the impact on the in-patient services may be less than that on accident and emergency.

The disproportionate increase in rate among males, particularly young males, poses an especially difficult problem for psychosocial assessment and care because they form a group whom clinicians and researchers have found difficult to engage and help.

B. What are the main implications of this study with regard to suicide prevention?

Non-fatal deliberate self-harm is known to be associated with greatly increased risk of subsequent suicide. Plainly a rise in self-harm seems likely to lead to increased incidence of suicide. This notion is supported by the correlational evidence here: the rise in annual rates of deliberate self-harm in young males and young females is correlated (not quite statistically significantly in females) with rises in suicides.

These findings do not bode well for the current public health strategies for reductions in suicide rates (for example in the *Health of the Nation* and in the *Our Healthier Nation* proposals).

C. What are the limitations of the findings regarding repetition rates?

Each person in the study is only followed up for one year after an episode (even though individuals may reappear in the data in a subsequent year). Repetition rate findings are thereby restricted to one-year maximum.

We are not told about rates of early repetition – for example within the first few days or weeks after an episode; this period has an important bearing on patient management and how quickly follow-up arrangements are needed.

D. In what way does the study provide evidence against effective primary prevention of deliberate self-harm?

If primary prevention of deliberate self-harm were effective then we might expect to see a decrease in raw numbers of lifetime first episodes of deliberate self-harm. Unfortunately no such fall was seen. There was a reduction in the proportion of cases due to 'first-timers' in the second five-year period of the study, but this is probably explained by a growth in the denominator of total episodes. The disproportionate increase in rates among young people may also suggest failure of primary prevention.

A CRITICAL REVIEW PAPER

Case–control study
Model answers by Simon Wessely

The psychiatric status of patients with the chronic fatigue syndrome

IAN HICKIE, ANDREW LLOYD, DENIS WAKEFIELD and GORDON PARKER

Straus (1988) stated that "ultimately, any hypothesis regarding the cause of the chronic fatigue syndrome must incorporate the psychopathology that accompanies and, in some cases, precedes it," emphasising the importance of assessing psychopathology both premorbidly and during the illness.

The frequency of neuropsychiatric and depressive symptoms in these patients (David et al, 1988; Straus, 1988) suggested the specific hypothesis that chronic fatigue syndrome (CFS) occurs in individuals with a premorbid vulnerability to depression.

In this paper we record the prevalence of psychiatric morbidity in patients with CFS both during and before the illness episode to determine whether the syndrome is associated with an increase in psychological disturbance, and whether subjects had a higher premorbid rate of psychiatric disturbance. We included a control group of patients with non-endogenous depression to assess whether CFS patients resembled patients with depression, either during the illness episode or on premorbid measures.

METHOD

We studied 48 subjects with marked and persistent fatigue who met the following operational criteria for CFS (Lloyd et al, 1988a).

To fulfil the criteria a patient must have chronic, persistent or relapsing fatigue of a generalised nature, causing major disruption of usual daily activities, present for more than six months, plus two major or one major and three minor criteria (symptoms, signs or assessments):

(a) Symptoms: persisting at least six months continuously, or relapsing on three or more occasions with a similar pattern over six months or more:

(i) Major: concentration/memory impairment

(ii) Minor: myalgia, arthralgia, depression, tinnitus, paraesthesia, headaches.

(b) Signs: present on at least one occasion subsequent to the initial illness:

(i) Major: lymphadenopathy

(ii) Minor: pharyngitis, muscle tenderness.

(c) Immunological assessment:

(i) Major: cutaneous anergy, T4 or T8 lymphopenia

(ii) Minor: hypoergy

The criteria that we have recommended since are a simplification of those original criteria (Lloyd et al, 1988b). Both of our sets of criteria emphasise the importance of a characteristic pattern of physical and neuropsychological impairment and the demonstration of impaired cell-mediated immunity.

All patients had been referred by their general practitioner to the immunology or infectious diseases department of a university teaching hospital for evaluation of their chronic fatigue. Patients referred to this service typically had been extensively investigated by their own practitioners and/or other consultant physicians. Additionally, many had been assessed previously by a psychiatrist. The patients in this report were drawn from a previously described sample of 200 patients (Lloyd et al, 1988b) who had been assessed rigorously to exclude other possible physical causes of fatigue (infectious diseases or thyroid, neurological, haematological, hepatic, renal or autoimmune dysfunction). Although the Centers for Disease Control (CDC) criteria were not established at the time our patients were enrolled, the process of physical evaluation and investigation we used was as extensive as that recommended by Holmes et al (1988).

Twenty-nine of the 48 patients had developed their persistent fatigue immediately after an acute infectious illness. Five of these illnesses had been documented serologically (four Epstein–Barr virus infections, one toxoplasmosis). Patients were approached to progress to a treatment trial on the basis of the persistence of their symptoms and their willingness to give informed consent to participate in a double-blind, placebo-controlled, treatment trial of intravenous immunoglobulin therapy (to be reported elsewhere). The extensive process of physical evaluation within a tertiary referral service, the application of strict clinical and laboratory criteria, and the delay between initial contact with the clinic and inclusion in the treatment trial, all limited the clinical heterogeneity that one might expect within such a sample.

Initially, each subject was asked by the psychiatrist (I.H.) to describe their 'key symptoms'. The interviewer recorded the frequency with which psychological and neuropsychological symptoms were reported spontaneously before administering a standardised psychiatric interview schedule (SCID–P; Spitzer & Williams, 1985) which generated DSM–III–R (American Psychiatric Association, 1987) diagnostic data. A relative of each patient was interviewed independently to corroborate the patient's report. Because of a delay in the commencement of the psychiatrist's involvement in the trial, 33 patients were interviewed before treatment, and the remaining 15 patients after completion of immunoglobulin infusions.

All subjects completed a number of psychometric measures, including the 30-item General Health Questionnaire (GHQ; Goldberg, 1979), the Zung Self-Rating Depression Scale (Zung, 1965), the Eysenck Personality Inventory (Eysenck & Eysenck, 1964) and the Illness Behaviour Questionnaire (Pilowsky & Spence, 1983). The latter scale generates scores on seven dimensions which indicate the subject's attitudes towards the illness. The 17-item Hamilton Rating Scale for Depression (Hamilton, 1960) and the Newcastle Depression Scale (Carney et al, 1965), used to identify patients with endogenous depression, were administered by the psychiatrist.

Forty-eight patients with non-endogenous depression (Newcastle Depression Scale score less than five) were selected from the in-patient and out-patient psychiatric services of the same hospital for comparison with the patients with CFS.

RESULTS

The mean age of the patients was 36 (range 15–63) years, and there were equal numbers of men and women. The mean duration of illness was 56 (median 46, range 12–156) months. The sample therefore contained patients with chronic illness with little prospect of spontaneous remission.

The control subjects suffering from non-endogenous depression were matched exactly for gender and similarly for age (36.1 $v.$ 37.8 years, $t=1.56$, NS) and social class (mean Congalton (1969) score: 3.69 $v.$ 3.89, $t=1.01$, NS). Of the 48 control patients, 28 met DSM–III–R criteria for major depression, while the remaining 20 had minor depressive disorders. None of these control patients had been depressed continuously for two years, so that there were no cases of dysthymic disorder. Nineteen were in-patients of a general hospital psychiatry unit, while 29 were from out-patient and liaison psychiatry clinics.

Of the 48 patients with CFS, 19 spontaneously reported psychological and 29 reported neuropsychological complaints among their key symptoms.

Twenty-four warranted a psychiatric diagnosis during the course of their illness. The most common disorder was major (non-endogenous) depression (8 men, 14 women). Six of these 22 patients with depression with CFS also experienced panic attacks, although these were frequent enough in only one case to justify an additional diagnosis of panic disorder. In addition, three non-depressed patients had experienced at least one panic attack and two of these subjects met criteria for panic disorder. Only one patient, who also met criteria for major depression, fulfilled criteria for somatisation disorder (Briquet's hysteria). There were no cases of generalised anxiety disorder and, although a number of patients reported simple phobias, none was associated with avoidant behaviour leading to significant impairment of daily functioning.

The overall concordance of subject/witness reports was very high (kappa= 0.87), with relatives reporting a psychiatric diagnosis in 23 of the patients, strongly supporting the accuracy of our estimate. In the 33 patients assessed before treatment, the prevalence rate of psychiatric disorder in the preceding month was 21% (7/33), all having major (non-endogenous) depression.

The GHQ scores of the 33 subjects assessed immediately before treatment established that 15 had a score of five or above, generally suggestive of psychiatric morbidity (Goldberg, 1979). In patients with known medical disorders, however, significant physical symptoms inevitably lead to positive responses on more of the GHQ items. Zung depression scores for the 33 subjects assessed before treatment showed that 19 scores above the recommended cut-off point of 40 (Zung, 1972) for identifying mild depression in community settings. As with the GHQ, the raw Zung score is known to be significantly elevated in medical patients (Zung et al, 1983). It is possible to overcome this effect, in part, by comparing the number of patients and depressive controls assigned to at least the moderately depressed range (48 or above) on the Zung scale. Using this higher cut-off point, a highly significant difference ($\chi^2=22.06$, $P<0.001$) remained between the number of patients with CFS (8/33) in comparison with the number of depressive controls (37/48). This established that depressive disorders of clinical severity were rare in the CFS sample.

This distinction was supported by the significant differences between the mean scores of the CFS patients and depressive controls on the Hamilton (10.6 $v.$ 19.0, $t=8.92$, $P<0.001$) and Zung (40.7 $v.$ 55.2, $t=7.67$, $P<0.001$) scales. Importantly, patients with CFS also reported significantly lower levels of neuroticism (7.3 $v.$ 15.8, $t=7.71$, $P<0.001$). This suggested that any psychiatric morbidity in the CFS sample was less severe, in addition to being less prevalent, than in depressed patients.

Table 1 records the patients', their relatives', and the depressives' estimates of prior psychological morbidity. Again there was substantial agreement between the patients' and relatives' estimates of overall premorbid psychiatric morbidity in the CFS group (kappa=0.81).

The scores of the patients with CFS on the seven dimensions of the Illness Behaviour Questionnare are shown in Table 2. Comparison of these data with previously reported Australian general practice samples (Pilowsky & Spence, 1983) and patients with Briquet's hysteria (Singer et al, 1988) suggests that the illness behaviour of patients with CFS is characterised by the strong conviction that they are physically ill (i.e. high scores on 'disease conviction': "an attitude of determined certainty as to the presence of disease, and a resistance to reassurance" (Pilowsky, 1988) and low scores on 'psychological $v.$ somatic concern', which is said to be indicative of "somatic focusing" (Pilowsky, 1988)).

In contrast to patients with Briquet's hysteria, who typically present their psychological concerns in a somatic form, patients with CFS are not hypochondriacal and are not inhibited in their expression of affectively laden topics. Patients with CFS do differ from general practice patients, however, principally in terms of their reluctance to accept psychological interpretations of their somatic symptoms. Further, they have somewhat higher scores on the 'denial' sub-scale, which purports to measure "the tendency to regard illness as the sole problem, whose resolution would result in a circumstance devoid of difficulties" and "the tendency to displace attention from psychosocial stressors onto physical problems" (Pilowsky, 1988).

DISCUSSION

Our findings do not confirm those of Taerk et al (1987), who suggested a much higher premorbid risk of depressive disorder in patients with CFS. The patients in that study were not as extensively evaluated as the patients in this study or that of Kruesi et al

Table I Numbers of patients and relatives reporting psychiatric morbidity before onset of CFS ($n=48$), and controls ($n=48$) before onset of depression

DSM–III–R	Patients		Depressive controls
	Self-report	Relatives' report	
Major depression	6 (12.5%)	6 (12.5%)	30 (62%)
Panic disorder	1 (2%)	1 (2%)	3 (6%)
Alcohol dependence	4 (8%)	4 (8%)	18 (38%)
Benzodiazepine dependence	–	–	5 (10%)
Psychotic episode	1 (2%)	1 (2%)	–
Total previous morbidity	12 (24.5%)	12 (24.5%)	43 (90%)

Table 2 Mean scores on dimensions of illness behaviour of patients with CFS as measured by the Illness Behaviour Questionnaire (IBQ)

IBQ subscale	CFS patients (n=44) mean (s.d.)	General practice[1] (n=147) mean	Briquet's syndrome[2] (n=17) mean
General hypochondriasis (range=0–9)	1.96 (1.9)	1.44	4.0
Disease conviction (range=0–6)	4.25 (1.2)	1.59	4.0
Psychological v. somatic focusing (range=0–5)	0.45 (0.8)	1.99	1.0
Affective inhibition (range=0–5)	1.98 (1.7)	2.46	4.0
Dysphoria (range=0–5)	2.00 (1.7)	2.31	5.0
Denial (range=0–5)	3.43 (1.6)	2.93	2.0
Irritability (range=0–6)	2.93 (1.8)	2.45	3.0

1. Pilowsky & Spence (1983).
2. Singer et al (1988).

(1989), so that it is likely that their sample was less homogeneous.

Although Taerk et al (1987) did not suggest that depression alone was the cause of their subjects' illnesses, they did suggest that "sporadic neuromyasthenia may be the result of an organic illness in psychologically susceptible (i.e. premorbidly depressed) individuals". By contrast, our results suggest that CFS patients are no more psychologically disturbed before the onset of their illness than members of the general population.

In conclusion, we have demonstrated that while depression and anxiety are common symptoms in patients suffering from CFS, there is no evidence from our well-defined sample to support the hypothesis that CFS is a somatic presentation of an underlying psychological disorder. In particular, there is no evidence that CFS is a variant or expression of a depressive disorder. Instead, our study supports the hypothesis that the current psychological symptoms of patients with CFS are a consequence of the disorder, rather than evidence of antecedent vulnerability. We are unable to say whether the psychological symptoms occur purely as a result of the fatigue, or as an integral symptom of the disease process. Comparisons between patients with CFS and patients who have fatigue on a peripheral basis (e.g. myasthenia gravis) or on a central basis (e.g. multiple sclerosis (Krupp

et al, 1988)) will be undertaken to clarify this issue further.

It is possible that the chronic production of cytokines, such as interferon, which is released by lymphocytes in response to viral infections, may account for the morbidity reported by these patients. These soluble products of lymphocytes may precipitate fatigue and neuropsychiatric syndromes in humans (Denicoff et al, 1987; McDonald et al, 1987) and, therefore, ongoing localised production of these substances within the central nervous system of patients with CFS constitutes a possible explanation for the diverse physical, neuropsychiatric, and psychological symptoms encountered in this syndrome (Wakefield & Lloyd, 1987).

REFERENCES

American Psychiatric Association (1987) Diagnostic and Statistical Manual of Mental Disorders (3rd edn, revised). Washington, DC: APA.

Carney, M. W. P., Roth, M. & Garside, R. F. (1965) The diagnosis of depressive symptoms and the prediction of ECT response. British Journal of Psychiatry, **III**, 659–674.

Congalton, A. R. (1969) Status and Prestige in Australia. Melbourne: F. W. Cheshire Publishing Pty Ltd.

David, A. S., Wessely, S. & Pelosi, A. J. (1988) Postviral fatigue syndrome: time for a new approach. British Medical Journal, **296**, 696–699.

Denicoff, K. D., Rubinow, D. R., Papa, M. Z., et al (1987) The neuropsychiatric effects of treatment with

interleukin-2 and lymphokine-activated killer cells. Annals of Internal Medicine, **107**, 293–300.

Eysenck, H. J. & Eysenck, S. B. (1964) Manual of the Eysenck Personality Inventory. London: Hodder & Stoughton.

Goldberg, D. P. (1979) Manual of the General Health Questionnaire. Windsor: NFER Publishing Co.

Hamilton, M. (1960) A rating scale for depression. Journal of Neurology, Neurosurgery and Psychiatry, **23**, 56–62.

Holmes, G. P., Kaplan, J. E., Gantz, N. M., et al (1988) Chronic fatigue syndrome: a working case definition. Annals of Internal Medicine, **108**, 387–389.

Kruesi, M. J. P., Dale, J. & Straus, S. E. (1989) Psychiatric diagnoses in patients who have chronic fatigue syndrome. Journal of Clinical Psychiatry, **50**, 53–56.

Krupp, L. B., Alvarez, L. A., LaRocca, N. G., et al (1988) Fatigue in multiple sclerosis. Archives of Neurology, **45**, 435–437.

Lloyd, A. R., Hales, J. P. & Gandevia, S. C. (1988a) Muscle strength, endurance and recovery in the post-infection fatigue syndrome. Journal of Neurology, Neurosurgery and Psychiatry, **51**, 1316–1322.

___, Wakefield, D., Boughton, C., et al (1988b) What is myalgic encephalomyelitis? Lancet, i, 1286–1287.

McDonald, E. M., Mann, A. H. & Thomas, H. C. (1987) Interferons as mediators of psychiatric morbidity. An investigation in a trial of recombinant α-interferon in hepatitis-B carriers. Lancet, ii, 1175–1177.

Pilowsky, I. (1988) Abnormal illness behaviour. In Handbook of Social Psychiatry (eds A. S. Henderson & G. Burrows). Amsterdam: Elsevier Science publishers.

___ & Spence, N. D. (1983) Manual for the Illness Behaviour Questionnaire (IBO) (2nd edn). Adelaide: University of Adelaide.

Singer, A., Thompson, S., Kraiuhin, C., et al (1988) An investigation of patients presenting with multiple physical complaints using the Illness Behaviour Questionnaire. Psychotherapy and Psychosomatics, **47**, 181–189.

Spitzer, R. L. & Williams, J. B. W. (1985) Structured Clinical Interview for DSM–III–R, Patient Version (SCID–P, 7/1/85). New York: Biometrics Research Dept, Psychiatric Institute.

Straus, S. E. (1988) The chronic mononucleosis syndrome. Journal of Infectious Diseases, **157**, 405–412.

Taerk, G. S., Toner, B. B., Salit, I. E., et al (1987) Depression in patients with neuromyasthenia (benign myalgic encephalomyelitis). International Journal of Psychiatry in Medicine, **17**, 49–56.

Wakefield, D. & Lloyd, A. (1987) Pathophysiology of myalgic encephalomyelitis. Lancet, ii, 918–919.

Zung, W. W. K. (1965) A self-rating depression scale. Archives of General Psychiatry, **12**, 63–70.

___ (1972) How normal is depression? Psychosomatics, **12**, 174–178.

___, Magill, M., Moore, J. T., et al (1983) Recognition and treatment of depression in a family medicine practice. Journal of Clinical Psychiatry, **44**, 3–6.

HICKIE *ET AL*

Please write your answers to questions I to III in the spaces provided.

I. **Methods**

A. Comment on how the study subjects were chosen. How could this have affected the results of this study? [10 marks]

....
....
....
....
....
....
....
....

B. Why do the authors tell us that not all patients were assessed by the psychiatrist at the same point in the trial? [5 marks]

....
....
....
....

C. (i) What was the purpose of choosing a control group with depression? [5 marks]

....
....
....
....

(ii) Was this the correct control group given the purpose of the study? What problems can you see with the chosen control group? [10 marks]

....
....
....
....
....
....
....
....

D. The interviewing psychiatrist was not blinded to the diagnoses of the patients he was interviewing. How might this have affected his evaluations of patients? [10 marks]

....
....
....
....
....
....
....
....
....
....

E. What can you say about the assessment of premorbid psychiatric disorder? Ideally, how should the rate of premorbid psychiatric disorder be assessed? [15 marks]

....
....
....
....
....
....
....
....

II. Results

A. The authors affirm that "depressive disorders of clinical severity were rare in the CFS sample". What evidence is presented to support this statement? Is there any evidence which does not support it? [15 marks]

....
....
....
....
....
....
....
....
....

III. Summary and further questions

A. What are the clinical implications of this study? [15 marks]

....
....
....
....
....
....
....
....
....
....

B. What are the main limitations of this study? [15 marks]

....
....
....
....
....
....
....
....
....
....

I. Methods

A. Comment on how the study subjects were chosen. How could this have affected the results of this study?

The 48 subjects were chosen from 200 patients referred to a specialist clinic and were those who agreed to take part in a randomised controlled trial of immunoglobulin therapy. Numerous biases operate between the commencement of illness and recruitment to the trial. Many had already been screened by a psychiatrist, suggesting that those with overt psychiatric disorder might already have been excluded. Patients willing to take part in the study may have differed from the other 160 in numerous ways. They could have a higher rate of immunological disorders, a higher rate of health anxiety, a higher or even lower rate of psychopathology, less or more premorbid psychiatric disorder and so on. In other words, the choice of the 48 from the 200 was not random, and was likely to be influenced by numerous factors relevant to those under investigation.

B. Why do the authors tell us that not all patients were assessed by the psychiatrist at the same point in the trial?

Most were assessed at the beginning, but some at the end. The purpose of a clinical trial is to treat patients – thus treatment or placebo effects may have caused a reduction in psychiatric symptoms in that subgroup.

C. (i) What was the purpose of choosing a control group with depression?

The study was concerned with the similarities or disimilarities between depression and CFS. A depressed control group would in theory provide comparisons for features such as symptoms, premorbid psychiatric disorder, treatment response and outcome.

(ii) Was this the correct control group given the purpose of the study? What problems can you see with the chosen control group?

The authors conclude that psychological symptoms in CFS are a consequence of disorder. This conclusion cannot be supported since the only valid comparison group would be patients with other chronic medical conditions, rather than controls who are all by definition chosen because they are depressed. Likewise, cause and effect can only be properly determined in a longitudinal design (see later).

To be a valid control group, cases and controls must come from the same population. Both cases and controls were attending hospital clinics, which reduces selection bias (since patients in the community or primary care differ from hospital patients on many variables), but 19 controls were actually psychiatric in-patients at the time of the study, suggesting severe illness. In contrast, many of the cases of CFS had already been assessed by a psychiatrist prior to referral, and it is possible that severely depressed CFS cases would have been excluded at that time. Likewise, patients with similar symptoms but who believed their problems were related to depression are unlikely to have attended this clinic, introducing a bias in favour of somatisation or somatic conviction in the cases. These are examples of selection bias.

D. The interviewing psychiatrist was not blinded to the diagnoses of the patients he was interviewing. How might this have affected his evaluations of patients?

The answer is observer bias, in that he may have been more likely to rate certain symptoms as present or absent according to the diagnostic status of the patient. Assessing such symptoms as anhedonia or avoidance in a person complaining of severe fatigue is extremely difficult and often subjective. Deciding whether or not loss of interest is true anhedonia, and hence a cardinal symptom of mood disorder, or due to the inability to undertake previously enjoyable tasks because of fatigue, is something even the most experienced interviewer finds difficult. However, it is worth pointing out that in practice it would have been very difficult indeed to ensure the interview stayed blind.

E. What can you say about the assessment of premorbid psychiatric disorder? Ideally, how should the role of premorbid psychiatric disorder be assessed?

Patients attending a psychiatric clinic, and their relatives, have by implication already agreed that their problems are 'psychiatric' in nature, and we can assume are in agreement that their problems are 'depression'. On the other hand, we know from the study that the CFS cases in this sample (but not necessarily elsewhere) are exactly the opposite, whether rightly or wrongly. Hence, there is likely to be considerable recall bias – the depressed controls are more likely to recall and admit to previous episodes of psychiatric disorder, the patients with CFS the opposite. Dating the onset of illness is also very problematic in retrospect, and is made more so by the overlap between the symptoms of depression and those of CFS. The CFS cases had been ill for a mean of nearly five years at assessment, suggesting that recall bias and search after meaning might now by a problem. Five years later 29 of the 48 patients with CFS reported an acute onset, of which only a small minority had been documented serologically. For the majority of the cases with CFS retrospective assessments of the onset of illness would have been difficult and probably unreliable. Thus a number of potential recall biases are operating.

The statement that CFS patients are "no more psychologically disturbed before the onset of their illness than members of the general population" could only be definitively established using longitudinal studies in which exposure (psychiatric disorder) is ascertained before outcome (CFS). This would be expensive, but failing that it would be necessary in a case–control design to compare randomly chosen samples of both the general population and CFS, preferably identified at the same time and by the same procedures.

II. Results

A. The authors affirm that "depressive disorders of clinical severity were rare in the CFS sample". What evidence is presented to support this statement? Is there any evidence which does not support it?

The main evidence to support this comes from the comparison between the psychiatric controls and the patients with CFS. The controls had higher scores on two rating scales (Hamilton and Zung). In addition, the authors show that using a higher cut-off for the Zung there was a substantial difference between the cases and controls.

Twenty-four out of 48 (50%) of the people with CFS fulfilled criteria for a psychiatric disorder at some stage of their illness. This suggests that psychiatric disorder is not uncommon in this sample. It is also plausible that this group of patients may be reluctant to endorse certain psychologically loaded items on these scales, because of their strong conviction that their problems are physically based. The control group was also selected to have 'non-endogenous' depression – probably reducing the number of somatic symptoms, which might be more congruent with those experienced in the CFS group.

III. Summary and further questions

A. What are the clinical implications of this study?

The authors have demonstrated that in a very selected sample of CFS patients there are many subjects who do not fulfil criteria for psychiatric disorders, and hence it is clear that CFS and formally diagnosed psychiatric disorders are not synonymous. On the other hand, psychological symptoms and disorders are common, and as these are potentially treatable, screening for such disorders should be routine. This conclusion is the same regardless of whether or not one accepts the authors' conclusion that psychological disorder is the consequence of illness. A second conclusion is that because the patients with CFS in this sample have high levels of disease conviction, and clearly do not accept there is a role for psychological factors in their illness, this screening needs to be performed with tact and sensitivity.

B. What are the main limitations of this study?

The answer to this question is bias. Selection bias may have reduced the association between psychological disorder and CFS, by excluding those with more serious disorder, or with different illness attributions, at an earlier stage. Bias was also introduced by the varying time of the clinical assessment. Recall bias concerning the timing of symptoms of CFS and depression, and the role of premorbid psychological factors, is likewise a problem.

A CRITICAL REVIEW PAPER

Case–control study
Model answers by Michael Sharpe

Cognitive deficits in patients suffering from chronic fatigue syndrome, acute infective illness or depression

UTE VOLLMER-CONNA, DENIS WAKEFIELD, ANDREW LLOYD, IAN HICKIE, JIM LEMON, KEVIN D. BIRD and REGINALD F. WESTBROOK

The main aims of this study were: (a) to provide a detailed assessment of cognitive performance in patients suffering from chronic fatigue syndrome (CFS); and (b) to compare the performance and the reports of workload of patients suffering from CFS with that of two relevant positive control groups (patients with major, non-melancholic depression and patients suffering from an acute infective illness), as well as healthy control subjects.

METHOD

Subjects

Patients who met our modified diagnostic criteria for CFS, which require six months or more of unexplained disabling fatigue and constitutional symptoms, but do not require demonstration of abnormal cell-mediated immunity (Lloyd et al, 1990) were selected from those referred to the Department of Immunology at the Prince Henry and Prince of Wales Hospitals, Sydney, for evaluation of chronic fatigue. Their mean duration of illness was five years (range eight months to 10 years). Twenty of the 21 patients reported developing CFS subsequent to an acute infectious illness. In 10 cases the illness had been documented serologically (eight Epstein–Barr virus infections, two Ross River fever). Patients with acute infective illness were recruited through the Casualty and the Infectious Disease Departments at the Prince Henry Hospital, general practitioners, and public notices in local newspapers and on radio. Five patients had documented acute Epstein–Barr virus infections, the remaining patients suffered from influenza-like illnesses. Patients with depression were recruited from in- and out-patient services at the Mood Disorders Unit, Prince Henry Hospital, and met DSM–III–R (American Psychiatric Association, 1987) criteria for major depressive episode (non-melancholic type). These control subjects were specifically chosen as they exhibit comparable socio-demographic characteristics to patients with CFS, including female

predominance and age at onset of symptoms between 20 and 40 years of age. Healthy control subjects were recruited from hospital staff and the general community.

Procedure

Subjects attended a 3–4 hour testing session. A structured interview was used to obtain relevant demographic information and medical history. Subjects completed the self-report Profile of Mood States (POMS) questionnaire (McNair et al, 1981) to obtain data from the tension/anxiety, depression, confusion, and fatigue sub-scales. A modified, computerised Rozelle Test Battery (Lemon, 1990) was used to assess cognitive performance. This battery consisted of six tests chosen to provide a relatively broad assessment of attention and concentration, while permitting an examination of specific difficulties previously described in patients with CFS, including a vulnerability to interference, slowed response execution, difficulties with sustained concentration, spatial orientation and short-term memory. The tests were: an auditory discrimination task; a pursuit-tracking task; a divided attention

task, which involved the concurrent performance of the first two tests; a task-shifting task, consisting of a Sternberg-type, short-term memory task (Sternberg, 1966) and an arithmetical task; a left–right discrimination/spatial orientation task; and the Mackworth clock, vigilance task (Mackworth, 1948). The order of the tests was counterbalanced across subjects. After the completion of each of the tasks, task-related subjective workload experience was assessed by visual analogue scales (0–9) with endpoint descriptions. Variables of interest were perceived mental demand, physical demand, time pressure, effort, fatigue, and frustration level (Hart & Staveland, 1988). Workload experience was assessed by a composite measure derived by summing a subject's scores on the separate workload variables.

RESULTS

There were no significant between-group differences in age ($F(3, 80) < 1$), education ($F(3, 80) < 1$) or measures of general intelligence: National Adult Reading Test (Nelson, 1982) ($F(3, 80) = 1.5$) and Raven's Matrices ($F(3, 80) < 1$). Descriptive statistics only for group performance on the different tasks are shown in Table 1. Comparative analyses were performed on summed error and reaction time data for each group.

Performance measures

Levels of performance

Overall, subjects in the three patient groups made significantly more errors ($F=9.69$) and

Table I Summary table of performance indices for five computerised tasks

	Beeps		STM		'Little Man'		Vigilance		Tracking
	Errors	RT	Errors	RT	Errors	RT	Errors	RT	
Patients with CFS	2.23	0.69	2.53	1.09	1.62	1.54	3.66	0.74	7.14
(n=21)	(1.6)	(0.3)	(1.3)	(0.2)	(1.3)	(0.5)	(2.1)	(0.1)	(0.68)
Patients with	1.89	0.56	1.20	0.95	1.21	1.34	1.90	0.70	6.54
infections (n=21)	(1.2)	(0.2)	(1.1)	(0.2)	(1.1)	(0.4)	(1.7)	(0.1)	(0.47)
Patients with	2.47	0.64	2.45	1.07	1.35	1.46	3.52	0.73	6.97
depression (n=21)	(1.9)	(0.2)	(1.4)	(0.2)	(0.9)	(0.3)	(1.7)	(0.1)	(0.61)
Healthy subjects	1.83	0.51	1.60	0.84	0.79	1.23	1.15	0.67	6.31
(n=21)	(1.2)	(0.5)	(1.4)	(0.1)	(0.6)	(0.3)	(1.1)	(0.1)	(0.4)

Mean log scores (s.d.) for tracking ability (as mean delay in screen movements, ms); and for error rates (Errors) and reaction times (RT) on tasks involving auditory discrimination (Beeps), short-term memory (STM), left–right discrimination ('Little Man'), and vigilance. Statistical tests were performed on summed data, or between different task components (e.g. easy v. difficult, see text).

took considerably longer to make their responses ($F=21.33$) than did healthy subjects on tests involving auditory discrimination, short-term memory, left–right discrimination and sustained attention. Patients with CFS and those with depression did not differ from each other ($Fs<1.0$), but were significantly slower ($F=9.49$) and less accurate ($F=10.88$) than those with an acute infective illness. Subjects in all patient groups were also less able to control the tracking display than were healthy subjects, both when this task was easy (performed in isolation, $F=17.29$) and difficult (in combination with the auditory discrimination task, $F=11.52$). The tracking performances of patients with CFS and with depression did not differ from each other, but were significantly worse than those of patients with acute infections under both easy ($F=8.38$) and difficult ($F=10.78$) task conditions.

Stability of performance

Tracking performance typically shows a negatively accelerated curve to the subject's maximal performance. This occurs because the test begins with a relatively large delay in screen movements (i.e. 80 ms). This delay is progressively reduced until the subject is making approximately one tracking error every five seconds. Healthy subjects tend to maintain maximal performance for the remainder of the 120 seconds. The performance of patients with CFS and depressive patients tended to vary cyclically throughout the session. Fourier analysis quantifies cyclic variation as the relative power (amplitude) of the sine wave components of that variation in successive frequency bands. The cut-off of 0.016 Hz was chosen to remove the component of variation which resulted from the normal decrease in delay to maximal performance. Table 2 shows the mean total power scores, summed across all frequency intervals, for each group of subjects under both task conditions. Higher

Table 2 Performance stability

	Task conditions	
	Easy	Difficult
Patients with CFS ($n=21$)	2.22	2.33
	(0.69)	(0.83)
Patients with infections ($n=21$)	1.65	1.69
	(0.66)	(0.54)
Patients with depression ($n=21$)	2.01	2.19
	(0.61)	(0.87)
Healthy subjects ($n=21$)	1.45	1.47
	(0.47)	(0.48)

Mean total log scores (s.d.) of subjects under easy and difficult (divided attention) tracking conditions.

scores signify greater instability in tracking performance.

Subjective workload

Subjects in all three patient groups generally reported higher levels of workload for the different tasks than did healthy subjects ($F=10.52$). No other between-group differences were evident ($Fs<3.34$). There was a linear increase in reported workload as a function of the number of completed tasks ($F=15.84$), but the rate of increase in perceived workload did not differ reliably between the four groups of subjects ($Fs<4.26$).

Measures of mood state

All three patient groups scored significantly higher than healthy subjects on each of the POMS factors (tension: $F=32.47$, depression: $F=28.32$, confusion: $F=42.23$, and fatigue: $F=111.13$). There were no significant differences between the three patient groups in the reported level of fatigue ($F=2.72$). However, the ratings of patients with depression were significantly higher than those

of patients with CFS and acute infective illness on the tension ($F=13.65$), depression ($F=39.41$) and confusion ($F=5.58$) sub-scales. The scores of patients with CFS and those with acute infective illness did not differ on any of the sub-scales ($Fs<4.0$).

Analysis of the multiple possible associations between subjects' scores on the four POMS sub-scales and three performance indices, in patients with CFS or depression, and healthy controls, revealed no significant relationships.

DISCUSSION

Our results demonstrate differences between a sample of healthy subjects and patients suffering from either CFS, major (non-melancholic) depression or acute infective illnesses in cognitive performance, workload experience and mood.

REFERENCES

American Psychiatric Association (1987) Diagnostic and Statistical Manual of Mental Disorders (3rd edn, revised) (DSM–III–R). Washington, DC: APA.

Hart, S. G. & Staveland, L. E. (1988) Development of NASA-TLX (task load index): Results from empirical and theoretical research. In Human Mental Workload (eds P. A. Hancock & N. Meshkati), pp. 139–183. Amsterdam: Elsevier.

Lemon, J. (1990) The Rozelle Test Battery: A Computerized Testing Instrument for Visuomotor and Cognitive Testing. (Technical report No. 9). Sydney: National Drug and Alcohol Research Centre.

Lloyd, A., Hickie, I., Boughton, C. R., et al (1990) The prevalence of chronic fatigue syndrome in an Australian population. Medical Journal of Australia, **153**, 522–528.

Mackworth, N. H. (1948) The breakdown of vigilance during prolonged visual search. Quarterly Journal of Experimental Psychology, **1**, 7–11.

McNair, D. M., Lorr, M. & Droppleman, L. F. (1981) Impaired attention in depressive states: a non-specific deficit? Psychological Medicine, **26**, 1009–1020.

Sternberg, S. (1966) High speed scanning in human memory. Science, **153**, 652–654.

VOLLMER-CONNA *ET AL*

Please write your answers to questions I to IV in the spaces provided.

I. Background

A. What are the components of the operational definition of CFS used in this paper? What were the main aims of the paper? [6 marks]

....
....
....
....
....

II. Method

A. What type of study have the authors used to address the question they have posed? State giving examples from the study, what biases may arise in the selection of subjects for such studies. What are the advantages and disadvantages of using hospital staff as 'healthy control subjects'? [10 marks]

....
....
....
....
....
....
....

B. What exclusion criteria would you have imposed on subjects? [10 marks]

....
....
....
....
....
....

C. Give the three categories of outcome measures used in the study, with one example of each. [6 marks]

....
....
....

D. List the advantages and disadvantages of the method of study. Suggest two other approaches to investigate this topic. [6 marks]

....
....
....
....
....
....

E. What method of statistical analysis is used in this study? What is the main assumption of this method? How could you transform the data, if necessary, to satisfy this assumption? [6 marks]

....
....
....

II. Results

A. Explain the meaning of the terms '$(F(3,80) < 1)$'. What is the difference between statistical and clinical significance? [6 marks]

....
....
....
....
....
....
....
....

B. (i) Give two examples of descriptive statistics used in this paper. [4 marks]

....
....

(ii) If a non-parametric approach was taken to the analysis what equivalent terms would be appropriate? [4 marks]

....
....

C. What do you observe from Table 1 concerning the difference between 'healthy subjects', and the rest, in relation to errors and response times? What is the meaning and importance of 's.d.' in the above text? What other statistical information would you have included in the table, and why? [6 marks]

....
....
....
....
....

D. What does Table 2 tell you about 'healthy subjects' in relation to other subject groups? Do you suspect the differences shown in Table 2 between subjects with depression and subjects with CFS are likely to be statistically significant? [6 marks]

....
....
....
....
....

E. How was fatigue measured? [6 marks]

....
....
....
....
....

F. Describe what is meant by visual analogue scale. What biases are inherent in the use of such scales and how may they be reduced? [6 marks]

....
....
....
....
....

G. What statistical corrections are available when multiple possible associations are tested? What precaution was taken in this regard by the authors? [4 marks]

....
....
....

IV. Summary

A. What are the main findings of this study? [6 marks]

....
....
....
....
....

B. What valid conclusions can be drawn from this study? [8 marks]

....
....
....
....
....
....

I.   Background

A.   What are the components of the operational definition of CFS used in this paper? What were the main aims of the paper?

Definition:

    (a) Symptoms of fatigue.
    (b) Disability.
    (c) Duration of six months or more.
    (d) Medically unexplained.

Aims:

    (a) Assess cognitive performance in CFS.
    (b) Compare this with major depression, acute infection and control subjects.

II.   Method

A.   What type of study have the authors used to address the question they have posed? State, giving examples from the study, what biases may arise in the selection of subjects for such studies. What are the advantages and disadvantages of using hospital staff as 'healthy control subjects'?

This is a descriptive 'case–control study' with multiple control or comparison groups.
  In relation to the true population from which each group is a sample the following biases may occur:

    (a) Hospital-referred patients may be biased by factors that determine referral – CFS group, depressed group, acute infections group.
    (b) They may be biased by willingness to take part and self-selection – acute infection group and 'healthy control subjects'.
    (c) They may be selected because they have or do not have the symptoms being measured in the study (all groups).

Hospital staff are convenient and likely to comply. However, they are likely to be a biased sample of the wider population and may be 'super healthy'.

B.   What exclusion criteria would you have imposed on subjects?

It is desirable to exclude patients who may be subject to confounding influences, that is, be susceptible to variables other than the illness that may influence the outcome measures.

    (a) All psychotropic medication (antidepressants and benzodiazepines in particular).
    (b) Substance misuse.
    (c) History of head injury.
    (d) Patients with more than one illness, for example, patients with depression who also have acute infection.

C.   Give the three categories of outcome measures used in the study, with one example of each.

    (a) Cognitive function – Rozelle test battery.
    (b) Mood – POMS.
    (c) Subjective workload – VAS.

D.   List the advantages and disadvantages of the method of study. Suggest two other approaches to investigate this topic.

Advantages to case–control with multiple comparison group method are:

(a) Easy to do.

(b) Control for several possible confounders at same time (depression and infection).

Disadvantages are:

(a) Very subject to observable (and non-observable) confounders, for example, medication.

(b) Assumes homogeneity of groups.

Alternatives are:

(a) Prospective method using cases of CFS as own controls.

(b) Experimental method – induce CFS or infection.

E. What method of statistical analysis is used in this study? What is the main assumption of this method? How could you transform the data, if necessary, to satisfy this assumption?

(a) Analysis of variance was used.

(b) This is a parametric test that assumes that the relevant variables are normally distributed.

(c) The data could be transformed using log, square or square-root equations.

III. Results

A. Explain the meaning of the terms 'F(3,80) < 1)'. What is the difference between statistical and clinical significance?

(a) F refers to the value of the F test or variance ratio test.

(b) 3 refers to degrees of freedom in variable 'groups'.

(c) 80 refers to degrees of freedom in variable 'subjects'.

(d) <1 refers to the value of F.

'Statistically significant' indicates that the difference observed would have been unlikely to have occurred by chance (conventionally on less than 5% of occasions). 'Clinically significant' means that the difference observed is of sufficient magnitude to be apparent and important in a clinical setting.

B. (i) Give two examples of descriptive statistics used in this paper.

(a) Mean.

(b) Standard deviation.

(ii) If a non-parametric approach was taken to analysis what equivalent terms would be appropriate?

(a) Median.

(b) Range or semi-interquartile range.

C. What do you observe from Table I concerning the difference between 'healthy subjects' and the rest, in relation to errors and response times? What is the meaning and importance of 's.d.' in the above context? What other statistical information would you have included in the table, and why?

In Table 1 the mean error scores of the healthy controls are consistently lower than those of the other groups.

The standard deviation indicated the spread of readings for each group and test. A measure of statistical significance is required (P value or confidence interval).

D. **What does Table 2 tell you about the performance of 'healthy subjects' in relation to the other subject groups? Do you suspect the differences in Table 2 between subjects with depression and subjects with CFS are likely to be statistically significant?**

Table 2 shows that the performance of healthy subjects is more stable than that of the other groups. The difference in scores between subjects with depression and those with CFS are unlikely to be statistically significant given the difference between the means and standard deviation shown.

E. **How was fatigue measured?**

Fatigue was measured by:

(a) Self-rating using POMS questionnaire.
(b) Objective impairment of performance using error scores on tests and reaction times.
(c) Subjective workload using visual analogue scale.

F. **Describe what is meant by visual analogue scale. What biases are inherent in the use of such scales and how may they be reduced?**

The visual analogue scale is a 10 cm line with an anchor term at each end. The subject is required to make a mark on the line at the point that indicates their response. Bias may be random (for example, marking the line without reading the question or responding idiosyncratically to the anchor term) or systematic (for example, tending to mark towards one end or in the centre).

It may be reduced by explicit instruction, for example, 'use all of the scale'. An idiosyncratic response to the anchor terms may be minimised by using several visual analogue scale scores using similar terms and summing them.

G. **What statistical corrections are available when multiple possible associations are tested? What precaution was taken in this regard by the authors?**

Multiple significance testing increases the chance that a test will show a significant difference by chance. This may be avoided by: (a) preselecting a limited number of tests to be done; (b) using the Bonferroni method; or (c) only accepting positive results at a higher than conventional level of statistical significance ($P < 0.01$).

The authors do not appear to have taken any precaution in this respect.

IV. Summary

A. **What are the main findings of this study?**

The subjects with CFS made more errors, had longer reaction times and reported higher subjective workload than the 'healthy controls'. There were no differences between the CFS group and either the group with infection or the subjects with depression on these measures. However, patients with CFS and patients with infection scored lower on depressed mood than patients with depression.

B. **What valid conclusions can be drawn from this study?**

On the tests of cognitive function employed, no statistically significant difference could be detected between patients selected from a hospital clinic meeting operational criteria for CFS, those with major depressive disorder and volunteers with acute infection. However, all three groups differed on these measures from selected 'healthy controls'. The difference in mood between depressed patients and the infection and CFS groups suggests that the deficit in patients with CFS may be related to factors other then depressed mood.

A CRITICAL REVIEW PAPER

Randomised controlled trial
Model answers by Max Marshall

London–East Anglia randomised controlled trial of cognitive–behavioural therapy for psychosis

I: Effects of the treatment phase

ELIZABETH KUIPERS, PHILIPPA GARETY, DAVID FOWLER, GRAHAM DUNN, PAUL BEBBINGTON, DANIEL FREEMAN and CLARE HADLEY

In this paper we present the results of the treatment phase of a three-centre study, based in London and East Anglia.

METHOD

Participants

The study was conducted at three major sites; at the Maudsley Trust, London; at Addenbrooke's Hospital Trust, Cambridge; and at Norfolk Mental Health Trust, Norwich. Participants were catchment area clients who were recruited by asking for referrals from community teams and in-patient units.

Criteria for referral were: at least one current positive psychotic symptom (such as delusions or hallucinations) that was distressing, unremitting (at least the past six months) and medication resistant, that is had not responded to a previous trial of at least six months of appropriate neuroleptic medication. Clients prescribed clozapine needed to have been stable on this for at least one year (to allow time for all benefit to occur). People who had drug, alcohol or organic problems as primary features were excluded.

Procedures and randomisation

Once referred, all possible participants were seen for a screening interview by an independent evaluator to establish whether they met our criteria. Once this was confirmed and informed consent had been obtained, randomisation was carried out separately within each treatment centre by the trial statistician (G.D.), using randomised permuted blocking (Pocock, 1983) and a block size of six. Participants then entered either the control condition or the treatment group, and baseline assessments were carried out. Considerable efforts were made to collect data from all participants in the trial from the time of randomisation onwards.

Prior power calculations, based on the results of the pilot study (Garety *et al*, 1994), had indicated that a trial with a total of 60 people would have a power of at least 0.80 to detect an effect size of 0.516 using a two-group *t*-test with a 0.05 two-tailed significance level.

Assessments

A wide range of assessments was administered to participants at baseline, three months, six months, and nine months (which was the end of the treatment condition).

Treatment condition

Participants randomised into the treatment group received up to nine months of individual cognitive–behavioural therapy (CBT) for psychosis. Sessions were conducted weekly initially, and then fortnightly, for up to an hour.

Therapists

Therapists in the trial were experienced clinical psychologists.

All clients in the treatment condition also received routine care from their clinical teams. In most instances, this included case management and medication. Clinical teams were asked, if at all possible, not to change clients' medication during the trial, and to inform us of changes that were unavoidable. This was monitored as closely as possible.

Control condition

Participants randomised into this condition received routine care from their clinical team, which as part of our entry criteria consisted of case management and medication.

RESULTS

Participants

One hundred and fifty-two people were referred for possible inclusion in the trial.

Table I Demographic data on participants who entered the therapy trial

Variable	CBT group			Control group		
	n	Mean	Range	*n*	Mean	Range
Age (years)	28	38.5	19–65	32	41.8	18–63
Duration of illness (years)	25	12.1	1–26	30	14.0	1–33
Number of admissions	24	5.2	0–30	29	4.3	0–12
Predicted IQ (NART)	25	102.9	69–129	25	98.7	71–131
Current IQ (Quick Test)	25	99.8	72–130	29	91.5	70–116
Gender						
Male	15			23		
Female	13			9		

NART, National Adult Reading Test (Nelson, 1982).

Table 2 Clinical data on participants who entered the therapy trial

Variable	CBT group			Control group		
	n	Mean	s.d.	*n*	Mean	s.d.
BPRS	27	26.4	6.5	26	24.5	7.1
BDI	27	23.6	10.1	26	20.0	10.1
BHS	27	11.6	4.8	27	9.8	5.2
BAI	27	17.5	11.0	26	17.3	14.8
Self-esteem	25	90.1	29.6	28	107.3	23.3
Social Functioning Scale	27	103.3	7.2	30	101.6	9.0

BPRS, Brief Psychiatric Rating Scale (Overall & Gorham, 1962); BDI, Beck Depression Inventory (Beck *et al*, 1961); BHS, Beck Hopelessness Scale (Beck *et al*, 1974); BAI, Beck Anxiety Inventory (Beck *et al*, 1988).

Table 3 Brief Psychiatric Rating Scale linear trends in each centre

Centre	CBT group			Control group		
	n	Mean	s.d.	n	Mean	s.d.
London	14	−1.49	1.57	12	0.18	1.66
Cambridge	6	−2.90	3.99	8	−0.35	3.08
Norwich	6	−2.37	1.60	7	−1.67	1.21
Combined	26	−2.02	2.31	27	−0.46	2.15

Significant difference between CBT and control groups (P=0.009).

Table 4 Mean Brief Psychiatric Rating Scale scores

Assessment	CBT group			Control group		
	n	Mean	s.d.	n	Mean	s.d.
Initial	27	26.4	6.5	26	24.5	7.1
Three-month	25	22.2	8.2	27	22.3	7.2
Six-month	25	21.2	7.3	27	22.9	6.2
Nine-month	23	19.9	8.5	24	22.7	7.6

Table 5 Medication levels based on chlorpromazine equivalents

	CBT group	Control group
Level of neuroleptic dose at start of trial		
None	2	1
Low	5	4
Medium	3	10
High	8	5
Changes in medication during trial		
No change	11	10
Fluctuating	1	2
Increasing	2	7
Decreasing	2	0
Level of neuroleptic medication throughout the trial		
None	4	0
Low	2	2
Medium	4	8
High	6	9

Levels of neuroleptic medication: Low: less than 300 mg chlorpromazine; medium: 300 to 600 mg chlorpromazine; high: greater than 600 mg chlorpromazine.
All available data on medication are included. These were predominantly from the London sample, which when considered on its own did not have a discernibly different pattern.

A total of 60 people met the criteria, consented, and were entered into the trial. Demographic and clinical information on participants in the two groups are presented in Tables 1 and 2.

Withdrawals

Out of the 60 people who gave their consent for the trial, a total of 11 people (18%) withdrew from assessments over nine months, four (14%) from the CBT condition and seven (22%) from the control group (five of whom withdrew immediately after randomisation). Of the four people who dropped out of the treatment condition by nine months, only three (11%) attended for fewer than 10 sessions.

Number of therapy sessions received

The median number of therapy sessions given to the treatment group was 15, and the mean was 18.6 (range 0–50). One person did not attend any therapy appointments, one had fewer than five sessions, six had 'brief therapy' (12 sessions or fewer). The rest of the treatment group (n=20) had what we defined as 'full therapy' (more than 12 sessions).

Outcome measures

Symptoms and functioning

The means for the Brief Psychiatric Rating Scale (BPRS (Overall & Gorham, 1962)) linear trends and raw scores can be seen in Tables 3 and 4.

The CBT group did significantly better than the controls ($F_{1,47}=7.41$; $P=0.009$). There was little evidence that the difference between the CBT and control groups depended on centre (the test for the group by centre interaction: $F_{2,47}=0.59$; $P=0.561$).

Medication

Medication regimes were complex and information was sometimes incomplete. We calculated chlorpromazine equivalents (CPZ) following the guidelines in the *British National Formulary*. Full data were available for the London participants, but data were more limited for East Anglia. We classified these into no medication, low (less than 300 mg CPZ/day), medium (300–600 mg CPZ/day) and high (more than 600 mg CPZ/day). We also divided participants into those receiving constant, fluctuating, decreasing or increasing doses. Four clients were switched to clozapine before the final assessment. Three of these were in the control group, and the change occurred between the three and six month assessments. One person was in the CBT group and the change only occurred after the six month assessment.

Inspection of the data at baseline in Table 5, suggests that there were no particular differences in medication between the treatment and control conditions.

DISCUSSION

The results of this trial show that at the end of nine months of CBT it is possible to improve the overall symptomatology of people with medication-resistant, distressing symptoms of psychosis.

REFERENCES

Beck, A. T., Ward, C. H., Mendelson, M., et al (1961) An inventory for measuring depression. *Archives of General Psychiatry*, **4**, 561–571.

— , Weissman, A. W., Lester, D., et al (1974) The assessment of pessimism: the Hopelessness Scale. *Journal of Consulting and Clinical Psychology*, **42**, 861–865.

— , Epstein, N., Brown, G., et al (1988) An inventory for measuring clinical anxiety: Psychometric properties. *Journal of Consulting and Clinical Psychology*, **56**, 893–897.

Garety, P., Kuipers, L., Fowler, D., et al (1994) Cognitive behavioural therapy for drug-resistant psychosis. *British Journal of Medical Psychology*, **67**, 259–271.

Nelson, H. E. (1982) *The National Adult Reading Test.* Windsor, Berkshire: NFER–Nelson.

Overall, J. E. & Gorham, D. R. (1962) The Brief Psychiatric Rating Scale. *Psychological Reports*, **10**, 799–812.

Pocock, S. (1983) *Clinical Trials.* Chichester: Wiley.

KUIPERS *ET AL*

Please write your answers to questions I to IV in the spaces provided.

I.   Background

A.   Define randomisation, stating its purpose, and illustrate your answer with different randomisation strategies. Describe, in your own words, the randomisation procedure adopted in this study and possible reasons for this approach. What checks would you introduce to establish that random allocation was achieved in this study?   [10 marks]

....
....
....
....
....
....
....
....
....
....

B.   List the essential features of informed consent, with particular reference to this study. What form of documentation of informed consent would be appropriate in this study? [5 marks]

....
....
....
....
....
....

C.   What is the rationale for the use of cognitive–behavioural therapy (CBT) for people with psychosis? Give examples of specific techniques that could, in principle, have a beneficial effect. What barriers are there to delivering CBT to people with psychosis?   [10 marks]

....
....
....
....
....
....
....
....

II.   Method

A.   Discuss critically biases introduced via the method of ascertainment used by the authors. What information would you require concerning the screening interview by an independent evaluator to satisfy you that the entry and exclusion criteria had been met?   [10 marks]

....
....
....
....
....
....
....
....

B.   Describe a power calculation. What is the purpose of a power calculation? What is meant by "a power of at least 0.80 to detect an effect size of 0.516"? What is a "two-group t-test with a 0.05 two-tailed significance level"?   [10 marks]

....
....
....
....
....
....
....
....
....
....

C.   State what is meant by 'blinding' in clinical trials, indicating what form of blinding, if any, was used by the authors. How could potential biases in treatment comparisons be lessened in this study?   [5 marks]

....
....
....
....
....
....

III. Results

A. What conclusions do you draw from Tables 1 and 2 about the differences between the CBT and control groups? Comment specifically about the possible impact on the trial results of differences in IQ and gender. [5 marks]

....
....
....
....
....
....
....
....

B. On the basis of the Beck Depression Inventory (BDI) group means, did the CBT and control groups have mild, moderate or severe symptoms of depression? Discuss the significance of the mean BDI scores at entry in this trial and the probable effect of CBT and control treatment on such symptoms, and on the trial results. [5 marks]

....
....
....
....
....

C. Describe the main features of the Brief Psychiatric Rating Scale (BPRS). Discuss why the results are reported in terms of linear trends and mean BPRS scores. What was the percentage improvement in the CBT and control groups? How would you assess whether or not the difference was clinically worthwhile? What form of statistical analysis was used by the authors? [10 marks]

....
....
....
....
....
....
....
....
....
....

IV. Summary and further questions

A. Accepting the results of the study at face value, what is the main conclusion and, in consequence, the main implication for clinical practice?   [5 marks]

....
....
....
....
....

B. List five main limitations of the study.   [5 marks]

....
....
....
....
....

C. Outline the further evidence that taken together would provide more definitive evidence of the clinical effectiveness of CBT for people with psychosis.   [10 marks]

....
....
....
....
....
....
....
....

D. Describe what is meant by an 'intention-to-treat' analysis. Based on the information provided to you, did the authors use such an analysis? Justify your answer.   [5 marks]

....
....
....
....
....
....

E. List five features of the CONSORT guidelines.   [5 marks]

....
....
....
....
....

I. Background

A. Define randomisation, stating its purpose, and illustrate your answer with different randomisation strategies. Describe, in your own words, the randomisation procedure adopted in this study and possible reasons for this approach. What checks would you introduce to establish that random allocation was achieved in this study?

Randomisation is a procedure that ensures all subjects recruited into a trial have equal chances of being allocated to the treatment or control groups. The purpose of randomisation is to eliminate the bias which occurs when experimenters are allowed to influence subject allocation. In this study, separate randomisation schedules were operated at each centre by the study statistician. The permuted block technique was used which, in this case, means that for every six subjects sequentially recruited three will be allocated to treatment and three to control. Within the block of six allocation would have been in random order. The investigators will have been unaware of the block size. Randomisation by block is to ensure that approximately equal numbers of subjects are allocated to each group. Separate randomisation schedules for each centre ensure that each centre contributes equally to treatment and control groups, this is both convenient (in terms of resource planning) and reduces bias that might arise from differing effectiveness of treatment in different centres. To establish that random allocation is achieved, the cards detailing allocation should be kept in numbered sealed envelopes. The number of envelopes left at the end of the study should be checked against the numbers of patients entering the study.

B. List the essential features of informed consent, with particular reference to this study. What form of documentation of informed consent would be appropriate in this study?

The patients should understand the nature and purpose of the study and any risks of intervention. They should understand that if they refuse to participate, their normal treatment will not be affected. They should know that they can withdraw from the study at any time without giving a reason. They should understand that they have an equal chance of being allocated to treatment or control group. The explanation should be given orally and in writing to the patient by an investigator. All documentation should have been scrutinised by an ethics committee. The patient should have the opportunity to ask questions and should have time (usually 48 hours or more) to consider participating. In this study a consent form signed by patient and investigator would be appropriate documentation. An information sheet explaining the study, which also gives the contact address of the investigator, should accompany it. The patient should retain the information sheet.

C. What is the rationale for the use of cognitive–behavioural therapy (CBT) for people with psychosis? Give examples of specific techniques that could, in principle, have a beneficial effect. What barriers are there to delivering CBT to people with psychosis?

There are two rationales. First, it is thought that many delusions are secondary phenomena that arise from attempts to cope with bizarre experiences and other consequences of psychosis – they should therefore be remedial through psychological interventions. Second, it is thought that patients can be taught better coping strategies to deal with abnormal perceptual experiences. Examples of cognitive techniques include: (a) inference chaining where the consequences of a delusion are examined and challenged; (b) Socratic questioning which uses a dialectical technique to help the patient explore the implications and consequences of their delusions; (c) reattribution of abnormal experiences; and (d) using signs of emotional distress to identify 'hot cognitions' that play a pivotal role in the patient's delusional system. Barriers to delivering CBT include: (a) patients who are too disabled to engage in the therapeutic process (for example owing to thought disorder) and (b) lack of suitably qualified therapists.

II. Method

A. Discuss critically biases introduced via the method of ascertainment used by the authors. What information would you require concerning the screening interview by an independent evaluator to satisfy you that the entry and exclusion criteria had been met?

Patients were recruited by asking for referrals from community mental health teams and in-patient units. The patients recruited are therefore not representative of people with severe mental illnesses as a whole. Possible biases might include a tendency for more cooperative patients or patients with less severe illnesses to be referred. Only 60 out of 152 referrals were actually accepted into the study. It is not clear why so many patients were excluded and the reasons for exclusion should be provided. The identity of the independent evaluator, their training and their relationship to the research team should be described. They should also describe the method by which the evaluator determined that entry and exclusion criteria were met (for example was a standardised interview used to elicit psychotic symptoms?)

B. Describe a power calculation. What is the purpose of a power calculation? What is meant by "a power of at least 0.80 to detect an effect size of 0.516"? What is a "two-group *t*-test with a 0.05 two-tailed significance level"?

A power calculation is used to determine how many subjects are required for a clinical trial to have a good chance of detecting a clinically significant difference on a particular outcome variable. To calculate power it is necessary to know the size of a clinically significant difference on the variable and the expected standard deviation of the variable. The power of the study is essentially determined by dividing the clinically significant difference by the standard deviation and then cross-referencing this ratio with a table of power for a given number of subjects. The statement means that the study has an 80% chance of detecting an effect size of approximately one-half of one standard deviation when such a difference is truly present. The second statement means that a *t*-test (a simple parametric statistical test) has been used to compare the means of two groups. A 0.05% significance level means that the chance of a Type 1 error is less than one in 20. 'Two-tailed' means that no assumption is made about which treatment will be superior *a priori* – a more stringent test than a one-tailed test.

C. State what is meant by 'blinding' in clinical trials, indicating what form of blinding, if any, was used by the authors. How could potential biases in treatment comparisons be lessened in this study?

Blinding may mean either that (a) the patient is unaware of whether they are in the treatment or control group; (b) the therapist/investigator is unaware of group allocation or (c) both are unaware (double-blind). Neither patients nor therapists were blind in this trial. It is not clear whether those conducting the outcome assessment were blind to group allocation. Biases could have been reduced by using raters blind to group allocation.

III. Results

A. What conclusions do you draw from Tables 1 and 2 about the differences between the CBT and control groups? Comment specifically about the possible impact on the trial results of differences in IQ and gender.

It is hard to judge the significance of any baseline differences without a statistical comparison. Scanning the data it is possible that the CBT groups were significantly more intelligent (and hence more likely to respond to therapy) and included a smaller proportion of males (who tend to have more severe illness and may be less cooperative). There do not appear to be major differences on the baseline data from the standardised instruments but again statistical tests are required to be certain.

B. On the basis of the Beck Depression Inventory (BDI) group means, did the CBT and control groups have mild, moderate or severe symptoms of depression? Discuss the significance of the mean BDI scores at entry in this trial and the probable effect of CBT and control treatment on such symptoms, and on the trial results.

The symptoms of depression are in the moderate–severe range of the BDI (tending towards the high end of moderate). It is possible that CBT is affecting mainly affective symptoms and that this explains the improvements in BPRS scores, rather than any specific effect on psychotic symptoms.

C. Describe the main features of the Brief Psychiatric Rating Scale (BPRS). Discuss why the results are reported in terms of linear trends and mean BPRS scores. What was the percentage improvement in the CBT and control groups? How would you assess whether or not the difference was clinically worthwhile? What form of statistical analysis was used by the authors?

The BPRS is a well-established standardised rating scale for measuring the severity of psychiatric symptoms. It consists of 18 questions and can produce subscores for affective, psychotic and negative symptoms. It is observer rated (and hence potentially prone to bias if the rater is not blind to group allocation). To determine whether the difference is worthwhile you should consult the appropriate papers that discuss what is widely considered to be a clinically significant difference on this scale. The authors will probably have given guidance on this matter. The authors have used an analysis of variance and have taken account of trends over time using a linear modelling technique.

IV. Summary and further questions

A. Accepting the results of the study at face value, what is the main conclusion and, in consequence, the main implication for clinical practice?

Accepting the results at face value, CBT may be a useful adjunct to medication in the treatment of an unknown proportion of people with treatment-resistant symptoms.

B. List five main limitations of the study.

The main limitation are:

(a) A lack of clarity over the method of randomisation (which should have been the sealed envelope method).
(b) The method of subject ascertainment (the sample was not representative of people with severe mental disorder so we do not know how many would actually benefit).
(c) A high rate of exclusion of potentially eligible subjects for reasons that are not clear.
(d) Lack of an active control treatment to control for the non-specific effects of spending time with an experienced therapist.
(e) Lack of information on the raters (particularly whether they were blind to group allocation).
(f) Lack of clarity over what type of symptoms were improved by the therapy and whether the difference seen was clinically significant.

C. Outline the further evidence that taken together would provide more definitive evidence of the clinical effectiveness of CBT for people with psychosis.

There needs to be a demonstration of a clinically significant change in key psychotic symptoms (hallucinations and delusions), as at present the findings could be explained by a non-specific effect on depressive symptoms. The therapy needs to be compared against an active control that takes account of the non-specific effects of seeing a therapist regularly.

D. Describe what is meant by an 'intention-to-treat' analysis. Based on the information provided to you, did the authors use such an analysis? Justify your answer.

In an intention-to-treat analysis, data on all randomised subjects are analysed within the groups to which they were assigned, regardless of whether they actually received the treatment to which they were allocated. This is probably not an intention-to-treat analysis because the authors state that 11 out of 60 people withdrew from assessments but in Table 4, at nine-month follow-up, data are presented on only 47 out of 60 patients. Two patients are not accounted for.

E. List five features of the CONSORT guidelines.

The CONSORT guidelines are guidelines for the reporting of data from clinical trials (CONsensus Statement On Reporting of Trials). They include that:

(a) All patients assessed for the trial should be accounted for and that the report should be accompanied by a diagram that explains what happened to all the patients involved in the trial.

(b) The randomisation procedure should be clearly specified.

(c) Inclusion and exclusion criteria should be clearly stated.

(d) Pre-study power calculations should be provided.

(e) The method of blinding should be specified.

(f) There should be an intention-to-treat analysis.

A CRITICAL REVIEW PAPER

Epidemiological follow-up study
Model answers by Glyn Lewis

The predictive validity of a diagnosis of schizophrenia

A report from the International Study of Schizophrenia (ISoS)
coordinated by the World Health Organization and the
Department of Psychiatry, University of Nottingham

PETER MASON, GLYNN HARRISON, TIM CROUDACE,
CRISTINE GLAZEBROOK and IAN MEDLEY

In the present study we aimed to test the predictive validity of three major diagnostic classifications of schizophrenia: DSM–III–R (American Psychiatric Association, 1987), ICD–10 (World Health Organization, 1992a) and ICD–9 (World Health Organization, 1978a), and a 'restrictive' CATEGO S+ definition of schizophrenia (which relies heavily upon Schneider's first rank symptoms). A 13-year follow-up was conducted with a complete and representative sample of first-onset psychoses. The contribution of a six-month duration criterion is specifically tested, and the stability of ICD–10 and DSM–III–R schizophrenia is also studied. The cohort under investigation was part of the International Study of Schizophrenia (ISoS), which is a transcultural investigation in 20 centres in 15 countries coordinated by the World Health Organization (WHO). It was designed to explain findings of previous WHO studies in this area; to identify patterns of long-term course and outcome of severe mental disorders in different cultures; to further develop methods for the study of characteristics of mental disorders and their course in different settings; and to strengthen the scientific basis for future international multidisciplinary research on schizophrenia and other psychiatric disorders seen in a public health perspective. The cohort described in this paper was identified in the WHO's Determinants of Outcome of Severe Mental Disorder Study (1978–1980) for which Nottingham was the UK field centre (Jablensky et al, 1992).

METHOD

The methods of case ascertainment, assessments and follow-up have been described previously (Harrison et al, 1994; Mason et al, 1995; Sartorius et al, 1996).

The sample

The sample comprised all patients (aged 15–54 years) making their first contact (out- and in-patients) from a defined catchment area (population 390 000) between 1 August 1978 and 31 July 1980. An over-inclusive screening schedule for psychosis identified the subjects, who were then assessed using several semi-structured interviews by the project team. Ninety-nine subjects were identified, comprising 65 men and 34 women, with a mean age of 29.60 (s.d. 10.12).

Follow-up information was available on 96% of the original sample. Four patients could not be traced and nine were dead. Sixty-nine subjects had full assessments, and for the remaining 17 subjects, high-quality information was available from records and informants. The 86 subjects available for follow-up did not differ significantly from those dead or lost to follow-up, with respect to their gender, age, type of onset, duration of symptoms and diagnosis (schizophrenia or not) for DSM–III–R, ICD–10, ICD–9 and CATEGO S+.

Initial assessments

All subjects were interviewed by a project psychiatrist using the Present State Examination (PSE; Wing et al, 1974) and the Psychological Impairments Rating Scale (PIRS; Jablensky et al, 1980). Other schedules covering the psychiatric, personal, family and social background (Psychiatric and Personal History Schedule (PPHS; World Health Organization, 1978b)) and social disability (Disability Assessment Schedule (DAS; Jablensky et al, 1980)) were completed by a different interviewer with a close relative of the patient, or other informant.

Follow-up assessment

Assessments were carried out with both patients and a key informant, and further information was elicited from general practice and hospital records. For comparability with earlier measures, assessments including the PSE, the PIRS and the DAS, and other instruments were developed by the WHO to measure long-term outcome (Life Chart Schedule; WHO, 1992c; Broad Rating Schedule; WHO, 1992b).

For the purposes of this paper, data from the Global Assessment of Functioning scales (GAF) for symptoms and disability, derived from the Global Assessment Scale (Endicott et al, 1976), were selected from the range of follow-up assessments. These scales rate the severity of symptoms and the severity of disability in the past month on an ordinal scale from one (most severe) to 90 (no symptoms/disability). Pre-study and maintenance reliability exercises were conducted (Mason et al, 1995). Pre-study intraclass correlation coefficients (ICC) for GAF symptoms and disability were 0.85 and 0.94, respectively. Maintenance ICC for GAF symptoms and disability were 0.96 and 0.89, respectively.

Diagnoses

ICD–9

On completion of the initial assessments (between 1978 and 1980), at least two project psychiatrists reviewed the available data and assigned a project ICD–9 diagnosis to each subject.

CATEGO S+

The CATEGO Diagnostic Program (Wing et al, 1974) was used to determine the subjects meeting the restrictive definition of S+ schizophrenia based upon the original PSE ratings.

DSM–III–R and ICD–10

A re-diagnosis exercise was conducted at the point of 13-year follow-up. The original schedules and narratives were reviewed by G. H., blind to outcome, who assigned a diagnosis according to DSM–III–R Research Diagnostic Criteria, using a diagnostic decision instrument which systematically checked criteria for every possible psychotic disorder in DSM–III–R and ICD–10 (available from the authors). The re-diagnosis exercise was possible given the extensive baseline clinical data collected at entry to the study. A reliability exercise was carried out with I. M., who independently diagnosed 20 cases, also blind to outcome. Pairwise agreement between G. H. and I. M. for a classification of schizophrenia versus other

Table I Concordance (Cohen's kappa) between standard and 'duration adjusted' definitions of schizophrenia, with 95% confidence intervals

Diagnosis	n	Male/female ratio	DSM–III–R	ICD–10	ICD–9	CATEGO S+	'Duration adjusted' DSM–III–R	'Duration adjusted' ICD–10	'Duration adjusted' ICD–9
DSM–III–R	31	20/11 (1.82)	–	–	–	–	–	–	–
ICD–10	56	37/19 (1.95)	0.52 (0.36–0.68)*	–	–	–	–	–	–
ICD–9	67	45/22 (2.05)	0.36 (0.18–0.54)*	0.77 (0.63–0.91)*	–	–	–	–	–
CATEGO S+	59	35/24 (1.46)	0.13 (−0.05–0.31)	0.32 (0.12–0.52)*	0.31 (0.11–0.51)*	–	–	–	–
'Duration adjusted' DSM–III–R	59	38/21 (1.81)	0.47 (0.31–0.63)*	0.90 (0.80–1.00)*	0.83 (0.71–0.95)*	0.37 (0.17–0.57)*	–	–	–
'Duration adjusted' ICD–10	27	16/11 (1.45)	0.85 (0.73–0.97)*	0.45 (0.27–0.63)*	0.30 (0.14–0.46)*	0.15 (−0.03–0.33)	0.37 (0.19–0.55)*	–	–
'Duration adjusted' ICD–9	31	20/11 (1.82)	0.77 (0.63–0.91)*	0.36 (0.18–0.54)*	0.36 (0.18–0.54)*	0.06 (−0.12–0.24)	0.28 (0.10–0.46)*	0.90 (0.80–1.00)*	–
'Duration adjusted' CATEGO S+	23	12/11 (1.09)	0.65 (0.47–0.83)*	0.26 (0.08–0.44)*	0.15 (−0.01–0.31)	0.34 (0.16–0.52)*	0.23 (0.05–0.41)*	0.73 (0.57–0.89)*	0.65 (0.47–0.83)*

*Confidence intervals that do not include zero are significant at $P < 0.05$.

psychotic disorder was 100% for both ICD–10 and DSM–III–R.

Duration criteria

To study the effects of six-month duration criteria, 'duration adjusted' definitions of schizophrenia were created for ICD–10, ICD–9, DSM–III–R and CATEGO S+. Information about duration, recorded in the PPHS, was used to add six-month duration criteria to the ICD–10, ICD–9 and S+ definitions. For DSM–III–R, the six-month duration criterion was removed by adding those subjects classified as having a schizophreniform disorder (meets criteria for schizophrenia, but episode lasts less than six months) to those meeting full DSM–III–R criteria for schizophrenia at intake into the study.

Diagnosis stability

For the purposes of assessing the stability of diagnosis over 13 years, a 'main overall diagnosis' for both DSM–III–R and ICD–10 was assigned to each subject. This diagnostic exercise was conducted by G.H. using the same diagnostic decision instrument as in the re-diagnosis exercise. The main overall diagnosis was made immediately after the re-diagnosis exercise and was based on all data collected at onset and at follow-up. This exercise attempted to assign an overall diagnosis taking into account the 13-year course of the disorder and the 'final' outcome in terms of symptoms and social disability. A reliability exercise was carried out with I.M. who independently diagnosed 20 cases. Pairwise agreement between G.H. and I.M. for a diagnosis of schizophrenia was 100% for both ICD–10 and DSM–III–R.

ANALYSES

The data were analysed using SPSS for UNIX. The degree of concordance between the eight definitions of schizophrenia was examined using Cohen's kappa, with 95% confidence intervals. To examine the predictive validity of a diagnosis of schizophrenia at 13 years, median scores and interquartile ranges were calculated for the two outcome measures (GAF symptoms and GAF disability) for each definition of schizophrenia. The median scores and interquartile ranges for those subjects not meeting criteria for schizophrenia were also calculated. Mann–Whitney U tests were used to test the null hypothesis that a diagnosis of schizophrenia is no better at predicting poor outcome than a non-schizophrenia psychotic disorder, for the eight definitions of schizophrenia.

The matrix of kappa values for diagnostic agreement between the diagnoses was subjected to exploratory, non-metric multidimensional scaling (using the ALSCAL procedure in SPSS). Since there were in total only eight diagnoses, a two-dimensional configuration was chosen.

Finally, kappa values were also calculated to demonstrate the degree of concordance between an onset diagnosis of schizophrenia and the final 'main overall diagnosis' of schizophrenia, for DSM–III–R and ICD–10. Sensitivities and specificities were calculated to determine their predictive relationships.

RESULTS

Diagnostic concordance

Table 1 shows the concordance between standard and 'duration adjusted' definitions of schizophrenia applied at first episode. There is high concordance between definitions sharing six-month duration criteria, and between ICD–9, ICD–10 and

Table 2 Prediction of symptoms (GAF) at 13 years by diagnosis

Diagnosis		n^1	Median (IQ range)	Mann–Whitney U test (corrected for ties)				Two-tailed P
				Mean rank	U	W	Z	
DSM–III–R	Schizophrenia	26	40 (34.25–70.25)	30.60	444.5	795.5	−3.0933	0.0020
	Other psychosis	59	75 (50–85)	48.47				
ICD–10	Schizophrenia	47	55 (35–80)	37.59	638.5	1888.5	−2.2623	0.0237
	Other psychosis	38	75 (50–85)	49.70				
ICD–9	Schizophrenia	57	60 (37.5–81)	40.48	654.5	1347.5	−1.3494	0.1772
	Other psychosis	28	72.5 (50–85)	48.13				
CATEGO S+	Schizophrenia	50	70 (40–82)	44.61	794.5	1424.5	−0.7229	0.4697
	Other psychosis	35	55 (35–81)	40.70				
'Duration adjusted' DSM–III–R	Schizophrenia	50	60 (38.75–80.25)	39.88	719.0	1661.0	−1.4009	0.1612
	Other psychosis	35	75 (50–85)	47.46				
'Duration adjusted' ICD–10	Schizophrenia	22	47.5 (31.5–72.5)	31.14	432.0	685.0	−2.6337	0.0084
	Other psychosis	63	70 (40–85)	47.14				
'Duration adjusted' ICD–9	Schizophrenia	25	50 (33.5–73)	32.18	479.5	804.5	−2.6238	0.0087
	Other psychosis	60	72.5 (41.25–85)	47.51				
'Duration adjusted' CATEGO S+	Schizophrenia	19	60 (35–80)	36.53	504.0	694.0	−1.3049	0.1919
	Other psychosis	66	70 (40–85)	44.86				

1. 14 cases missing (nine dead, four lost and one cerebrovascular accident).

Table 3 Prediction of disability (GAF) at 13 years by diagnosis

Diagnosis		n^1	Median (IQ range)	Mann–Whitney U test (corrected for ties)				Two-tailed P
				Mean rank	U	W	Z	
DSM–III–R	Schizophrenia	27	45 (40–75)	32.41	497.0	875.0	−2.8026	0.0051
	Other psychosis	59	75 (45–85)	48.58				
ICD–10	Schizophrenia	48	55 (40.25–80.75)	37.55	626.5	1938.5	−2.4967	0.0125
	Other psychosis	38	80 (50–85)	51.01				
ICD–9	Schizophrenia	58	58 (44–81)	39.94	605.5	1424.5	−1.9138	0.0556
	Other psychosis	28	77.5 (51.25–85)	50.88				
CATEGO S+	Schizophrenia	51	75 (45–81)	43.95	869.5	1499.5	−0.2033	0.8389
	Other psychosis	35	61 (45–81)	42.84				
'Duration adjusted' DSM–III–R	Schizophrenia	51	55 (45–81)	39.55	691.0	1724.0	−1.7813	0.0749
	Other psychosis	35	80 (50–85)	49.26				
'Duration adjusted' ICD–10	Schizophrenia	23	45 (40–75)	32.61	474.0	750.0	−2.4578	0.014
	Other psychosis	63	75 (45–85)	47.48				
'Duration adjusted' ICD–9	Schizophrenia	26	45 (38.75–75)	32.15	485.0	836.0	−2.7895	0.0053
	Other psychosis	60	75 (46.25–85)	48.42				
'Duration adjusted' CATEGO S+	Schizophrenia	20	72.5 (40.25–78.75)	38.28	555.5	765.5	−1.0742	0.2827
	Other psychosis	66	67.5 (45–85)	45.08				

1. 13 cases missing (nine dead and four lost).

'duration adjusted' DSM–III–R. Table 1 also shows that inclusion of six-month duration criteria restricts the diagnosis to between 23 and 31 cases. Of the standard diagnoses, DSM–III–R provides the most restrictive definition of schizophrenia, with only 31 subjects fulfilling DSM–III–R criteria compared with 56 and 67 subjects fulfilling ICD–10 and ICD–9 criteria for schizophrenia, respectively.

Predictive validity of diagnosis

Tables 2 and 3 show that a diagnosis of schizophrenia has significantly greater predictive validity at 13 years, in terms of symptoms and disability, than a non-schizophrenia psychotic disorder, for the DSM–III–R and ICD–10 systems of classification. An ICD–9 diagnosis of schizophrenia is less discriminating (especially for symptoms), and a CATEGO S+ definition of schizophrenia has no predictive validity. Tables 2 and 3 also show that the addition of six-month duration criteria improves the predictive validity of ICD–10 and ICD–9, but this improvement is much less for CATEGO S+. Removing the duration criterion from DSM–III–R makes it a much broader diagnosis, but reduces its predictive validity, particularly for symptomatic outcome.

Stability of diagnosis

For DSM–III–R an onset diagnosis of schizophrenia proved to be very stable over 13 years, with all 31 subjects retaining schizophrenia as a main overall diagnosis (specificity 100%). ICD–10 proved to be less specific (specificity 88.64%), with five subjects who were given an onset diagnosis of schizophrenia changing to a non-schizophrenia main overall diagnosis. These included four subjects with a main overall diagnosis of bipolar affective disorder, and one subject with a psychotic disorder due to use of alcohol (schizophrenia-like). In terms of the ability to predict a main overall diagnosis of schizophrenia, DSM–III–R proved to be considerably less sensitive than ICD–10

(60.78 and 92.73%, respectively). In addition to the 31 subjects meeting DSM–III–R criteria at onset, an additional 20 subjects received a main overall diagnosis of schizophrenia. Of these, 17 were initially assigned a diagnosis of schizophreniform psychosis, one a bipolar disorder (manic with psychotic features), one had a psychotic disorder 'not otherwise specified', and the last had major depression (single episode with psychotic features). For ICD–10, an additional four subjects given a non-schizophrenia diagnosis at onset received a main overall diagnosis of schizophrenia. Of these, one was initially assigned a diagnosis of acute polymorphic disorder with symptoms of schizophrenia, one had a schizoaffective disorder (manic type), one had an unspecified non-organic psychosis, and one had a severe depressive episode (with psychotic symptoms). For DSM–III–R there were 48 subjects who received a non-schizophrenia diagnosis at onset who retained this as a main overall diagnosis, and for ICD–10 there were 39. The concordance (Cohen's kappa) between onset diagnoses and main overall diagnoses (schizophrenia and non-schizophrenia) was 0.60 (95% CI 0.44–0.76) for DSM–III–R and 0.82 (95% CI 0.70–0.94) for ICD–10.

REFERENCES

American Psychiatric Association (1987) *Diagnostic and Statistical Manual of Mental Disorders* (3rd edn, revised) (DSM–III–R). Washington, DC: APA.

Endicott, J., Spitzer, R. L., Fleiss, J. L., et al (1976) The Global Assessment Scale. A procedure of measuring overall severity of psychiatric disturbance. *Archives of General Psychiatry*, **33**, 766–771.

Harrison, G., Mason, P., Glazebrook, C., et al (1994) Residence of incident cohort of psychotic patients after 13 years of follow-up. *British Medical Journal*, **308**, 813–816.

Jablensky, A., Schwarz, R. & Tomov, T. (1980) WHO collaborative study on impairments and disabilities associated with schizophrenic disorders. *Acta Psychiatrica Scandinavica* **62**, (suppl. 285), 152–163.

__ , Sartorius, N., Ernberg, E., et al (1992) Schizophrenia: manifestations, incidence and course in different cultures. A World Health Organisation Ten Country Study. *Psychological Medicine*, Monograph Supplement 20. Cambridge: Cambridge University Press.

Mason, P., Harrison, G., Glazebrook, C., et al (1995) Characteristics of outcome in schizophrenia at 13 years. *British Journal of Psychiatry*, **167**, 596–603.

Sartorius, N., Gulbinat, W., Harrison, G., et al (1996) Long term follow-up of schizophrenia in 16 countries. A description of the International Study of Schizophrenia conducted by the World Health Organization. *Social Psychiatry and Psychiatric Epidemiology*, **31**, 249–258.

Wing, J. K., Cooper, J. E. & Sartorius, N. (1974) *The Measurement and Classification of Psychiatric Symptoms.* Cambridge: Cambridge University Press.

World Health Organization (1978a) *Mental Disorders: Glossary and Guide to their Classification in Accordance with the Ninth Revision of the International Classification of Diseases.* Geneva: WHO.

__ **(1978b)** *Psychiatric and Personal History Schedule.* Geneva: WHO.

__ **(1992a)** *The ICD–10 Classification of Mental and Behavioural Disorders.* Geneva: WHO.

__ **(1992b)** *Broad Rating Schedule.* Geneva: WHO.

__ **(1992c)** *Life Chart Schedule.* Geneva: WHO.

MASON *ET AL*

Please write your answers to questions I to IV in the spaces provided.

I.   Background

A.   What is the study design?   [2 marks]

....

....

....

B.   How can you establish the validity of psychiatric diagnosis? What is meant by the term predictive validity? Is predictive validity important for clinicians?   [6 marks]

....

....

....

....

....

....

C.   What is the difference between reliability and validity? Are they related to each other in any way?   [6 marks]

....

....

....

....

....

....

II.   Method

A.   Explain the terms DSM–III–R, ICD–9, ICD–10 and CATEGO S+. What is the main difference between ICD–9 and DSM–III–R in relation to the diagnosis of schizophrenia?   [4 marks]

....

....

....

....

....

....

....

....

B.   The authors put a lot of effort into obtaining all the new cases. They also achieved a 96% follow-up. Which of these are the most important in achieving their study aims? [6 marks]

....
....
....
....
....
....

C.   What is meant by the phrase 'stability of ICD–10 and DSM–III–R schizophrenia'? Is this the same as predictive validity?   [2 marks]

....
....
....
....
....
....

D.   The authors have chosen a sample of new presentations. What would be the advantages and disadvantages of using a cross-sectional sample rather than new presentations?
                                                                                             [6 marks]

....
....
....
....
....
....

E.   Was the Present State Examination (PSE) a good choice to assess psychopathology?
                                                                                             [4 marks]

....
....
....
....
....
....

F.   What does kappa measure? Is it a measure of reliability or validity?   [6 marks]

....
....
....
....
....
....

G.   Is it helpful to have asterisks indicating statistical significance in Table 1?   [6 marks]

....
....
....
....
....
....

III.   Results

A.   What is the concordance between CATEGO S+ and ICD–9? How do the confidence
      intervals help the interpretation of this value?   [4 marks]

....
....
....
....
....
....

B.   Why did the authors use the Mann–Whitney U test? Why did they use the median and not
      the mean? Why did they omit confidence intervals from Tables 2 and 3?   [6 marks]

....
....
....
....
....
....

C.   What were the null hypotheses for the P values given in Tables 2 and 3?   [4 marks]

....
....
....
....
....

D.   In Table 3 for the ICD–9 results, the P value is greater than 0.05. How should this finding
      be interpreted? Is it a non-significant result?   [6 marks]

....
....
....
....
....
....
....

E. For what diagnoses are the differences between schizophrenia and other psychoses the greatest in Tables 2 and 3?   [2 marks]

....

....

....

F. The authors have compared diagnoses at study outset to those at follow-up 13 years later. Define the terms 'sensitivity' and 'specificity'. Are the terms sensitivity and specificity appropriate for these comparisons? What is most important for clinicians – sensitivity or specificity? What is the positive predictive value of the DSM–III–R diagnoses?   [8 marks]

....

....

....

....

....

....

IV Discussion

A. In the full version of this paper, the authors conclude that "DSM–III–R and ICD–10 definitions of schizophrenia are good predictors of outcome at 13 years". Can this be supported by their evidence?   [6 marks]

....

....

....

....

....

....

B. What is a confounder? Should the authors have considered the possibility of confounding? What variables might have confounded the relationship described in the paper? [8 marks]

....

....

....

....

....

....

C.   In the full version of this paper, the authors conclude that diagnoses that rely on certain characteristic cross-sectional symptoms of schizophrenia (CATEGO S+) are unable to define an illness with poor prognosis. Does their evidence support this?   [8 marks]

....

....

....

....

....

....

I. Background

A. What is the study design?

It is a longitudinal or cohort study where the main outcome is the disability associated with schizophrenia.

B. How can you establish the validity of a psychiatric diagnosis? What is meant by the term predictive validity? Is predictive validity important for clinicians?

Various criteria have been suggested that help to establish the validity of psychiatric diagnoses. There is, however, no gold standard criterion in psychiatry (along with many other areas of medicine). Suggested criteria include genetic evidence that a psychiatric diagnosis is heritable, that outcome can be predicted with a diagnosis and that diagnoses define a group responsive to a particular treatment.

Validity refers to the property that an assessment measures what it intends to measure. Predictive validity is meant to refer to the ability to predict outcome. In this case the predictive validity of various diagnostic criteria for schizophrenia are being studied. It is important to clinicians as it helps in informing them, patients and relatives about the prognosis.

C. What is the difference between reliability and validity? Are they related to each other in any way?

Reliability is an estimate of the extent to which a measure of an attribute agrees with itself. In contrast, validity is the extent to which a measure assesses what it intends to measure. Reliability can be thought of as repeatability whereas validity assumes that there is a 'gold standard' with which to compare a measure. Reliability and validity are related to each other because an unreliable measure cannot be valid. If a measure cannot agree with itself then it cannot really be a valid measure of the construct it is intending to measure.

II. Method

A. Explain the terms DSM–III–R, ICD–9 and ICD–10 and CATEGO S+. What is the main difference between ICD–9 and DSM–III–R in relation to the diagnosis of schizophrenia?

DSM–III, ICD–9 and ICD–10 are diagnostic manuals issued by the American Psychiatric Association and the World Health Organization respectively. CATEGO S+ is a computer-generated diagnostic system that puts emphasis on the presence of Schneider's first-rank symptoms and is used in association with the ninth version of the Present State Examination (PSE–9). The main difference in the diagnostic criteria for schizophrenia between ICD–9 and DSM–III–R is that DSM–III–R requires a six-month duration of illness and this can include a prodromal phase of illness.

B. The authors put a lot of effort into obtaining all the new cases. They also achieved a 96% follow-up. Which of these are the most important in achieving their study aims?

For a cohort study it is more important that the subjects are followed-up than to ensure a representative sample. It is possible, but unlikely, to have selection bias in a cohort study, in the sense that the initial selection of the subjects at cohort entry can influence the results. However, incomplete follow-up can introduce serious bias in a cohort study. These authors have accomplished both with a sample of new cases representative of those in that geographical area and 96% follow-up. Biases due to selection of cases or incomplete follow-up will be very unlikely to affect the conclusions in this study.

C. What is meant by the phrase 'stability of ICD–10 and DSM–III–R schizophrenia'? Is this the same as predictive validity?

There seems to be an assumption in this paper that a patient retaining the same diagnosis for 13 years is a sign of the validity of the diagnosis. The authors are therefore assuming that the stability of the diagnoses is the same as predictive validity. This is the conventional view at present, but it is perfectly possible that diagnoses change over time. Someone presenting with schizophrenia might, many years later, have predominantly affective symptoms, or vice versa.

D. The authors have chosen a sample of new presentations. What would be the advantages and disadvantages of using a cross-sectional sample rather than new presentations?

The advantage of a cross-sectional sample is that it would contain a representative mixture of old and new cases. Statements about outcome could then be generalised to the cases currently seen by a psychiatrist at any one time. One could not, however, generalise from a cross-sectional sample to a new case of schizophrenia. In contrast, an incident sample of new cases enables the outcome to be generalised to a new case. One could argue that a cross-sectional sample would be of more use to clinicians as there are few new cases of schizophrenia presented to a single psychiatrist in a year.

E. Was the Present State Examination (PSE) a good choice to assess psychopathology?

The PSE is a semi-standardised structured interview. It specifies some of the questions to be asked in the mental state examination and includes a precise glossary of terms for the various aspects of psychopathology. However, it allows the interviewer discretion in the use of supplementary questions. This kind of approach is very appropriate for the definition of psychotic symptoms. It improves the reliability of clinical diagnoses performed without any form of standardisation.

F. What does kappa measure? Is it a measure of reliability or validity?

The kappa is a chance corrected measure of agreement. It is primarily a measure of reliability. It could also be used to measure the agreement with a 'gold standard' measure and would then be assessing validity.

G. Is it helpful to have asterisks indicating statistical significance in Table I?

We are not primarily interested in whether two diagnostic schemes agree with each other more than one would expect by chance. The main aim of Table 1 is to look at the extent of the agreement. Therefore, the kappa value and confidence intervals are of most value. There are also a large number of statistical tests so one would expect one or two significant results by chance (or Type 1 errors) in a table of this size.

III. Results

A. What is the concordance between CATEGO S+ and ICD–9? How do the confidence intervals help the interpretation of this value?

The kappa value for CATEGO S+ and ICD–9 is 0.31 and the confidence intervals are between 0.11 and 0.51. The confidence intervals give a range of values with which the empirical data are consistent, having taken account of the sampling variation. It is therefore perfectly reasonable to expect that in a large enough study the agreement between CATEGO S+ and ICD–9 could be as low as 0.11 indicating very low agreement or as high as 0.5 indicating quite good agreement.

B. Why did the authors use the Mann–Whitney U test? Why did they use the median and not the mean? Why did they omit confidence intervals from Tables 2 and 3?

The authors do not state this but the Mann–Whitney U test is a non-parametric test and so the data for the GAF must be non-normally distributed. For the same reason medians are given rather than the mean as the median and mean only have the same value in a symmetrical distribution such as the normal distribution. You cannot calculate confidence intervals using non-parametric tests.

C. What were the null hypotheses for the P values given in Tables 2 and 3?

The null hypothesis was that the GAF symptom and disability scores are the same for those given a diagnosis of schizophrenia and those given other psychotic diagnoses.

D. In Table 3, the ICD–9 results, the *P* value is greater than 0.05. How should this finding be interpreted? Is it a non-significant result?

The value is given as 0.0556. To have the *P* value expressed to three decimal places seems unnecessary though they are correct in giving exact *P* values rather than using the term 'NS'. One would usually round this figure to 0.06. Although 0.05 is taken as a conventional level of significance, there is not much difference between 0.05 and 0.06 and it is most appropriate to interpret all such values as of borderline statistical significance rather than 'non-significant'. An additional problem, however, is the multiple testing that has been carried out. There are 16 tests presented in Tables 2 and 3 so the possibility of Type 1 error is increased. In that light it is best to ignore findings of borderline statistical significance unless there are strong *a priori* grounds for supporting a real effect. As there is also a non-significant finding for ICD–9 in Table 2 there is not much evidence here to support the idea that ICD–9 diagnosis of schizophrenia is associated with poor outcome.

E. For what diagnoses are the differences between schizophrenia and other psychoses the greatest in Tables 2 and 3?

The differences are the greatest for DSM–III–R with a median difference of 35 on symptoms and 30 on disability. Duration adjusted ICD–10 also has a median difference of 30 on disability and 22.5 on symptoms.

F. The authors have compared diagnoses at study outset to those at follow-up 13 years later. Define the terms 'sensitivity' and 'specificity'. Are the terms sensitivity and specificity appropriate for these comparisons? What is most important for clinicians – sensitivity or specificity? What is the positive predictive value of the DSM–III–R diagnoses?

The authors are assuming that the overall diagnosis made at the end of the study is the most accurate diagnosis. In that sense they are using this as the 'gold standard' with which to compare the original diagnoses. However, there will probably be some unreliability in the final diagnosis so in that sense it is inappropriate to use these terms, although it is a reasonable shorthand. Sensitivity is the proportion of true positives correctly identified. Specificity is the proportion of true negatives correctly identified.

Clinicians probably would prefer more specific diagnoses that reduce the proportion of false positives. Schizophrenia is still a stigmatising term with profound consequences for the individual. Most clinicians tend to reserve it for cases where there is little doubt of the diagnosis. For other diagnoses, clinicians might wish for a more sensitive diagnosis. For example, if a cheap, effective and safe treatment were available for a condition, most clinicians would tend to use it more freely and include potential false positives for a trial of treatment.

The positive predictive value is the probability that someone is a true positive given a positive test result. In this case, it is the probability that the person was given a diagnosis of schizophrenia 13 years later. The authors do give figures to calculate the positive predictive value but it is a bit confusing to extract the values. DSM–III had a positive predictive value of 100% as all the 31 cases remained cases at follow-up. The figures for ICD–10 are not given in this excerpt.

IV. Discussion

A. In the full version of this paper, the authors conclude that "DSM–III–R and ICD–10 definitions of schizophrenia are good predictors of outcome at 13 years". Can this be supported by their evidence?

It is not clear what is meant by a good predictor. The interquartile ranges given in Tables 2 and 3 indicate a large overlap between the outcomes of those with schizophrenia and the remaining psychotic diagnoses. The proportion of people diagnosed with schizophrenia differs between the various diagnostic categories so each diagnostic category is being compared with a different group of 'other psychoses'. It is not surprising that the diagnostic criteria that give the smallest number of cases also identify the poorest prognostic group. It is more remarkable that ICD–10 identifies a similar number to CATEGO S+ but is better at predicting outcome. The outcome measures here are not clinically very meaningful and so the statement these are 'good predictors' does not seem very meaningful. Just because they show statistically significant differences on a scale is not enough to support the idea they are good predictors. The authors would need a more clinically relevant measure of outcome to justify this conclusion.

B.   What is a confounder? Should the authors have considered the possibility of confounding? What variables might have confounded the relationship described in the paper?

A confounder is a characteristic that is associated with both the outcome of a study (disease in epidemiological terminology) and the independent variables of interest (the exposure). Confounding should always be considered in interpreting results especially in non-randomised or observational studies such as this one. There are a number of factors that are known to be associated with a poor prognosis in schizophrenia including early age of onset, insidious onset, absence of affective symptoms and poor insight. If these happened to be associated with one or other of the diagnostic criteria they could lead to the apparent differences in prognosis. Ideally, the authors should have considered confounders and performed an analysis which would have taken them into account. They might also have used statistical techniques to model the individual criteria used in the different diagnostic schemes in order to draw conclusions about which particular criteria are associated with a poor outcome.

C.   In the full version of this paper, the authors conclude that diagnoses that rely on certain characteristic cross-sectional symptoms of schizophrenia (CATEGO S+) are unable to define an illness with poor prognosis. Does their evidence support this?

The authors did not find statistically significant differences between those diagnosed with CATEGO S+ schizophrenia versus the remaining psychotic patients in either the disability or symptom scale. However, a non-significant difference does not mean there is no difference between the categories. In both Tables 2 and 3 the people with CATEGO S+ schizophrenia scored more highly on the symptom (median difference 15) and disability (median difference 14) scale of the GAF. Confidence intervals are not given because of the use of non-parametric tests, but in any case it is difficult to decide whether the differences found between CATEGO S+ are of any clinical importance or whether the study had sufficient statistical power to be able to detect a clinically important difference. The authors can probably conclude that DSM–III–R and ICD–10 are better at predicting poor prognosis than CATEGO S+. However, it is difficult to conclude that CATEGO S+ cannot identify a poor prognosis group.

A CRITICAL REVIEW PAPER

Randomised controlled trial
Model answers by Stephen Lawrie

Controlled trial of exposure and response prevention in obsessive–compulsive disorder

MERRAN LINDSAY, ROCCO CRINO and GAVIN ANDREWS

Obsessive–compulsive disorder (OCD) is a complex and debilitating disorder with a lifetime prevalence of about 2% (Karno & Golding, 1991). It is not rare. Two treatments are effective: one is behaviour therapy using exposure and response prevention, the other is pharmacotherapy with selective serotonin reuptake inhibitors. The aims of the present study were threefold: to replicate the seminal work of Rachman, Hodgson and Marks at the Maudsley Hospital in a different setting with a credible placebo; to examine the specific contribution of exposure and response prevention to outcome in OCD; and to examine the contribution of non-specific therapy factors, such as therapist supportiveness, to treatment outcome.

METHOD

Subjects

Eighteen subjects were recruited from a population of adult out-patients referred for treatment of OCD. All met DSM–IV diagnostic criteria for a primary diagnosis of OCD. The average duration of OCD was 11 years (range 1–26 years). Five subjects were taking clomipramine or fluoxetine and all had been on these medications for at least 12 months without improvement.

Assessment

The outcome measures used to assess the severity of obsessions, compulsions, anxiety and depression were:

The Padua Inventory

A 60-item self-report questionnaire (Sanavio, 1988) assessing the severity of obsessive–compulsive thoughts and behaviours. Each item is rated on a five-point scale (from 0 to 4), giving a maximum possible score of 240.

The Maudsley Obsessional–Compulsive Inventory (MOCI)

A 30-item self-report questionnaire (Rachman & Hodgson, 1980) assessing the presence of common OCD symptoms. Each item is answered 'true' or 'false', giving a maximum possible score of 30. The MOCI has four subscales: checking, cleaning, slowness and doubting.

The Yale–Brown Obsessive–Compulsive Scale (Y–BOCS)

This is a clinician-rated scale (Goodman et al, 1989a,b) with 10 items. It was designed to assess severity of OCD symptoms independent of the type or number of obsessions or compulsions present. Severity is assessed in terms of time, interference, distress, resistance and control. Each item is rated on a five-point scale (0 to 4) giving a maximum possible score of 40.

The State–Trait Anxiety Inventory (STAI; Spielberger et al, 1970) and the Beck Depression Inventory (BDI; Beck et al, 1961) were also used. They are scales with well established psychometric characteristics.

Interference rating scale

In addition to the above measures, each subject was asked to rate the extent to which OCD interfered with their life and activities. The scale was numbered 1 to 7, where 1 represented 'not at all', 3 represented 'a little', 5 represented 'a lot' and 7 represented 'totally'.

Therapist variables

In order to rule out the possibility that any observed differences in treatment outcome were due to differences in therapist variables, patients were contacted following treatment and asked to rate their therapist for two qualities: supportiveness and understanding. These interviews were conducted over the phone by an independent assessor. Ratings were made on a four-point scale, where 0=not at all, 1=somewhat, 2= moderately and 3=highly.

Treatment

Subjects were randomly assigned to one of two treatment conditions: exposure and response prevention or anxiety management (control). Both treatments involved approximately 15 hours of face-to-face therapy over a three-week period with experienced clinical psychologists. All subjects received a treatment manual which outlined in detail a rationale for treatment and treatment guidelines.

Exposure and response prevention

Treatment consisted of graded exposure to situations previously associated with obsessional thoughts or impulses coupled with self-imposed prevention of compulsive rituals (for treatment manual see Andrews et al, 1994). In addition to attending out-patient therapy sessions in the clinic, these subjects were required to complete homework exposure tasks each day.

Anxiety management

In the light of our views about the common neurotic syndrome (Andrews et al, 1994) general anxiety management techniques were seen to provide a credible and possibly effective placebo treatment condition. Treatment sessions focused on teaching the subjects anxiety management techniques, including breathing techniques for the management of hyperventilation, progressive muscle relaxation and structured problem-solving about non-OCD life stressors.

RESULTS

The demographic characteristics are shown in Table 1.

Post-treatment ratings of therapists

Patients in both treatment groups rated their therapists as highly supportive and understanding.

Pre-treatment dependent variables

Pre-treatment scores on all seven dependent variables were compared using a series of one-way ANOVAs (with Bonferroni adjustment). There was no significant difference between the groups on any of these measures (see Table 2).

Table 1 Demographic characteristics of patients

	Exposure and response prevention (n=9)	Anxiety management (n=9)
Gender		
Male	5	1
Female	4	8
Mean age (years) (s.d.)	31.6 (8.9)	34.0 (9.3)
Duration of complaints (years) (s.d.)	9.0 (8.7)	12.9 (8.9)
Marital status		
Single	44%	22%
Married or de facto	44%	78%
Divorced or widowed	11%	0%
Educational standard		
Low	22%	22%
Medium	33%	11%
High	45%	67%

Table 2 Group means (s.d.) pre- and post-treatment

	Exposure group		Control group	
	Pre	Post	Pre	Post
Interference	5.9 (0.93)	3.4 (0.88)	6.4 (0.88)	6.3 (0.87)*
Y–BOCS total	28.70 (4.56)	11.00 (3.81)	24.44 (6.98)	25.89 (5.80)*
Obsessions	14.11 (2.71)	6.33 (1.80)	11.56 (4.06)	12.89 (3.18)*
Compulsions	14.56 (2.12)	4.67 (2.35)	12.89 (3.22)	13.00 (2.83)*
MOCI total	17.00 (4.06)	9.56 (4.59)	20.33 (4.06)	17.89 (4.23)*
PADUA total	84.56 (28.36)	41.44 (22.54)	95.78 (39.44)	81.22 (35.15)*
STAI state	51.89 (12.18)	44.33 (8.97)	53.11 (11.38)	52.11 (13.77)
STAI trait	58.00 (10.08)	49.89 (8.71)	58.22 (12.03)	55.89 (12.89)
BDI total	21.33 (10.45)	13.11 (8.30)	19.22 (9.28)	18.33 (9.66)

Y–BOCS=Yale–Brown Obsessive–Compulsive Scale; MOCI=Maudsley Obsessional–Compulsive Inventory; PADUA=Padua Inventory; STAI=State–Trait Anxiety Inventory; BDI=Beck Depression Inventory.
*$P < 0.05$ Exposure v. control at same time point

Table 3 Principal components: variable loadings and eigenvalues

Variable	Component 1 weight	Component 2 weight
Interference	0.897	0.176
Y–BOCS	0.808	0.196
MOCI	0.826	0.315
PADUA	0.716	0.509
STAI state	0.315	0.799
STAI trait	0.218	0.899
BDI depression	0.238	0.907
Eigenvalue	4.38	1.17
% Variance explained	62.6	16.7

Y–BOCS=Yale–Brown Obsessive–Compulsive Scale; MOCI=Maudsley Obsessional–Compulsive Inventory; PADUA=Padua Inventory; STAI=State–Trait Anxiety Inventory; BDI=Beck Depression Inventory.

Treatment effects

Scores on the different outcome measures were likely to be highly correlated, so treatment effects were examined using a principal components analysis of dependent variable scores followed by a two-way analysis of variance. Treatment effects were also examined on the seven outcome measures individually, giving a total of nine two-way ANOVAs with Bonferroni adjustment for multiple comparisons (critical value=0.5/9=0.0056).

Principal components analysis (with varimax rotation) yielded two components with an eigenvalue greater than one. The first of these components accounted for 62.6% of the variance in scores on individual measures. As can be seen in Table 3, this component provides a combined measure of OCD symptom severity, with high loadings for the Y–BOCS, MOCI, PADUA and the interference measure. The second component accounted for a further 16.7% of the variance, and appeared to be a more general measure of anxiety and depression, with high loadings for both of the STAI measures and the BDI.

When scores on the first principal component were combined across groups, there was an overall reduction in scores following treatment ($F(1,32)=27.8$, $P < 0.0056$). Likewise scores on this component were lower for the exposure and response prevention group than for the anxiety management group when combined across measurement occasions ($F(1,32)=35.0$, $P < 0.0056$). However, there was also a significant interaction between component scores for each group over time, indicating that the reduction in obsessional symptoms following treatment was specific to patients in the exposure and response prevention group ($F(1,32)=20.3$, $P < 0.0056$). There was no change in scores following treatment for patients in the anxiety management group.

By comparison, there were no significant differences between the groups ($F(1,32)=0.002$, NS) or following treatment ($F(1,32)=0.434$, NS) in scores on the second principal component, and no significant interaction effects ($F(1,32)=0.031$, NS). Analysis of variance in individual measures showed similar results. When scores for both groups were combined, there was a significant reduction from pre-treatment to post-treatment in scores on the Y–BOCS ($F(1,32)=20.1$, $P < 0.0056$) and the MOCI ($F(1,32)=12.2$, $P < 0.0056$), and in subjective ratings of the degree to which OCD interfered with life and activities ($F(1,32)= 18.6$, $P<0.0056$). When pre-treatment and post-treatment scores were combined there were significant differences between the groups in scores on the MOCI ($F(1,32)= 17.0$, $P<0.0056$) and in subjective ratings of inter-ference ($F(1,32)=33.7$, $P<0.0056$). More importantly, the interactions between group scores over time were significant using the Y–BOCS ($F(1,32)=27.9$, $P<0.0056$), and subjective ratings of interference ($F(1,32)=15.5$, $P<0.0056$). These results show that the reduction in Y–BOCS and in-terference scores from pre-treatment to post-treatment was specific to the exposure and response prevention group, with no change in scores for the anxiety management group. This is illustrated using Y–BOCS scores in Fig. 1.

DISCUSSION

The results of the present study provide con-siderable evidence for the specificity of change associated with exposure and re-sponse prevention techniques. The failure of the control group to show any significant changes in OCD symptoms following treat-ment with general anxiety management techniques is further evidence for the specific effects of exposure and response prevention in the reduction of obsessional symptoms. The absence of change in this group cannot

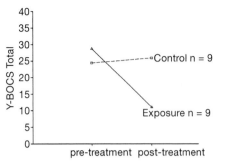

Fig. I Mean Y–BOCS total scores.

be attributed to differences in treatment ex-pectations since considerable effort was made to design a control treatment package which would have good face validity for pa-tients. This is supported by the high compli-ance with monitoring tasks in the control group and the fact that no patients dropped out of treatment.

The results of the present study suggest that while therapist variables may be impor-tant in maximising treatment outcomes with behaviour therapy, they make little differ-ence to obsessional symptoms in the absence of exposure and response prevention.

In summary, by evaluating the contribu-tion of non-specific therapy factors to treat-ment outcomes with obsessional patients, the current investigation adds further evi-dence to the efficacy of exposure and re-sponse prevention in the treatment of

OCD. The findings clearly show that the therapeutic benefits associated with expo-sure and response prevention are a function of the specific procedures involved. Support-ive and understanding therapists offering face valid treatments with a comprehensive rationale make little difference to OCD in the absence of exposure-based treatment.

REFERENCES

Andrews, G., Crino, R., Hunt, C., et al (1994) *The Treatment of Anxiety Disorders.* New York: Cambridge University Press.

Beck, A., Ward, C., Mendelson, M., et al (1961) An inventory for measuring depression. *Archives of General Psychiatry,* **4**, 561–571.

Goodman, W., Price, L., Rasmussen, S., et al (1989a) The Yale–Brown obsessive compulsive scale: development, use and reliability. *Archives of General Psychiatry,* **46**, 1006–1011.

—, —, —, et al (1989b) The Yale–Brown obsessive compulsive scale: validity. *Archives of General Psychiatry,* **46**, 1012–1016.

Karno, M. & Golding, J. (1991) Obsessive Compulsive Disorder. In *Psychiatric Disorders in America–The Epidemiological Catchment Area Study* (eds L. Robins & D. Regier), pp. 204–219. New York: Macmillan.

Rachmans, S. & Hodgson, R. (1980) *Obsessions and Compulsions.* New Jersey: Prentice Hall.

Sanavio, E. (1988) Obsessions and compulsions: the Padua inventory. *Behavior Research and Therapy,* **26**, 169–177.

Spielberger, C. D., Gorsuch, R. L. & Lushene, R. E. (1970) *STAI Manual for the State–Trait Anxiety Inventory.* Palo Alto, CA: Consulting Psychologists Press.

LINDSAY *ET AL*

Please write your answers to questions I and II in the spaces provided.

I.   Methods

A.(i) Comment on the adequacy of the description of the subjects recruited for the trial.

[10 marks]

....
....
....
....
....
....

(ii)   Comment on the description of how the sample was chosen from the clinic
population.   [15 marks]

....
....
....
....
....
....

B.   Why was it important to control for therapist contact time?   [5 marks]

....
....
....
....

C.   Why do we need to know the length of time that the five drug-treated patients had been
taking their drugs?   [5 marks]

....
....
....
....

D.(i) What is meant by variance? [5 marks]

....
....
....
....

(ii) What is a principal components analysis? [5 marks]

....
....
....
....

E.(i) Why was the assessment of therapist variable carried out after treatment? [5 marks]

....
....
....
....

(ii) Why was an independent assessor used for this purpose? [5 marks]

....
....
....
....

II. Results and further questions

A. List three main clinical implications of this study. [15 marks]

....
....
....
....
....
....
....
....
....
....

B.   List three main limitations of this study.   [15 marks]

....

....

....

....

....

....

....

....

....

....

C. (i) The authors emphasise the credibility of the control group. What is the basis of their
        confidence in its credibility?   [10 marks]

....

....

....

....

....

....

....

....

(ii)   How could this credibility have been assessed?   [5 marks]

....

....

....

....

I. Methods

A. (i) Comment on the adequacy of the description of the subjects recruited for the trial.

The description of the subjects is very limited, mentioning only the long duration of illness. Table 1 reveals that two-thirds of the subjects were female. Educational standard in Table 1 is not defined or explained, but is presumably a proxy for intelligence and/or social class in those who may not be working because of illness. Therefore, the overall description of subjects is poor. This is an important issue as some of the demographic characteristics may reveal biases in the referral or recruitment process, and may also have some bearing on treatment response.

(ii) Comment on the description of how the sample was chosen from the clinic population.

The description of sample recruitment is again very limited. All that we are told is that subjects were out-patients referred for treatment of OCD who met DSM–IV criteria for a primary diagnosis of OCD. No mention is made of the number of potential subjects in the clinic population or the number who were approached to participate in the trial – patients who participate in treatment trials are likely to differ from those who do not give consent and this affects the extrapolation of results to everyday clinical practice. Simply meeting DSM–IV criteria for a particular disorder is not a particularly reliable diagnosis unless the results are based on a structured psychiatric interview. Some patients could, in theory at least, have been 'squeezed' into the desired diagnostic category. Similarly, simply stating that the primary diagnosis was OCD could hide several comorbid disorders that could have an impact on the trial results. For example, patients with comorbid depression or substance use or personality disorder, if over-represented in the treatment or control groups, could adversely affect the treatment response in that arm of the trial.

B. Why was it important to control for therapist contact time?

Controlling for therapist contact time is important so as to ensure that any differences between those getting different treatments is not attributable to non-specific factors. Any therapeutic intervention is associated with a placebo response which is itself likely to be a result of attention from someone else, the chance to discuss problems ('a problem shared is a problem halved'), reassurance and general emotional support.

C. Why do we need to know the length of time that the five drug-treated patients had been taking their drugs?

The length of drug treatment is important as antidepressants take some time (usually weeks) to exert a therapeutic response, so that if some patients had only recently started the drugs and were over-represented in one of the treatment arms, this could have confounded the comparison of treatments in the trial. Similarly, given the usual dose–response relationship in antidepressant treatment, it would be important to know that the dose had not been recently changed.

D. (i) What is meant by variance?

Variance refers to the spread or variation in the distribution of the values of a measured variable. It is usually quoted as a standard deviation or a range.

(ii) What is a principal components analysis?

A principal components analysis is that part of a factor analysis which tries to identify underlying commonalities in a large number of variables or, in other words, groups together measures which are relatively highly and selectively correlated with one another. The number of components is usually determined by those which have eigenvalues greater than one (and/or by a 'scree plot'). The varimax rotation is designed to make the principal components more interpretable.

E. (i) Why was the assessment of therapist variable carried out after treatment?

The assessment of therapist was carried out after treatment so that the patient could give an opinion after all aspects of treatment were completed and would be able to comment on the potential importance of any non-specific therapeutic factors as mentioned above.

(ii) Why was an independent assessor used for this purpose?

An independent assessor was used for this purpose for several reasons. Ratings by the therapists themselves – who could not be blind to the treatment they were giving – could have been biased by their belief or lack of it in the particular treatment given or encouraging patients simply to say that they were always highly supportive and understanding. Finally, depending on how the assessment was done, the independent assessor could have ensured that the patients would not simply say their therapist was very supportive and understanding (rather than professional, for example) simply because they were feeling better as a result of the treatment.

II. Results and further questions

A. List three main clinical implications of the study

Three clinical implications are:

(a) Exposure and response prevention is an effective treatment of the symptoms of OCD.
(b) Anxiety management is not an effective treatment of the symptoms of OCD.
(c) Exposure and response prevention is not an effective treatment for anxiety and depression symptoms in OCD.

B. List three main limitations of the study.

Three limitations are that:

(a) The number of subjects in the trial is very small.
(b) The lack of information about subject referral and recruitment means that the results may not apply in everyday clinical practice.
(c) The method of randomisation is not explicit.

C. (i) The authors emphasise the credibility of the control group. What is the basis of their confidence in this credibility?

The credibility of the control group is based on the fact that they received a generic intervention from an 'experienced therapist' that controlled for therapist time and any non-specific/placebo response. It does appear that the patients thought that they were getting an effective treatment from their compliance with symptom ratings and the treatment as a whole (that is, no drop-outs). Although it could be argued that the two treatments were not as well controlled as the authors suggest – progressive muscle relaxation may not be the best form of relaxation treatment and those receiving exposure spent more time in treatment if homework is included – the trial is generally well controlled.

(ii) How could this credibility have been assessed?

Credibility could have been assessed by directly asking patients whether they thought they were in the treatment or control groups.

A CRITICAL REVIEW PAPER

Randomised, double-blind, placebo-controlled trial
Model answers by John Cookson

Paroxetine in the treatment of panic disorder

A randomised, double-blind, placebo-controlled study

S. OEHRBERG, P. E. CHRISTIANSEN, K. BEHNKE, A. L. BORUP, B. SEVERIN,
J. SOEGAARD, H. CALBERG, R. JUDGE, J. K. OHRSTROM and P. M. MANNICHE

The efficacy of paroxetine as an antidepressant is well established (Feighner & Boyer, 1989). The purpose of the present study was to evaluate the efficacy and tolerability of the highly selective serotonin reuptake inhibitor (SSRI), paroxetine, in the treatment of patients with panic disorder.

METHOD

This study was a double-blind, placebo-controlled, parallel-group comparison. An initial three-week placebo period was followed by a 12-week treatment period with either paroxetine or placebo, after which patients underwent a two-week placebo period. Seven Danish centres participated in the study.

To be included in the study, patients of either gender had to be aged 18–70 years and have a diagnosis of panic disorder according to DSM–III–R (American Psychiatric Association, 1987), with or without agoraphobia, and have to have had at least three full panic attacks during the four weeks before entry in the study. A baseline score of 14 or less on the Hamilton Depression Scale (Hamilton, 1969), 17-item version, was also required.

Among the exclusion criteria were primary diagnosis of major depression (DSM–III–R) or generalised anxiety disorder (DSM–III–R), schizophrenia or dementia, organic brain disease, alcohol or drug abuse, concomitant treatment with psychotropics, monoamine oxidase inhibitors, anticoagulants or benzodiazepines. In the case of benzodiazepines, patients were excluded if they were still receiving these drugs at entry to the three-week placebo period, or if there was an emergence of benzodiazepine-withdrawal symptoms in the placebo period.

All patients received placebo tablets in the first three weeks (placebo period), followed by random allocation to either paroxetine or placebo treatment. Regardless of the magnitude of improvement seen in the placebo period, patients could enter the active treatment period as long as they satisfied the inclusion criteria. In the first two weeks of study treatment, paroxetine doses were gradually increased from 10 to 20 mg/day ('low dose'). From Week 3 onward, the dosage was flexible, either 20 mg/day ('low dose') or 40 mg/day ('medium dose'), and from Week 4 onward dosage could be further increased to 60 mg daily ('high dose') according to efficacy and tolerability. In both treatment groups, all daily doses consisted of two visually identical tablets. Patient compliance was assessed at each visit by tablet counts. Urinalysis was done to determine whether patients had been taking concomitant benzodiazepines. In addition to pharmacological treatment, all patients received standardised psychotherapy according to the principles developed by Hawton et al (1989).

Patients were assessed at weekly intervals during the placebo period; at the end of Weeks 1, 2, 3, 4, 6, 9, and 12, and at the end of the two-week placebo period. Throughout the study period, regular joint rating sessions with the participating psychiatrists were arranged to minimise interrater variability on the observer rating scales. Assessment of response was based on consecutive three-week intervals.

The principal measure of outcome was the reduction in the number of panic attacks, as recorded by the patient in a daily diary. A reduction equal to or more than 50% from baseline was considered to be beneficial. In addition, the percentage of patients who had their panic attacks reduced to zero, or one, in a three-week interval was determined, and the mean change in the number of panic attacks from baseline in each group was evaluated from the diary assessments. The daily diary card was used to document the severity of each panic attack, the duration of each attack, whether or not there were any precipitating factors, and the severity of agoraphobia, if present, for each attack.

Secondary measures of outcome included:

(a) A reduction in score equal to or greater than 50% on the Hamilton Anxiety Scale (HAM–A) (Hamilton, 1969).

(b) A response on the Clinical Global Impression (CGI) scale (Guy, 1976) where a response was defined as a score of two (borderline illness) or less at the assessments for patients whose baseline score was three (mildly ill) or more.

(c) The mean reduction on the Zung Self-Rating Scale for Anxiety (Zung, 1971).

The sample size was based upon the assumption that response rates in the paroxetine and the placebo groups would be 70% and 40%, respectively ($\alpha=0.05$, $1-\beta=0.80$). To allow for a 30% attrition rate, we considered it necessary to recruit 120 patients in total. Data analysis of the efficacy variables was based on the Cochran–Mantel–Haenszel χ^2 test, adjusting for centre, categorical data, the Breslow–Day test for homogeneity over centres, and analysis of variance with the factors treatment, centre, and treatment/centre interaction for continuous variables. In all cases, a two-tailed significance level of 5% was used to determine presence of statistical significance.

RESULTS

In the analysis of this study, two populations were considered – the intention-to-treat and the per protocol. Within these populations, the analyses used the observed cases data set, consisting of each patient's observations at each interval and the endpoint, which was generated from the observed cases data set by taking the last valid result between Weeks 3 and 12. Results are presented for the intention to treat population (consisting of each patient's observations at each interval) only, as the other analyses yielded similar results.

Demographic data and patient history

A total of 129 patients were enrolled, nine patients dropped out during the placebo period, and the remaining 120 patients were equally allocated to receive either paroxetine or placebo. Thus, 60 patients in each group comprised the intention-to-treat

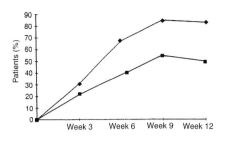

Fig. I Panic attack response rates. Percentage of patients with at least 50% reduction from baseline number of panic attacks per three-week period. Statistically significant differences in favour of paroxetine were seen at 6, 9, and 12 weeks (*P*=0.006, *P*=0.001, and *P*=0.001, respectively). ◆—◆: paroxetine; ■—■: placebo.

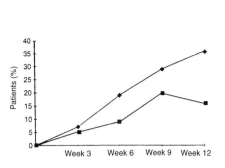

Fig. 2 Panic attack response rates – percentage of patients with number of panic attacks reduced to one or zero per three-week period. Statistically significant difference in favour of paroxetine was seen at 12 weeks (*P*=0.024). ◆—◆: paroxetine; ■—■: placebo.

Fig. 3 Panic attack response rates – mean changes from baseline total number of panic attacks per three-week period. Differences were not statistically significant at any time point (*P* > 0.05). ◆—◆: paroxetine; ■—■: placebo.

analysis. The two treatment groups were comparable with respect to demographic variables. Eighty per cent of the paroxetine group and 72% of the placebo group were female, the mean ages being 37.7 years and 37.0 years for paroxetine and placebo, respectively; the age range was 21–69 years for the population. Familial disposition to panic disorder was seen in 33% of the paroxetine group and 25% of the placebo group. Almost all of the patients had panic attacks which were rated as moderate or severe at baseline. Only seven patients in the paroxetine group and nine patients in the placebo group did not report any agoraphobic avoidance at baseline. Of those that did report agoraphobic avoidance, 66% and 63% reported the severity as moderate or severe in the paroxetine and placebo groups respectively.

Patient withdrawals

Of the 120 patients entering the 12-week treatment period, 55 (92%) paroxetine patients and 52 (87%) placebo patients completed the 12-week treatment period. Five patients on paroxetine were withdrawn, as compared with eight on placebo: one paroxetine patient was withdrawn for lack of efficacy plus adverse events, three were withdrawn because of adverse events, and one was withdrawn for lack of compliance. The adverse events leading to withdrawal in this group were abdominal pain, confusion, decreased appetite, depression, dizziness, headache, incoordination, decreased libido, nausea, and unintended pregnancy. Three placebo patients were withdrawn for lack of efficacy/relapse, one for lack of compliance, three for protocol violations, and one for uncertain diagnosis.

Efficacy

The primary efficacy evaluations were based on measures of changes in the frequency of panic attacks occurring in three-week intervals (see Figs 1–3). The number of patients with at least 50% reduction from baseline in number of panic attacks (Fig. 1) was significantly greater in the paroxetine group at six weeks, at nine weeks (*P*=0.006 and *P*=0.001, respectively), and at 12 weeks (*P*=0.001) when 82% (*n*=42) of the paroxetine patients as compared with 50% (*n*=25) of the placebo patients, had responded.

Evaluation of the reduction in number of panic attacks to one or zero (Fig. 2) showed similar differences in favour of paroxetine, although statistical significance was not seen until week 12 when 36% (*n*=19) of paroxetine patients, as compared with 16% (*n*=8) of the placebo patients, had responded (*P*=0.024).

As this study employed flexible dosing, it is not possible to determine a minimally effective dose. However, in the paroxetine group, most patients (75%) were treated with a 40 or 60 mg dose and 47% of patients received the 60 mg dose at some point in the study.

Adverse events

The number of patients reporting at least one adverse event was 46 (77%) in the paroxetine group and 33 (55%) in the placebo group: this difference between groups was statistically significant (*P*=0.012). In this study, all patients who completed 12 weeks of active treatment then received two weeks

of placebo, thus enabling adverse events occurring after discontinuation of paroxetine or placebo to be compared. In this placebo period only 19 patients out of 55 (34.5%) who had received paroxetine reported any adverse event on discontinuation, as compared with seven out of 52 (13.5%) patients who had received placebo.

Overall, paroxetine was well tolerated and most patients were able to discontinue abruptly without ill effect, even from the higher doses (40 and 60 mg).

DISCUSSION

Significant improvement was seen in panic disorder (DSM–III–R) patients treated with paroxetine, as compared with placebo, for both the primary and secondary outcome measures. In the paroxetine group, clear improvement for the primary outcome measures was seen at three weeks, and statistical significance, as compared with placebo, was seen from Week 6 onward. With regard to the primary outcome measures, the response in the paroxetine group increased and was maintained over the 12-week treatment period, while in the placebo group, deterioration, after initial improvement up until nine weeks, was seen during the last three-week period. Of particular clinical significance is the fact that from a baseline mean of 21.2 panic attacks in the paroxetine group, at week 12, 36% of these patients had become almost free of panic attacks in that their panic-attack frequency had been reduced to zero or one over the last three weeks of the study.

Placebo response rates can be quite high for panic disorder patients – up to 40%

Table I Secondary efficacy measures, Hamilton Anxiety Scale (HAM–A), Clinical Global Impression (CGI), and Zung Patient Self-Rating Scale for Anxiety (ZUNG): summary of statistically significant differences between treatment groups

HAM–A	Mean baseline score	Percentage of patients with at least 50% reduction from baseline score	
		Week 6	Week 12
Paroxetine	24.3	59%	85%
Placebo	23.5	38%	51%
P value	–	0.021	< 0.001

CGI		Percentage of patients with severity of illness $\leqslant 2$ (mildly ill)	
	Baseline	Week 6	Week 12
Paroxetine	0%	42%	71%
Placebo	0%	38%	40%
P value	–	0.023	0.003

ZUNG	Mean baseline score	Mean change from baseline score	
		Week 6	Week 12
Paroxetine	42.1	−6.0	−6.5
Placebo	41.6	−3.4	−4.3
P Value	–	0.013	0.042

P values for mean changes from baseline in ZUNG rating scale were obtained with F-tests in analysis of variance adjusting for centre. All other P values were obtained with Cochran–Mantel–Haenszel χ^2 tests.

being reported in some studies (Maier *et al*, 1991; Rosenberg *et al*, 1991). The placebo response seen in this study was higher, but that was to be expected since both treatment groups received standardised cognitive therapy.

Generally, unspecific treatment factors are probably responsible for high response rates on placebo; for example, patients receive more attention and explanation. These factors are also an inherent part of behaviour/cognitive therapies.

Panic disorder appears to be a chronic condition in most patients. Although a minority of patients have a short episode, the rest have either recurrent episodes of varying severity or chronic, persistent symptoms (Uhde *et al*, 1985). Thus long-term treatment appears to be indicated for many patients, and therefore a safe and well tolerated treatment regimen is essential. Such long-term studies are under way with paroxetine.

This study is the first comparison of an SSRI with placebo in which both groups received standardised cognitive therapy. A clear advantage for combination therapy, such as paroxetine plus cognitive therapy, in the treatment of panic disorder, was demonstrated.

REFERENCES

American Psychiatric Association (1987) *Diagnostic and Statistical Manual of Mental Disorders* (3rd edn, revised) (DSM–III–R). Washington, DC: APA.

Feighner, J. P. & Boyer, W. F. (1989) Paroxetine in the treatment of depression: a comparison with imipramine and placebo. *Acta Psychiatrica Scandinavica*, **80** (suppl.), 125–129.

Guy, W. (1976) *ECDEU Assessment Manual for Psychopharmacology*. US Department of Health, Education, and Welfare, Public Health Service, Alcohol, Drug Abuse, and Mental Health Administration.

Hamilton, M. (1969) Diagnosis and rating of anxiety. *British Journal of Psychiatry*, **3**, 76–79.

Hawton, K., Salkowski, P., Kirk, J., et al (1989) *Cognitive Behaviour Therapy for Psychiatric Problems*. Oxford: Oxford University Press.

Maier, W., Roth, M., Argyle, N., et al (1991) Avoidance behaviour: a predictor of the efficacy of pharmacotherapy in panic disorder. *European Archives of Psychiatry and Clinical Neuroscience*, **241**, 151–158.

Rosenberg, N. K., Andersch, S., Kullingslio, H., et al (1991) Efficacy and safety of alprazolam, imipramine and placebo in treating panic disorder. *Acta Psychiatrica Scandinavica*, (suppl. 365), 18–27.

Uhde, T. W., Boulenger, J. P., Roy Byrne, P. P., et al (1985) Longitudinal course of panic disorder: clinical and biological considerations. *Progress in Neuropsychopharmacology and Biological Psychiatry*, **9**, 39–51.

Zung, W. W. K. (1971) A rating instrument for anxiety disorders. *Psychosomatics*, **12**, 371–379.

OEHRBERG *ET AL*

Please write your answers to questions I to III in the spaces provided.

I. Background

A. Why were there placebo periods at the beginning and end of the 12-week treatment period? [5 marks]

....
....
....
....

B. What hypotheses were being tested in this study? [10 marks]

....
....
....
....
....
....
....
....
....

C. What is meant by "a two-tailed significance level of 5%"? [5 marks]

....
....
....
....

D.(i) By what criteria do you assess the validity of a therapeutic trial? [15 marks]

....
....
....
....
....
....
....
....
....
....
....
....

(ii)   How well were these criteria met in this study?   [5 marks]

....
....
....
....

E.   What further information about psychotherapy treatment would be helpful for interpreting the results?   [5 marks]

....
....
....
....

II.   Results

A.   In the results section, why was it important to carry out an intention-to-treat and per protocol analysis?   [10 marks]

....
....
....
....
....
....
....
....

B.   What are the main advantages and disadvantages of employing a flexible dosing regime?   [10 marks]

....
....
....
....
....

C.   Why is it important to report on adverse events in a trial like this?   [5 marks]

....
....
....
....
....
....
....

III. Summary

A.   List and discuss the main clinical implications of this study.   [15 marks]

....
....
....
....
....
....
....
....
....
....
....
....

B.   List and discuss the main limitations of this study.   [15 marks]

....
....
....
....
....
....
....
....
....
....

I.   Background

A.   Why were there placebo periods at the beginning and end of the 12-week treatment period?

The placebo run-in should help to reduce the size of the placebo response during the randomised phase: placebo response rates in panic disorder of 60% or more have been reported.

The placebo run-in was also intended to help to exclude the patients with benzodiazepine dependency which itself exacerbates panic disorder.

The two-week placebo phase at the end of the study could explore the durability of the benefits, the possibility of rebound exacerbation on discontinuation and the phenomena of paroxetine withdrawal.

B.   What hypotheses were being tested in this study?

(a)   Does paroxetine differ from placebo in its effect upon the frequency of panic attacks in patients with panic disorder who are also receiving cognitive therapy? Does it differ in its effect on anxiety or on the global clinical impression of severity of the illness?

(b)   Is there any evidence for panic disorder worsening in the early stages of treatment with paroxetine?

(c)   Are there problems with the discontinuation of paroxetine at the end of the study?

(d)   Do adverse events occur more commonly with paroxetine or placebo in this context?

C.   What is meant by "a two-tailed significance level of 5%"?

This tests whether a difference in favour of either treatment would be significant rather than a difference in favour only of paroxetine. For instance, it allows for the possibility that paroxetine may exacerbate the condition in the early stage of treatment while improving it later. Five per cent means there is less than a one in 20 probability of the finding occurring by chance.

D.   (i) By what criteria do you assess the validity of a therapeutic trial?

The authors used standard diagnostic criteria and described the exclusion criteria.

They recruited patients from a wide range of ages, both genders (more female than male), some of whom had underlying physical illness requiring concomitant medication, but not psychotropic drugs.

Patients were randomly assigned to receive either paroxetine or placebo. The randomised part of the study was conducted double-blind, so that neither the patient nor the rater were aware of which treatment the patient was receiving.

The authors treated both groups the same, by requiring that all patients received cognitive therapy with a standardised technique. They performed a power calculation to determine how many patients would be needed to test the main hypothesis.

Successful randomisation was confirmed in that the two treatment groups were comparable with respect to demographic variables at the outset.

(ii)   How well were these criteria met in this study?

The authors do not describe the method of randomisation but the procedure is standard in psychopharmacological studies and is likely to have been clearly defined and scrutinised by the company sponsoring this study.

The authors do not state the sources of information about response rate upon which the power calculation is based.

Blindness was achieved by making the active and placebo tablets look identical. There was the possibility of side-effects revealing the nature of the treatment to patients (especially if they had previously received an SSRI) and to the rater. This is a potential weakness in the study, in common with many placebo-controlled studies of drugs with characteristic side-effects.

E. What further information about the psychotherapy treatment would be helpful for interpreting the results?

No information is given about training the individual doctors had in the use of cognitive therapy, and it is possible that the cognitive therapy which they received was sub-optimal.

II. Results

A. In the results section, why was it important to carry out an intention-to-treat and per protocol analysis?

It is important that all patients should be accounted for. Information was provided about all patients, including those who dropped out of the study. 'Intention-to-treat' analysis is generally considered preferable, on the basis that if patients discontinue treatment because of adverse effects of the drug, their last score before dropping-out is carried forward and tends, therefore, to lower the average response rate as they will not have been on the treatment sufficiently long for full benefits to develop. This method of analysis would be weakened (in favour of the drug) if there were many more drop-outs on placebo (for instance due to lack of efficacy). In this study there were slightly more drop-outs on paroxetine than on placebo; the 'intention-to-treat' analysis is therefore the more rigorous one, and that is what the authors present. The per protocol analysis gives results for the patients who do complete the treatment at each time point and so provides the most optimistic view of the drug's effects.

B. What are the main advantages and disadvantages of employing a flexible dosing regime?

Flexible dosing allowed the medication to be increased gradually according to the needs of each patient individually, in a way that could minimise side-effects including the exacerbation of anxiety at the start of treatment. However, the dose may have been sub-optimal for some patients. A study with a range of fixed doses would be needed to determine any dose–response relationship.

C. Why is it important to report on adverse events in a trial like this?

The description of adverse events in a placebo-controlled trial gives a measure of the excess frequency due to drug treatment, which can be tested for significance statistically. The excess adverse event rate on treatment was 22%. The severity of adverse events can also be gauged by the number of early drop-outs, which would limit the usefulness of the drug in routine practice.

III. Summary

A. List and discuss the main clinical implications of this study.

(a) Paroxetine may be useful to reduce the severity of panic attacks in patients with panic disorder including those receiving cognitive therapy.

(b) Paroxetine may bring about a global improvement in panic disorder in patients also receiving cognitive therapy.

(c) When the dose of paroxetine is increased slowly towards 60 mg daily, there is no evidence of worsening of the condition at the start of treatment.

(d) The improvement in panic disorder with paroxetine develops over a period of 12 weeks, with significant improvement on most measures by six weeks.

(e) Up to 92% of patients with panic disorder may be able to tolerate 12 weeks of treatment with paroxetine in this dose schedule.

(f) By 12 weeks the number needed to treat (NNT) for a 50% reduction in frequency of panic attacks was 3.1 (82 v. 50%; Fig. 1): for reduction to one or zero panic attacks in the previous three weeks, the NNT was 5.0 (36 v. 16%; Fig. 2). For reduction of 50% in the HAM–A score the NNT was 2.9 (85 v. 51%); and for reduction of the CGI score to two or less the NNT was 3.2.

(g) Twenty-two per cent of patients on paroxetine in this dose schedule will experience at least one adverse event more than they would have done on placebo.

(h) Withdrawal symptoms occurred with a 21% difference between groups corresponding to a NNT of 4.8. The main symptom was dizziness.

(i) On the most rigorous measure of improvement (having one or no panic attacks in the previous three weeks) the NNT is 5.0 (only 36% of patients on paroxetine achieved this and 16% on placebo).

B. List and discuss the main limitations of this study.

(a) The study was of only 12 weeks' duration and the study does not show how long treatment should continue.

(b) No information is provided about confidence intervals.

(c) Side-effects were reported numerically but no statistical tests were reported.

(d) Details of the sponsorship are not explicit. Unsurprisingly, as there may be a conflict of interest, the paper is reticent in its analysis of adverse events and withdrawal effects.

(e) Although the patients in this study were from a demographically broad range there is no information about ethnic groups. Patients with comorbid conditions such as major depression were excluded although panic disorder often has comorbidity. This limits the generalisability of the findings. Likewise, patients with benzodiazepine dependence were excluded.

(f) Sometimes authors present information about the proportion of patients who are able correctly to guess whether they are on an active drug or placebo by the end of the study.

(g) Other approaches to treatment are not discussed, and there is no active comparator drug.

A CRITICAL REVIEW PAPER

Systematic review
Model answers by John Geddes

Discontinuation rates of SSRIs and tricyclic antidepressants: a meta-analysis and investigation of heterogeneity

MATTHEW HOTOPF, REBECCA HARDY and GLYN LEWIS

The serotonin-specific reuptake inhibitors (SSRIs) and tricyclic or heterocyclic antidepressants have been compared in 105 randomised controlled trials (RCTs), but there is little consensus as to which class of drug should be given as first-line treatment in depression (Paykel, 1989; Effective Health Care, 1993; Drugs and Therapeutic Bulletin, 1993).

Much of the present controversy has focused on the acceptability of SSRIs, assessed by discontinuation rates in RCTs. Meta-analyses suggest that those treated with SSRIs in RCTs have lower discontinuation rates than those treated with tricyclic antidepressants. However, tricyclics differ in their side-effect profiles and most RCTs have compared SSRIs with 'reference' antidepressants (i.e. imipramine and amitriptyline) which are said to have the worst side-effects (Henry & Martin, 1987). Some of the newer antidepressants are among the most commonly prescribed in the UK but cost little more than imipramine and amitriptyline. The present meta-analysis investigated whether the advantage in discontinuation rates of SSRIs was present when compared with newer tricyclics or heterocyclics.

METHOD

Literature search

All RCTs reported in the previous meta-analyses, where the SSRIs were fluoxetine, sertraline, paroxetine or fluvoxamine, were used. These studies are all relatively short-term comparisons of SSRIs with tricyclic or heterocyclic antidepressants in treatment of depression. Studies of these compounds for other indications have not been included. A MEDLINE search was performed checking all papers that used the drug name in the title, abstract or keywords. In addition, owing to the failure of electronic searches to detect all relevant references (Adams et al, 1994), two journals which contained a high proportion of the trials, International Clinical

Psychopharmacology and Acta Psychiatrica Scandinavica, were searched manually. If studies did not produce full details of overall discontinuation rates, the first author was contacted and asked for details. The same duplicated studies were excluded as in Anderson & Tomenson (1995). This systematic review is part of an ongoing Cochrane Collaboration review.

Studies were classified according to three criteria:

(a) the SSRI used;

(b) the type of tricyclic or heterocyclic used: reference compounds (imipramine and amitriptyline), newer tricyclics (dothiepin, nortriptyline, desipramine, clomipramine and doxepin) and heterocyclic antidepressants (bupropion, mianserin, trazodone, maprotiline, amineptine and nomifensine);

(c) whether or not the treated group was defined as elderly in the RCT (cut-off points varied from 60 to 70 years of age).

Data analysis

The odds ratio and relative risk were calculated for each study, together with the relevant standard errors. A fixed-effect meta-analysis method (Woolf, 1955) was used to obtain the estimate of overall effect in terms of the odds ratio (empirical logits were used since some studies had small or zero drop-outs). Heterogeneity of treatment effects between studies was formally tested using the Q statistic (Der Simonian & Laird, 1986). However, since the test is known to have low power (Berlin et al, 1989), possible sources of heterogeneity were considered and investigated with the aid of a Galbraith plot (Galbraith, 1988). A random-effects estimate, which takes account of any additional between-study variation, was calculated using a moment estimator of the between-study variance (Der Simonian & Laird, 1986) as a sensitivity check on the

fixed-effect estimate. Since the data are sparse, and some RCTs report no drop-outs in at least one group, the methods described above may be unreliable as they are based on asymptotic assumptions. Hence, the analyses were checked using an approach based on the exact distribution of the 2×2 contingency tables, as described by van Houwelingen et al (1993), providing both fixed-effect and random-effects estimates of the overall odds ratio, as well as a likelihood ratio test of the null hypothesis of homogeneity of effects across studies. There was little difference between the results obtained from the two approaches, hence, the results from the simple weighted average method using empirical logits are presented here, although where results do differ a comment is made.

An overall estimate of the relative risk was also calculated, in order to compare results with previous papers and to express the difference as a percentage reduction in risk. A Mantel–Haenszel-type estimator proposed by Nurminen (1981) and Kleinbaum et al (1982), which is suitable for sparse data, was used, together with the relevant confidence interval (CI; Greenland & Robins, 1985).

Finally, a separate meta-analysis, both in terms of odds ratio and relative risk, was carried out for each of the pre-defined tricyclic/heterocyclic groups compared with SSRIs.

RESULTS

A funnel plot (Fig. 1) (Wilson & Henry, 1992) showed no evidence of publication bias being a problem in the data collected. Table 1 summarises the odds ratios and 95% CIs for each study. Most estimates are close to one, with CIs including one. Three studies were omitted from the analysis as they had no drop-outs in either group and thus provide no information about a difference in effect.

The estimate of the overall odds ratio for drop-outs in the SSRI group compared with drop-outs in the tricyclic/heterocyclic group indicates significantly fewer drop-outs on SSRIs (odds ratio 0.86, 95% CI 0.78–0.94). The test statistic for heterogeneity indicated evidence of homogeneity ($Q=113.62$, d.f.$=91$, $P=0.05$) and the likelihood ratio test for heterogeneity gave a more significant value of $P=0.033$. Furthermore, the estimate of the between-study

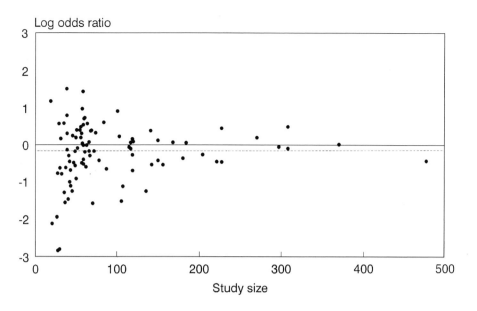

Fig. I Funnel plot of estimated logarithmic odds ratio against the size of the study. Broken horizontal line represents the overall estimate of the logarithmic odds ratio (-0.15).

Table 2 Fixed-effect meta-analysis results using odds and risk ratios as outcome measurements

Meta-analysis (number of studies)	Odds ratio (95% CI)	Risk ratio (95% CI)	Test statistic for heterogeneity (P)
Overall (92)	0.86 (0.78–0.94)	0.91 (0.86–0.96)	113.62 (0.05)
Old tricyclics (51)	0.82 (0.72–0.92)	0.88 (0.82–0.94)	70.50 (0.03)
Newer tricyclics (24)	0.89 (0.74–1.06)	0.92 (0.81–1.03)	27.48 (0.24)
Heterocyclics (17)	1.02 (0.78–1.35)	1.02 (0.83–1.25)	13.35 (0.65)

variance was greater than zero. Possible sources of heterogeneity were therefore investigated.

A Galbraith plot (Fig. 2) is a plot of the standardised effect (z statistic) of each study against the reciprocal of the standard error. The standardised effect is the logarithmic odds ratio for the study, divided by its standard error. The gradient of the plot is therefore equivalent to the treatment effect, and in this study the overall fixed-effect estimate of the logarithmic odds ratio may be represented by a line with gradient equal to -0.15 [$=\ln(0.86)$]. A negative z statistic indicates fewer drop-outs in the SSRI group, whereas a positive statistic indicates fewer drop-outs in the comparison tricyclic/heterocyclic group. Parallel lines at $+2$ and -2 standard deviations either side of this line may be used as an aid to interpreting the heterogeneity within these data, since the further a study's estimate is away from this line the greater the contribution it makes to the test statistic for heterogeneity.

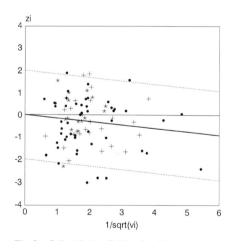

Fig. 2 Galbraith plot. Solid inclined line represents the fixed-effect estimate, bounded by plus and minus two units (broken inclined lines). ●, old tricyclics; +, newer tricylcics; *, non-tricyclic antidepressants.

It is noticeable that four out of the five points with a z statistic of < -2 units from the overall estimate are comparisons of SSRIs with older tricyclics, and the largest trial that is also highly negative on the plot is a comparison with an old tricyclic. On

the other hand, two of the four with a z statistic of $> +2$ units from the overall estimate are comparisons with new tricyclics. This may suggest that the reference tricyclics perform less well compared with SSRIs than the newer ones, although the pattern within the limits is less clear.

Separate overall odds ratios were calculated for the three groups of trials with different types of comparison antidepressants (reference tricyclics, newer tricyclics and non-tricyclics). Table 2 shows that there is a significant difference in drop-out rates between SSRIs and reference tricyclics. However, there is also evidence of heterogeneity within this group of study estimates ($Q=60.50$, d.f.$=50$, $P=0.05$). The CIs of the random-effects estimates still did not include one (overall odds ratio 0.86, 95% CI 0.76–0.96). Conversely, the overall estimate of difference in drop-out rates for both the newer tricyclics and the heterocyclics do not suggest any significant differences. There is far less heterogeneity within these two subgroups ($P=0.24$ and 0.65 for the newer tricyclics and the heterocyclics, respectively). The relative risk estimates show a similar pattern (Table 2).

There were only 11 RCTs on elderly populations and the results of these did not appear to differ from the results of trials on younger populations. There appears to be some variation in the results for different SSRIs, with fluvoxamine producing a more homogeneous set of results than either fluoxetine or paroxetine. Furthermore, the overall estimate for fluvoxamine is closer to one than those for either fluoxetine or paroxetine. There are only six studies using sertraline, so any conclusions regarding this drug are tentative. Hence, the type of SSRI used does not explain much of the heterogeneity present in these data, but it appears that the drugs that produce the greatest overall effect are also those with the greatest variation in individual effect estimates across studies. Furthermore, within each comparison group (older tricyclics, newer tricyclics and heterocyclics) each SSRI (excluding sertraline) is represented reasonably consistently. Hence, it is not the case that each comparison group is compared with one particular SSRI.

DISCUSSION

The estimate of effect for the heterocyclics compared with SSRIs is very close to one, with no evidence of heterogeneity between the estimates from the different trials. The CI is wider than for the other comparisons because of the smaller number of trials (17) included, and suggests that the increase in risk of using SSRIs versus heterocyclics could be as much as 25%, or the decrease in risk could be 17%. Further information, preferably in terms of a large clinical trial, is required before a definite conclusion can be made. The inclusion of these compounds in Song *et al*'s (1993) meta-analysis may have led to their negative result.

REFERENCES

Adams, C. E., Power, A., Frederick, K., et al (1994) An investigation of the adequacy of MEDLINE searches for randomized controlled trials (RCTs) of the effects of mental health care. *Psychological Medicine*, **24**, 741–748.

Anderson, I. M. & Tomenson, B. M. (1995) Treatment discontinuation with selective serotonin reputake inhibitors compared with tricyclic antidepressants: a meta-analysis. *British Medical Journal*, **310**, 1433–1438.

Berlin, J. A., Laird, N. M., Sacks, H. S., et al (1989) A comparison of statistical methods for combining event rates from clinical trials. *Statistics in Medicine*, **8**, 141–151.

Der Simonian, R. & Laird, N. (1986) Meta-analysis in clinical trials. *Controlled Clinical Trials*, **7**, 177–188.

Drugs and Therapeutic Bulletin (1993) Selective serotonin reuptake inhibitors for depression. *Drugs and Therapeutic Bulletin*, **31**, 57–58.

Effective Health Care (1993) The treatment of depression in primary care. *Effective Health Care Bulletin*, **5**, 1–12.

Galbraith, R. F. (1988) A note on graphical presentation of estimated odds ratios from several clinical trials. *Statistics in Medicine*, **7**, 889–894.

Greenland, S. & Robins, J. M. (1985) Estimation of a common effect parameter from sparse follow-up data. *Biometrics*, **41**, 55–68.

Henry, J. A. & Martin, A. J. (1987) The risk–benefit assessment of antidepressant drugs. *Medical Toxicology*, **2**, 445–462.

Kleinbaum, D. G., Kupper, L. L. & Morgenstern, H. (1982) *Epidemiologic Research: Principles and Quantitative Methods.* Belmont, CA: Lifetime Learning Publications.

Nurminen, M. (1981) Asymptotic efficiency of general noniterative estimators of common relative risk. *Biometrika*, **68**, 525–530.

Paykel, E. (1989) The background: extent and nature of the disorder. In *Depression: An Integrative Approach* (eds. K. Herbst & E. Paykel), pp. 3–17. Oxford: Heinemann.

Song, F., Freemantle, N., Sheldon, T. A., et al (1993) Selective serotonin reuptake inhibitors: meta-analysis of efficacy and acceptability. *British Medical Journal*, **306**, 683–687.

van Houwelingen, H. C., Zwinderman, K. H. & Stijnen, T. (1993) A bivariate approach to meta-analysis. *Statistics in Medicine*, **12**, 2273–2284.

Wilson, A. & Henry, D. A. (1992) Meta-analysis. Part 2. Assessing the quality of published meta-analyses. *Medical Journal of Australia*, **156**, 173–187.

Woolf, B. (1955) On estimating the relation between blood group and disease. *Annals of Human Genetics*, **19**, 251–253.

HOTOPF *ET AL*

Please write your answers to questions I to IV in the spaces provided.

I.   Background

A.   Compare and contrast the pharmacological modes of action of SSRIs and tricyclic antidepressants.   [4 marks]

....
....
....
....

B.   What are the main arguments in favour of the use of SSRIs as first-time treatment for people with depression?   [4 marks]

....
....
....
....

C.   Identify the main selection bias in this study.   [4 marks]

....
....
....
....

D.   What do you understand by the term discontinuation rate? Why might SSRIs have an advantage over 'reference' antidepressants in this respect?   [4 marks]

....
....
....
....
....
....

E.   List the features of a randomised controlled clinical trial.   [6 marks]

....
....
....
....
....

II.   Method

A.   How can a meta-analysis be distinguished from a systematic review?   [4 marks]

....
....
....
....

B.   What steps have these authors taken to improve the validity of their
      meta-analysis?   [4 marks]

....
....
....
....

C.   Indicate ways in which the authors could have improved their meta-analysis.   [4 marks]

....
....
....
....

D.   What is the Cochrane Collaboration? Can you give two examples of Cochrane
      Collaborations?   [4 marks]

....
....
....
....

E. Define odds ratio, relative risk, standard error, z statistic and 2×2
    contingency table.   [10 marks]

....
....
....
....
....
....
....
....
....

F. What does the term heterogeneity mean in this study? What methods were applied to
    evaluate heterogeneity?   [4 marks]

....
....
....
....

G. Define the term confidence interval. Give an example derived from this study,
    demonstrating the value of using confidence intervals.   [4 marks]

....
....
....
....

III. Results

A. In your own words, state why Fig. 1 shows no evidence of publication bias being a problem
    in the data collected. What is the significance of the logarithmic transformation? [4 marks]

....
....
....
....

B. Table 1 is not shown but its content is referred to. What is the significance of the
    authors' phrase, concerning Table 1: "Most estimates are close to one, with CIs
    including one."?   [4 marks]

....
....
....
....

C. In your own words, describe the Galbraith plot. What is your evaluation of the authors' suggestion that reference tricyclics perform less well than newer ones when compared with SSRIs?   [6 marks]

....

....

....

....

....

D. What are the main findings based on the contents of Table 2? Give examples to justify your answer.   [6 marks]

....

....

....

....

....

IV. Summary of study

A. What do you consider are the three main findings of this study?   [6 marks]

....

....

....

....

....

B. What do you consider to be the three main clinical implications arising from this work?   [6 marks]

....

....

....

....

....

C. List the methodological issues arising from antidepressant trials that might have led the authors to reach erroneous conclusions.   [6 marks]

....

....

....

....

....

D. Does this study provide statistical evidence of a benefit for SSRIs over tricyclic or heterocyclic antidepressants? Justify your answer from the results.   [6 marks]

....

....

....

....

....

I.   Background

A.   Compare and contrast the pharmacological modes of action of SSRIs and tricyclic antidepressants.

Tricyclic antidepressants block presynaptic reuptake of noradrenaline and serotonin (5-HT) and therefore increase the availability of these neurotransmitters. Tricyclics also have anticholinergic effects. SSRIs specifically inhibit the presynaptic 5-HT transporter.

B.   What are the main arguments in favour of the use of SSRIs as first-time treatment for people with depression?

The main arguments in favour of SSRIs are that they are less toxic in overdose, have fewer side-effects (and are therefore more acceptable) and that the therapeutic dose is more easily achieved.

C.   Identify the main selection bias in this study.

The main selection bias is in the selection of studies for inclusion in the systematic review. Only MEDLINE was searched – this database has a bias towards English language, especially North American, literature. The authors should have considered using EMBASE, a European database which has good coverage of pharmacological studies. The Cochrane Controlled Trials Register is possibly the best source of randomised controlled trials. The authors manually searched only two journals and made no attempt to identify unpublished studies.

D.   What do you understand by the term discontinuation rate? Why might SSRIs have an advantage over 'reference' antidepressants in this respect?

The discontinuation rate is the total number of participants dropping out (for whatever reason) from a clinical trial prior to the planned end point. It is assumed to give a reasonable overall estimate of the acceptability of the treatment. If SSRIs have fewer side-effects, it might be anticipated that they would be more acceptable to patients who would then be more likely to remain in the trial.

E.   List the features of a randomised controlled clinical trial.

A defined group of participants with a defined problem are randomly allocated to one of two or more comparative treatment conditions. The outcomes after a defined period are then compared between the groups. The randomisation should be concealed. The internal validity of a trial is increased if both patient and clinician are blind as to the treatment condition.

II.   Method

A.   How can a meta-analysis be distinguished from a systematic review?

A systematic review is a literature review which has been done according to an explicit protocol in order to avoid bias. A meta-analysis is a statistical summary of the results of several studies. A systematic review may include a meta-analysis if statistical summary is possible. Meta-analyses done without systematic review are potentially very misleading.

B.   What steps have these authors taken to improve the validity of their meta-analysis?

The authors correctly included only randomised controlled trials. They tested for heterogeneity between the individual studies and used both fixed and random effects models as appropriate. They used several methods of calculating the pooled odds ratio to investigate whether the results were method-dependent.

C. Indicate ways in which the authors could have improved their meta-analysis.

(a) They could have attempted to estimate comparative efficacy of the drugs.
(b) They could have examined the effect of tricyclic dose.
(c) They could have examined the effect of severity of depression.
(d) They could have done further sensitivity analyses.
(e) As they were interested in the possibility of a difference between older tricyclics and new tricyclics, they could have formally tested this.

D. What is the Cochrane Collaboration? Can you give two examples of Cochrane Collaborations?

The Cochrane Collaboration is a rapidly expanding international organisation undertaking systematic reviews of the effectiveness of health care interventions. The systematic reviews are published in the Cochrane Library, a quarterly, regularly updated electronic publication which also contains the Database of Abstracts of Reviews of Efficiency, the Cochrane Controlled Trials Register and the Cochrane Review Methodology Database.

E. Define odds ratio, relative risk, standard error, z statistic and 2 × 2 contingency table.

(a) An odds ratio is the ratio of the odds of an outcome in the experimental group divided by the odds of the outcome in the other group.
(b) The relative risk is the ratio of the risk of an outcome in one experimental group divided by the risk of the outcome in the other group.
(c) The z statistic is the standardised normal deviate. It represents the deviation from the mean value in standard deviation units.
(d) A 2 × 2 contingency table is a cross-tabulation of the possible outcomes on two variables. One variable defines the rows and one the columns. Individuals are assigned to the appropriate cell of the table on the basis of their scores on two variables.

F. What does the term heterogeneity mean in this study? What methods were applied to evaluate heterogeneity?

Heterogeneity means that the observed variation in the study-specific results is greater than would be expected by chance alone. In this study, the authors used the Q statistic and the Galbraith plot.

G. Define the term confidence interval. Give an example derived from this study, demonstrating the value of using confidence intervals.

A confidence interval of an estimate expresses the uncertainty around the estimate. For example, a 95% confidence interval is the range of values within which we can be 95% confident that the true value exists. In this paper, the overall odds ratio for drop-out is 0.86 (95% confidence interval 0.78 to 0.94). This means that the most likely value is 0.86, but that we are 95% confident that the true value lies between 0.78 and 0.94.

III. Results

A. In your own words, state why Fig. I shows no evidence of publication bias being a problem in the data collected. What is the significance of the logarithmic transformation?

If publication bias was present, one might expect to see a gap in the area of small studies with no or negative effects. In this example, because most of the studies were Phase III studies undertaken by the drug industry, it is possible that they would have been reluctant to publish studies in which more patients dropped out on SSRIs than on the reference compound. In the presence of publication bias, there would be a gap in the top left hand corner of the figure. The logarithmic transformation in this instance is to make the plot symmetrical.

B. Table I is not shown but its content is referred to. What is the significance of the authors' phrase, concerning Table I: "Most estimates are close to one, with CIs including one."?

This means that there is little evidence of any difference between the two drugs – if the confidence intervals include 1, the result is not statistically significant.

C. In your own words, describe the Galbraith plot. What is your evaluation of the authors' suggestion that reference tricyclics perform less well than newer ones when compared with SSRIs?

The Galbraith plot is a way of identifying which studies contribute most to the overall heterogeneity between studies. These studies can then be examined to see whether there is any reason why their results might be different. In this case, the majority of trials which find a much higher drop-out rate for TCAs than SSRIs use older TCAs as the reference compound. The authors argue that this may mean that older TCAs perform less well than SSRIs. However, it is perhaps more likely that another factor may explain this finding because there is heterogeneity within the older TCA versus SSRI comparison ($P = 0.03$, Table 2).

D. What are the main findings based on the contents of Table 2? Give examples to justify your answer.

The main finding is that the odds of dropping out are 14% lower for SSRIs than for TCAs. There is some evidence that, compared with SSRIs, the odds of dropping out are lower on newer TCAs (e.g. dothiepin, clomipramine, odds ratio 0.89) than on older drugs (imipramine and amitriptyline, odds ratio 0.82), but the difference is small and of uncertain clinical relevance. There is heterogeneity in the older TCA groups: this may mean that there is a difference between imipramine and amitriptyline, or that these studies investigated different patients or used different doses, etc. Heterocyclic drugs (e.g. bupropion, mianserin) may have similar drop-out rates to SSRIs.

IV. Summary of study

A. What do you consider the three main findings of this study?

(a) Due to shortcomings in the primary studies, the authors were unable to compare the effectiveness of the drugs. There are significant limitations in the primary evidence – large-scale, long-term trials of alternative approaches to the treatment of depressive disorders are required.

(b) On the basis of the current best evidence, SSRIs lead to fewer drop-outs from therapy than other antidepressant drugs. The difference is relatively small and of uncertain clinical significance.

(c) The difference may be even smaller for the newer tricyclics (such as dothiepin and clomipramine) and some of the heterocyclics such as mianserin and trazodone may have similar drop-out rates to SSRIs.

B. What do you consider to be the three main clinical implications arising from this work?

Clinical interpretation would require information on comparative efficacy which is not provided by this study. However:

(a) Overall, SSRIs are associated with a lower drop-out rate from treatment than TCAs and so, on average, they are likely to be more acceptable. The difference is small and it is not clear how clinically significant it is.

(b) The difference may be even smaller for the newer tricyclics (such as dothiepin and clomipramine) and some of the heterocyclics such as mianserin and trazodone may be equally as acceptable as SSRIs.

(c) On the basis of acceptability, therefore, there is no reason to use the more expensive SSRIs as a first-line treatment for depressive disorder.

C. List the methodological issues arising from antidepressant trials that might have led the authors to reach erroneous conclusions.

(a) No information is provided on the comparative efficacy of the drugs.

(b) Discontinuation rates are a crude indicator of overall acceptability.

(c) The trials are very short.

(d) They may include unrepresentative groups of patients.

(e) The doses of drugs used in the trials are not reported – but may have been inadequate.

(f) Blinding in the trials may have been inadequate: the patients and clinicians may have known which drug they were taking and this may have led to bias.

D. Does this study provide statistical evidence of a benefit for SSRIs over tricyclic or heterocyclic antidepressants? Justify your answer from the results.

There is statistical evidence of an advantage for using SSRIs compared with other antidepressants. There is heterogeneity between the results of the studies – which makes the fixed effect pooled odds ratio of uncertain reliability. However, the confidence interval of a random effects estimate, which makes no assumption of a common underlying treatment effect, also excludes one – this means that there probably really is a difference. In a planned subgroup analysis, the authors found that SSRIs were no better than newer tricyclics or heterocyclics. The study provided no evidence of a difference in the effectiveness of the drugs.

The single case study
Anne Farmer

This critical review of the single case study does not include a worked example. None the less, the single case or small series report provides an important aspect of scientific endeavour and this chapter will discuss the strengths and weaknesses of this methodology. In addition a summary will be given of how to review a single case report critically.

Strengths of the single case method: the generation and refutation of hypotheses

The single case has an important contribution in two main areas, first in the generation of hypotheses and second in their refutation.

Generation of hypotheses

In contributing to the generation of hypotheses the single case or small series can lead to important novel conjecture which can open up or redirect a whole area of scientific thinking. In a clinical context, single cases observed and reported by both Parkinson and Alzheimer led to the identification of two previously unrecognised diseases that now bear their names. Similarly, much of our present understanding of the structure and function of the cerebral cortex has been based on the intensive study of single cases or small series of subjects with unique localised lesions caused by trauma or tumour (Weinstein *et al*, 1956; Piercy, 1964). Technological developments such as those that have recently occurred in neuroimaging have facilitated the identification of cerebral pathology previously only rarely noted, here again the single case or small series study can highlight this. For example, central pontine myelinolysis is a rare complication of chronic alcohol misuse which generally has a poor outcome and previously could only be diagnosed at post-mortem. A single case report pointed out that it is now possible to identify this lesion at an early stage via the use of magnetic resonance imaging scans, which can then facilitate more rapid treatment and improved prognosis (Joseph & Farmer, 1995).

Genetic research is also an area where the single case or family can provide important 'leads'. In particular, linkage between known chromosomal abnormalities with other diseases in a single case or family has contributed to the localisation of genes. One such successful example was the description of a patient with a minor deletion on the short arm of the X chromosome which ultimately led to the localisation of the gene for Duchenne muscular dystrophy on that chromosome (Francke *et al*, 1985).

In other settings, the astute observer may also notice an unusual event and be able to generate new hypotheses on the basis of that single observation. Again, there are a number of well-known examples, including Fleming's discovery of the antibacterial effects of penicillin, and the chance discovery of the psychotropic effects of a number of drugs, for example, chlorpromazine, iproniazid and imipramine, which were initially developed to treat other conditions (Healy, 1996). A recent example is that of the drug sildenafil, whose well-known properties in the treatment of impotence were originally noted as a result of its development to treat angina. The above examples have been termed "serendipity" (Charlton & Walston, 1998) since the discoveries apparently occurred by lucky chance. However, little in science occurs merely by chance. Noticing the unexpected often requires considerable mental preparation and for the clinician or researcher to show considerable astuteness and acumen.

Refutation of hypotheses

A single example can also be used to refute a hypothesis. Popper stated that science should advance by the method of refutation and that the correct test of the proposition 'all swans are white' is to find a black individual (Magee, 1973). Single case reports are like the black swans in Popper's example. Although it is possible to come across a black swan purely by chance, it is probable that only an alert and questioning observer will recognise the importance of a black individual. A more clinically relevant example is that of identical triplets who were non-identical with respect to psychotic disorder. McGuffin *et al* (1982) suggested that this single set of triplets provided a refutation of the Kraepelian dichotomy that proposed separate genetic bases for schizophrenia and manic–depressive disorder.

Returning to Popper's example, it is also possible to undertake a systematic search for a black swan, both among white swans or among other black birds. In this case, a careful experimental design is required in order to detect the 'single case'. Systematic searching methods have been termed the 'formal case study' approach (Charlton & Walston, 1998). In this method, large numbers of subjects need to be screened in order to find 'pure' individual cases where there are no other confounding variables. Charlton & Walston (1998) provided such an example. They wished to test the hypothesis proposed by Frith & Corcoran (1996) that subjects with persecutory delusions had impairment of their 'theory of mind'. Charlton & Walston screened a number of subjects with psychotic symptoms to find a few who had 'pure' persecutory delusions and no other mental state abnormalities. They then examined four such individuals using tests of 'theory of mind' and demonstrated that none had any impairment on these tests. They therefore concluded that their four cases represented four single refutations of the Frith & Corcoran hypothesis (Charlton & Walston, 1998; Walston, 1997).

Clearly the methodology of such a study requires as much care, time and thought as studies that have been undertaken on larger numbers. Despite this, single case methods have a number of methodological weaknesses.

Weaknesses

The single case report has been much denigrated as a valid and legitimate scientific approach. It is certainly the case that far fewer such reports are now published in mainstream journals such as the *British Journal of Psychiatry* (Farmer, 1999). The main criticisms are that such reports are anecdotal and the individual unusual case may also misrepresent more typical presentations of a disorder. Because of their unique nature, they are also often unrepeatable. At a procedural level they have also been criticised for their susceptibility to misdiagnosis, measurement error, observer bias and subjective interpretation. They may have been devised with an inadequate protocol, and statistical analysis is not possible. Thus, case study methods are often regarded as 'soft' and somewhat unscientific. Indeed, in terms of evidence-based medicine the single case report represents the lowest level of evidence (type five).

Conclusions

Like other methodologies the single case report method has its strengths and weaknesses. The single case method is merely the starting point for other approaches and this is particularly the case in a clinical setting. It is also important to remember that although the anecdote cannot be extended to create general principles, it is also the case that grouped frequencies are not always applicable to the individual (Allport, 1961). A well-known example cited by Allport is that of the recidivist from a broken home whose chances of reoffending are given as 80%. Allport points out that this is meaningless, since the delinquent has a 100% certainty of either going straight or repeating his crimes.

Finally, innovative thinking is essential if science is to progress. It is often the individual unusual case that provides the spark for such new ideas.

Summary of how to review a single case report critically

(a) If the report describes an identifiable subject, written consent must have been obtained before publication.

(b) The report should be clearly, yet succinctly, written. The important key aspects of the case must be highlighted, including noteworthy features that are absent.

(c) The report should clearly state whether the authors are presenting a novel hypothesis or refuting a prior one.

(d) The authors should have made every effort to remove bias from their account. This includes using objective means for assigning diagnosis such as using a structured interview and computerised scoring system, the use of objective rating scales including self-report measures, obtaining objective assessments from a 'blind' third party or using consensus findings from an 'expert panel'.

(e) The authors should also have made some statement regarding the applicability and generalisability of their findings to other cases and settings.

(f) The authors should have made a clear statement about the limitations of their study and should suggest the direction that further research should take.

References

Allport, G. W. (1961) *Pattern and Growth in Personality*. New York: Holt, Rinehart and Winston.

Charlton, B. G. & Walston, F. (1998) Individual case studies in clinical research. *Journal of Evaluation in Clinical Practice*, **4**, 147–155.

Farmer, A. E. (1999) The demise of the published case report? Is resuscitation necessary? *British Journal of Psychiatry*, in press.

Francke, U., Ochs, H. D., de Martinville, B., *et al* (1985) Minor Xp21 chromosome deletion in a male associated with expression of Duchenne muscular dystrophy, chronic granulomatous disease, retinitis pigmentosa and McLeod syndrome. *American Journal of Human Genetics*, **37**, 250–267.

Frith, C. D. & Corcoran, R. (1996) Exploring "theory or mind" in people with schizophrenia. *Psychological Medicine*, **26**, 521–530.

Healy, D. (1996) *The Psychopharmacologists*. London: Altman.

Joseph, A. P. & Farmer, A. E. (1995) An unusual case of central pontine myelinolysis. *Alcohol and Alcoholism*, **30**, 423–425.

Magee, B. (1973) *Popper*. London: Fontana.

McGuffin, P., Reveley, A. & Holland, A. (1982) Identical triplets: non-identical psychosis? *British Journal of Psychiatry*, **140**, 1–6.

Piercy, M. (1964) The effects of cerebral lesions on intellectual function: a review of current research trends. *British Journal of Psychiatry*, **110**, 310–348.

Walston, F. (1997) *The Cognitive Neuropsychiatry of Paranoid Delusions*. BMedSci thesis. Newcastle upon Tyne: University of Newcastle upon Tyne.

Weinstein, S., Semmes, J. & Ghent, L. (1956) Spatial orientation in a man after cerebral injury. II. Analysis according to concomitant defects. *Journal of Psychology*, **42**, 249–493.

Appendix 1
MRCPsych Part II Examination
Critical Review Paper Spring 1999

Please read the instructions carefully before going further.

Instructions

1. This examination lasts for 90 minutes.
2. The paper has TWO questions. You must attempt ALL parts of BOTH questions.
3. A total of 100 marks has been allocated to the whole paper. Each part of each question is worth 10 marks. Therefore, Question A is worth 70 Marks and Question B is worth 30 marks.
4. In answering Question A, candidates may wish to glance briefly at the questions they are asked to answer (on pages 134–136 of the paper), before reading the details of the research (described on pages 130–133).
5. You are advised to bring a calculator to the examination hall. You are permitted to take a noiseless, cordless, pocket-sized non-programmable calculator WITHOUT printout or graphic/word display facilities.

Question A

A brief primary care intervention for problem drinkers

Scenario

You are working in a general psychiatry service within an inner city catchment area, characterised by a multi-cultural and fairly mobile population, and higher than average levels of unemployment. Talking with Dr Patel, one of the local general practitioners who also works as a clinical assistant in the acute hospital's accident and emergency department, you learn that there appear to be a disproportionately high number of attendances in the accident and emergency department attributable to alcohol-related problems. Dr Patel queries whether it would be possible for general practitioners to detect some of these problems earlier and, if so, whether they could intervene to reduce the levels of problem drinking and thus reduce the number of accident and emergency department attendances. Dr Patel has done a literature search, and has found the following paper, which he offers you for your opinion:

Fleming, M. F., Barry, K. L., Manwell, L. B., *et al* (1997) Brief physician advice for problem alcohol drinkers: a randomized controlled trial in community-based primary care practices. *Journal of the American Medical Association*, **277**, 1039–1045.

Read through the summary of the methods and results below, and then answer the questions which follow.

The paper

This paper describes a brief intervention for problem drinkers by primary care physicians in one mid-western state of the USA. The main aim was to determine whether a brief intervention by primary care physicians was better than an information booklet in reducing problem alcohol use among people attending their general practitioner.

Methodology

Background

The physicians who participated (*n*=64) had an average of 13 years of practice after qualification, and worked in a variety of primary care settings, from single-handed rural practices to large suburban clinics, but none in built-up urban areas. Over a two-year period, all their adult patients (aged 18–65 years) with scheduled appointments were asked by the practice receptionists to complete a screening questionnaire. Refusal rates varied considerably between clinics (mean 13%, range 2–30%). The questions were phrased in general terms to minimise the possible intervention effects of asking directly about alcohol use. Those patients who screened positive on the questionnaire were invited to participate in a 'Research Lifestyle Interview', conducted in the general practice clinic by one of 10 trained research interviewers. The interview was designed to gather information not only about alcohol use, its possible consequences and any previous treatment, but also about illicit drug use, past psychiatric history and family history. Patients who completed the interview procedures were each paid the equivalent of £30.

Eligibility criteria

Patients were eligible for the intervention if they consumed above threshold amounts of alcohol (13 drinks or 168 g alcohol per week for men, and 11 drinks or 132 g of alcohol per week for women). Exclusion criteria were:

(a) age below 18 or above 65 years;

(b) pregnancy;

(c) attendance at an alcohol treatment programme in the previous 12 months;

(d) reported symptoms of alcohol withdrawal in the previous 12 months;

(e) having received advice from their doctor about their drinking in the previous three months;

(f) consumption of more than 50 drinks per week;

(g) being judged suicidal on the basis of reported symptoms.

Patient sample

The age profile of those recruited reflected that of the community in which they lived. Eighty-eight per cent were Caucasian, 62% were married or cohabiting and 61% had received more than the compulsory level of education.

Patient allocation to the treatment groups

Patients who were eligible for inclusion in the study were randomised into either an experimental or a control group. Randomisation was carried out separately for men and women in each participating practice, using a computer-generated allocation method. Neither the doctors nor the practice staff knew which patients had been randomised to the control group.

Interventions

All patients who were recruited into the study received a booklet about general health matters. The patients in the control group received no other intervention for their drinking. Those randomised into the experimental group were invited to participate in two 15-minute interviews, one month apart with their own doctor, plus a follow-up telephone call from the practice nurse two weeks after the second interview. The intervention used a standard format, based on a workbook, and focused on general health as well as drinking alcohol and its effects. The doctors who took part in the study were all trained to use the intervention prior to the start of the research, and received at least two further 'booster' training sessions during the study.

Outcome assessments

Patients recruited into the study were followed up by telephone interviews six and 12 months after the intervention. For these follow-up interviews, the interviewers were rotated so that they did not interview the same patients as they had screened initially. The interviews focused on changes in alcohol use, health care utilisation and changes in health status. Family members were also contacted at 12 months to corroborate the patients' accounts. After the interviews, the patients' medical records were reviewed.

Results

Recruitment and follow-up

The patient flows are shown in Figure 1.

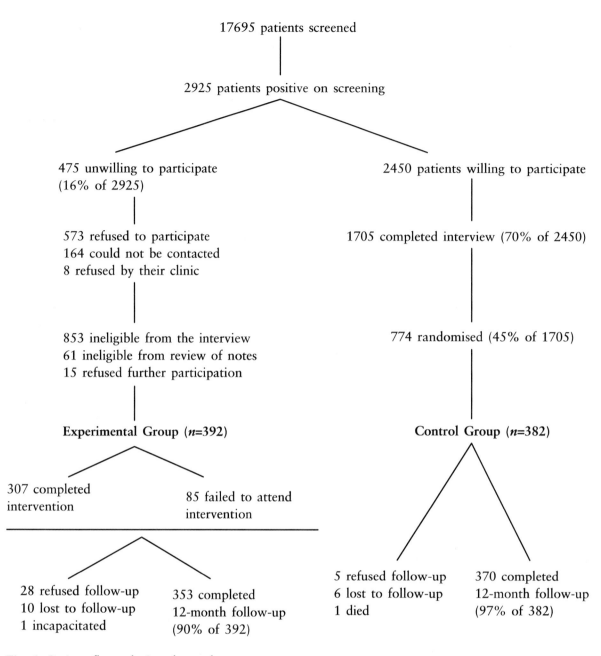

17695 patients screened

2925 patients positive on screening

475 unwilling to participate
(16% of 2925)

573 refused to participate
164 could not be contacted
8 refused by their clinic

853 ineligible from the interview
61 ineligible from review of notes
15 refused further participation

Experimental Group (*n*=392)

307 completed
intervention

85 failed to attend
intervention

28 refused follow-up
10 lost to follow-up
1 incapacitated

353 completed
12-month follow-up
(90% of 392)

2450 patients willing to participate

1705 completed interview (70% of 2450)

774 randomised (45% of 1705)

Control Group (*n*=382)

5 refused follow-up
6 lost to follow-up
1 died

370 completed
12-month follow-up
(97% of 382)

Fig. 1. Patient flows during the study

Identification by general practitioners of problem drinkers

At 12-month follow-up, only 50 control patients (13% of the group) reported that they had received an intervention for problem drinking from their general practitioner.

Alcohol consumption

Table I shows the number of episodes of binge drinking in the 30 days prior to each assessment (binge drinking was defined as >4 drinks for women and >5 drinks for men on a single occasion). Note that information in all the tables is given in the same format as in the published paper.

Table 2 shows the number of episodes of excessive drinking in the seven days prior to each assessment (excessive drinking was defined as >20 drinks per week for men and >13 drinks per week for women).

Table 1. Participants who were binge drinking in the 30 days prior to each assessment

| | Treatment (n=392) | | Control (n=382) | | | |
	n	%	n	%	χ^2	P
Baseline	288	85	317	87	0.44	NS
6 months	200	59	266	73	3.77	<0.001
12 months	188	56	261	71	4.33	<0.001

Table 2. Participants who drank excessively in the seven days prior to treatment

| | Treatment (n=392) | | Control (n=382) | | | |
	n	%	n	%	χ^2	P
Baseline	160	47	176	48	0.26	NS
Six months	67	20	115	31	3.52	<0.001
12 months	60	18	119	33	4.53	<0.001

Accident and emergency department attendance

Self-reported accident and emergency department attendance is shown in Table 3.

Table 3. Number of participants who reported attending the accident and emergency department in the six months prior to each assessment

| | Treatment (n=392) | | Control (n=382) | | | |
	n	%	n	%	χ^2	P
Baseline	75	58	80	65	2.45	>0.10
6 months	47	40	70	56		
12 months	60	47	62	50		

Question A

NOTE: Each question is worth 10 marks. There are a total of 100 marks for the whole paper, 70 marks for Question A and 30 marks for Question B.

Question A1

List five features of the design of this study which contribute to the strengths of its methodology.

....
....
....
....
....
....

Question A2

For each feature listed above, explain briefly how it contributes to the strengths of the study design.

....
....
....
....
....
....
....
....
....
....

Question A3

List four potential or actual weaknesses of the study design.

....
....
....
....
....
....

Question A4

Although 85 patients assigned to the intervention group failed to participate in the intervention, they were included as part of the intervention group in the analyses. Why was this done? What is this method of analysis called?

....
....
....
....
....
....
....
....
....
....

Question A5

Summarise as precisely and as accurately as you can the main results as they have been given in the tables.

....
....
....
....
....
....
....
....
....

Question A6

Considering only excessive drinking at 12 months (Table 2).

(i) What is the relative rate reduction (RRR) due to the intervention? (As well as giving the RRR, show how you calculate this.)

....
....
....

(ii) What is the absolute rate reduction (ARR) and how do you calculate this?

....
....
....

(iii) If you were a Wisconsin general practitioner introducing this intervention, to how many people would you need to offer it to have one patient with a successful outcome?

....
....
....

Question A7

Dr Patel's original query was whether local practitioners might be able to detect alcohol-related problems earlier and intervene to reduce alcohol-related accident and emergency visits. What would you say to him about the applicability of this paper to his query?

....
....
....
....
....
....
....
....
....
....
....

Question B

The following table is taken from a study of 521 patients admitted to medical or orthopaedic wards of a single general hospital. The ability of the CAGE questionnaire to predict alcohol-related problems (alcohol misuse or alcohol dependence, both operationally defined) was compared using a rigorous diagnostic interview as the 'gold standard'.

No. of positive CAGE responses	Alcohol misuse/dependence		Sensitivity	Specificity	Positive predictive value
	Present	Absent			
0	18	358	—	—	—
1	11	28	0.85	0.89	0.62
2	26	14	0.73	0.93	0.82
3	37	1	0.51	0.997	0.99
4	23	0	0.20	1.00	1.00
Total	117	401			

Question B1

The chairman of your local Community Health Council (a lay person with little medical knowledge) has been given a copy of this table during a discussion on alcohol problems. He wants to know what the results mean. How would you briefly summarise the table for him, and interpret its results?

....
....
....
....
....
....
....
....
....

Question B2

To use the questionnaire, you need to define how many positive responses the patient needs to give before being classified as having alcohol-related problems in screening. If you were applying the CAGE questionnaire as a screening tool in clinical practice in a general hospital setting, what cut-off point would you select?

....
....
....
....
....
....
....
....
....

Question B3

What would be the consequences of choosing this cut-off point, in terms of people without alcohol-related problems screening positive on the CAGE, and people with alcohol-related problems being missed?

....
....
....
....
....
....
....
....
....

MRCPsych Part II Examination
Critical Review Paper Autumn 1999

Question A
Long-term prognosis in schizophrenia

Mr Alan James, an 18-year-old man, is admitted to hospital with a six-week history of third person auditory hallucinations, agitation and passivity feelings. He had previously been well, with no past history of psychiatric disturbance. He denies any drug abuse and a drug screen following admission proves negative. The working diagnosis is schizophrenia. Mr James's parents ask for an interview with you to discuss their son's prognosis. The first question they want to ask is: 'what is the overall outcome likely to be over the next 10 years?' A second question concerns the effects of negative symptoms on the outcome. Through a colleague at work, Mr James's father has made contact with another family who have a son with schizophrenia. Apparently, this young man has shown negative symptoms and has remained unwell for some years. When the parents come to see you, they bring with them a copy of a paper they have found via the internet. Read through the summary of the paper below, then answer the questions which follow.

Mason, P., Harrison, G. Glazebrook, C., *et al* (1995) Characteristics of outcome of schizophrenia at 13 years. *British Journal of Psychiatry*, **167**, 596–603.

Background

The patients studied in this paper were first identified in the International Pilot Study of Schizophrenia, which examined the determinants of outcome of schizophrenia in 15 countries. Nottingham, where the present study is based, was the UK centre for the International Pilot Study.

Sample
Original sample

During the two-year period 1 August 1978–31 July 1980, all patients between the ages of 15 and 54 years making first-ever contact with psychiatric services in Nottingham (population 390 000) were screened. Screening included not only those who were admitted as in-patients, but also every other type of contact with services. All eligible patients were interviewed by a research psychiatrist, using (among other assessment instruments) the Present State Examination. After the assessments had been completed, at least two project psychiatrists together with the researchers who had conducted the interviews discussed all the available information on each patient to reach a consensus diagnosis, using ICD–9 criteria. This procedure identified 67 patients (22 women, 45 men) who could be assigned a project diagnosis of schizophrenia. The investigators also checked the Nottingham Psychiatric Case Register, general practitioners and private psychiatric hospitals near Nottingham to identify patients who should possibly have been included in the study but were not identified by the procedures used. Of nine such cases identified, only three were judged to fall into 'certain' or 'very likely' categories of schizophrenia.

Follow-up sample

Most patients in the original sample were traced using the Nottingham Psychiatric Case Register and the Medical Records Department at Mapperley Hospital, Nottingham. Others were found using the Electoral Register and the Registrar for Births, Deaths and Marriages. Use was also made of the National Health Service Central Register and various family health services authorities throughout the country. It was possible to trace 63 of patients in the original sample (94%). Of the patients traced, five (8%) had died, three following suicide and another under circumstances suggesting suicide. Of the remaining 58 patients, high quality information could be obtained either by face-to-face interview or through records and informants on 54 patients (94%).

Face-to-face interviews were conducted with 48 patients (83% of 58) and two further patients (3%) were interviewed by telephone. No significant differences were found between the 58 patients who completed follow-up, those lost to follow-up (n=4) and those who died (n=5) in age, sex, marital status, type of onset, or initial Present State Examination profile.

Assessments

The following instruments were used:

(a) Present State Examination (PSE): the CATEGO computer programme was used to determine the number of subjects who met the restrictive definition of schizophrenia (CATEGO Class S+), at entry and at follow-up.

(b) Scale for the Assessment of Negative Symptoms (SANS): The SANS was used to determine the number of patients who had negative symptoms during the month before the follow-up assessment. A SANS summary score of greater than two indicates the presence of negative symptoms.

(c) Life Chart Schedule (LCS): This codes symptoms, treatment, residency and employment history for the two years prior to the assessment, and for the entire follow-up period.

(d) Disability Assessment Schedule (DAS): The information used from this scale included the adjusted score for Dysfunctional Overall Behaviour (derived from scores for social withdrawal and self-care).

Information for each assessment was gathered from both the patient and a key informant, and further information was elicited from general practice records and hospital records.

Results
Symptoms

At entry to the study, 70% of the patients were classified according to the CATEGO programme as S+ (i.e. meeting a restrictive definition of schizophrenia). At follow-up, only 19% of those assessed were classified at S+. Of the patients assessed at follow-up with the SANS, 48% had summary scores greater than two (i.e. showed clinically important negative symptoms in the months prior to follow-up). Twenty-seven of those assessed at follow-up (47%) showed evidence of negative symptoms in the two years prior to the follow-up assessment.

Course of the illness

Table I summarises the course of the illness in the two years prior to the follow-up assessment, separately for the whole sample and for those patients (n=27) who had shown negative symptoms in the two years prior to the follow-up assessment.

Table I. Course of illness and negative symptoms in the two years prior to the follow-up assessment (percentages in parentheses)

Type of course	Total sample	Negative symptoms in the 2 years prior to the follow-up assessment	
		Present	Absent
Episodic	6 (10)	3 (50)	3 (50)
Continuous	20 (34)	16 (80)	4 (20)
Neither episodic nor continuous	2 (3)	2 (100)	1 (0)
Never psychotic	30 (52)	6 (20)	24 (80)
Total	58	27 (47)	31 (53)

Disability

Information from the Disability Assessment Schedule was available on 55 subjects. Of these, 24 (44%) showed no dysfunction in overall behaviour and 23 (43%) showed no dysfunction in their social roles.

Complete recovery

If this is defined as meaning that the patient is alive at follow-up with no symptoms, no disability and on no treatment, then 11 (17%) of the sample available for follow-up had recovered completely at 13 years.

Associations between negative and other symptoms

Table 2 shows the association between negative symptoms at follow-up assessment, and: (a) overall psychotic symptoms at follow-up; (b) psychotic symptoms which had been continuous during the two years prior to the follow-up assessment.

Table 2. Association between negative symptoms and overall psychotic symptoms at follow-up

	Negative symptoms at follow-up assessment		Total	Odds ratio (95% CI)[1]	(P)
	Present	Absent			
Overall psychotic symptoms at follow-up					
Present	17	8	25	6.0 (1.5–26.2)	6.9 (P<0.01)
Absent	6	17	23		
Total	23	25	48		
Continuous psychotic symptoms for 2 years prior to follow-up					
Present	16	5	21	9.1 (2.1–43.9)	10.0 (P<0.01)
Absent	7	20	27		
Total	23	25	48		

1. 95% CI, 95% confidence interval of odds ratio.

Question B

Mortality of a cohort of patients with schizophrenia

The following data are taken from Anderson et al, British Journal of Psychiatry, **159** (suppl. 13), 30–33, 1991.

All patients discharged from in-patient or day patient care at Northwick Park Hospital near London in the 11-year period 1 January 1975–1 January 1985 were followed up between two to five years after discharge. The case notes were examined and those that fulfilled the St Louis criteria for schizophrenia formed the study sample. After this procedure 532 cases were identified, of which 291 were men and 241 were women.

At the time of enquiry on 1 January 1989, 382 of these patients were known to be alive, 69 were dead and 81 could not be traced. Of the 69 deaths, 40 died of natural causes whereas 24 deaths were unnatural. The five remaining deaths could not be clearly classed as natural or unnatural. However, only seven of the 24 deaths were adjudged to be due to suicide with 15 recorded as an open verdict (no decision made about cause) in the Coroner's Court. Two patients had no inquest and no decision was made about the cause of death in these individuals.

The frequency of all causes of death, including suicide and myocardial infarction recorded separately, is shown in Table 3. The expected mortality of the general population living in the same district health authority during the period under enquiry was calculated separately. The subject-years method was used to calculate the expected number of deaths among the cohort with schizophrenia.

Table 3. Standardised mortality rates (SMR) for all causes of death, death due to myocardial infarction and death attributed to suicide

Cause of death	Women			Men		
	Deaths (n)	SMR	95% CI[1] of SMR	Deaths (n)	SMR	95% CI[1] of SMR
All causes of death	30	2.57	1.73–3.64	39	2.44	1.75–3.34
Death due to myocardial infarction	7	2.83	1.14–5.83	6	1.42	0.52–3.09
Suicide (whole sample)[2]	2	12.77	1.53–46.13	5	19.5	6.22–44.7
Suicide (patients aged 15–44 years)	2	29.25	3.51–105.6	4	27.85	7.5–71.3
Suicide (patients aged over 44 years)	0	–	–	1	8.51	0.21–47.4

1. 95% confidence interval.
2. Using suicide verdicts only.

Question A

NOTE: Each question is worth 10 marks. There are a total of 100 marks for the whole paper, 70 marks for Question A and 30 marks for Question B.

Question AI

What type of study design is used in the study described in the paper?   [2 marks]

....
....
....
....

Give one advantage and one disadvantage of its use.   [2 marks]

....
....
....
....

Why are alternative designs unsuitable to answer this question?   [2 marks]

....
....
....
....

Please given an example of a plausible alternative study design.   [2 marks]

....
....
....
....

Explain why one of these is not suitable.   [2 marks]

....
....
....
....

Question A2

List three strengths of the execution of this study. Take care to distinguish between the study *design* and its execution; only the latter is relevant here. Do not include any points you may have mentioned in answering Question AI. For two of the points you list, explain why it is a strength.

[6 marks]

....
....
....
....
....
....

For two of the points you list, explain why it is a strength.

[4 marks]

....
....
....
....
....
....

Question A3

Only 54 of the 67 patients in the original cohort could be assessed at follow-up by 'high quality information'. How far does this affect the conclusions in the paper?

[2 marks]

....
....
....
....

Give two reasons for your answer.

[8 marks]

....
....
....
....
....
....
....
....

Question A4

Summarise five points from the results (excluding results in Table 2, i.e. the relationship between negative symptoms and psychosis) which can contribute to answering the first question posed by Mr James's parents (what is the longer term outcome likely to be)? [10 marks]

....
....
....
....
....
....
....
....
....

Question A5

The results in Table 1 show that over 50% of those followed up from the original cohort where not psychotic during the two-year period before follow-up assessment. Please give five possible reasons to explain these results. [10 marks]

....
....
....
....
....
....
....
....
....
....

Question A6

What do the results of Table 2 show about the relationship between outcome and the presence or absence of negative symptoms? Please state two main findings. [6 marks]

....
....
....
....
....
....

What information in the table allows you to judge how certain you can be about these findings?

[4 marks]

....
....
....
....
....
....

Question A7

Assume that, instead of being admitted to a psychiatric unit, Mr James had been taken to see his general practitioner who had decided to treat Mr James himself with an antipsychotic drug, because Mr James and his family were very resistant to referral to psychiatric services. In this event, how far are the results of the present study applicable? Give two reasons for your answer.

[2 marks]

....
....
....
....

Give two reasons for your answer.

[8 marks]

....
....
....
....
....
....

Question B

Question BI

Define standardised mortality rate (or ratio) (SMR).

[6 marks]

....
....
....

Using the data in Table 3, how many deaths would have been expected among (a) *all* men and (b) *all* women, of the same age distribution as the study sample with schizophrenia, in the catchment area of the district health authority in which the patients resided?   [4 marks]

....
....
....
....

Question B2

The mortality rate in women from myocardial infarction appears greater than in men. Is this difference statistically significant?   [2 marks]

....
....

Explain the reasons for your choice.   [3 marks]

....
....
....
....

Is the mortality rate in women from myocardial infarction significantly different statistically from that of the general population?   [2 marks]

....
....

Explain your reasonsing.   [3 marks]

....
....
....
....
....
....

Question B3

Twenty-four deaths were considered unnatural. The majority was given open verdicts (no decision made about cause). In the light of this, comment on the use of suicide verdicts only in the calculation of SMR for patients with schizophrenia. [4 marks]

....
....
....
....
....
....

Summarise the results concerned with suicide verdicts shown in Table 3. Please list three main findings. [6 marks]

....
....
....
....
....
....
....
....
....

MRCPsych Part II Examination
Critical Review Paper Spring 2000

Question A

Detecting mood disorders in general practice

Scenario

A local general practitioner asks you for advice about how to improve her ability to detect depression and anxiety in routine clinical practice. She and her partners have recently completed an audit of their management of patients whom they eventually refer to a psychiatrist for advice about depression. They have discovered that such patients have been frequent surgery attenders prior to referral, but with physical symptoms. She wonders if she and her partners have been missing depression in the earlier consultations, particularly in view of a recent paper she has found. She asks for your comments on the paper, which is:

Kessler, D., Lloyd, K., Lewis, G., et al (1999) Cross sectional study of symptom attribution and recognition of depression and anxiety in primary care. *British Journal of Psychiatry*, **318**, 436–440.

The paper

The paper evaluates the ability of general practitioners to identify anxiety and depression in attenders at routine surgeries. In this paper the diagnosis of depression or anxiety by the general practitioner is regarded as the test to be applied against the gold standard of the General Health Questionnaire (GHQ) score. The study also describes characteristics of the patients, which might have an influence on the judgement of general practitioners in detecting mood disorder.

Methodology

Setting

The study was undertaken in the UK, in a single urban general practice with eight partners, serving a population of 12 800 patients.

Sample

Consecutive attenders at surgery who were aged over 16 years.

Measures

1. The 12-item General Health Questionnaire (GHQ–12) was administered to all patients while they were waiting to see the doctor. A score of $\geqslant 3$ was used to identify people who were

probable cases of depression or anxiety, although this information was not made available to the doctor at the time of the consultation. This score was chosen because, in an earlier study undertaken in primary care in the UK, it had been the optimal threshold for 'caseness' when compared with a more detailed psychiatric assessment.

2. At the same time, the patients completed the Symptom Interpretation Questionnaire (SIQ). In this instrument, patients are presented with a list of 13 common symptoms. They are asked to rate whether each symptom usually has a *somatic* cause, a *psychological* cause, or whether it is a feature of *normal* bodily function. The Questionnaire therefore yields three scores, according to how many symptoms the patients attributes to each of these three causes. The three scores sum to 13. If the patient attributes the majority (seven or more) of symptoms to any one cause, he or she is described as predominantly *somatising, psychologising* or *normalising* in style, depending on which attribution is most used. If no attribution is used for the majority of symptoms, then the patient is described as having no predominant attributional style.

3. After the consultation, the general practitioners were asked to give each patient a psychiatric diagnosis if appropriate, and to say whether any anxiety or depression was new or already known.

Results

1. Of 355 consecutive attenders, 26 (7%) refused to participate and 24 (6.8%) returned incomplete questionnaires. In the remaining 305, there were 225 women and 80 men. The average age of the patients was 44 years (range 16–90). Men were slightly older than women (49 years *v.* 42 years).

2. The GHQ–12 identified 157 (52%) people as cases using the cut-off $\geqslant 3$.

3. The general practitioners diagnosed 71 (24%) people as cases of anxiety, depression or both.

4. Results on the SIQ showed that 145 (48%) of patients were predominantly 'normalisers', 71 (23%) were predominantly 'psychologisers', and only 16 (5%) were predominantly 'somatisers', 72 (24%) had no predominant attributional style.

5. Other results are shown in Tables 1 and 2.

Table 1. Ability of general practitioners (GPs) to identify cases of depression or anxiety (as defined by GHQ–12 score)

	GHQ–12 defined case	GHQ–12 defined non-case	Total
GP diagnosed case	57	14	71
GP diagnosed non-case	100	134	234
Total	157	148	305

Table 2.   Detection by general practitioner of anxiety and depression in 305 patients according to style of symptom attribution

	Predominant attribution type (score 7 or more)			
	Psychologising	Normalising	Somatising	No predominant score
Total sample				
Number of patients	71	146	16	72
Number of women (%)	61 (86)	99 (68)	9 (56)	56 (78)
Mean age (years)	43.4	40.4	58.6	48.8
Number (%)	55 (77)	54 (37)	6 (38)	42 (58)
General Health Question- naire (GHQ) cases				
Number not detected[1]	21	46	5	29
Percentage not detected	38	85	83	69
95% CI[2]	25–52	73–93	36–100	53–82

1. 'Not detected', patients classified as cases according to the GHQ–12 but not diagnosed as such by the general practitioner.
2. 95% CI, 95% confidence interval of percentage of GHQ cases not detected.

Question B

Early life family disadvantages and major depression in adulthood

Table 3 has been modified from:

Sadowski, H., Ugarte, B., Kolvin, I., et al (1999) Early life family disadvantages and major depression in adulthood. *British Journal of Psychiatry*, **174**, 112–120.

Table 3 reports results from a study which followed a cohort of children into adult life. The main aim of the study was to determine whether disadvantages in early family life were associated with major depression later in adulthood. From the original cohort (n=781) a sample was taken (n=301) and assessed at 33 years of age. The presence of major depression in the year before assessment was the main outcome. For the analysis, the sample was divided into those who had experienced 'multiple disadvantage' in childhood, and those who had not.

Table 3.   One-year prevalence of major depressive disorder at 33 years of age in relation to 'multiple disadvantage' experienced in the first 5 years of life

	No multiple disadvantage group	Multiple disadvantage group	Odds ratio	95% confidence interval
Sample population				
Total	16/223 (7.2%)	11/39 (28.2%)	5.1	2.1–12.0
Females	12/108 (11.1%)	7/22 (31.8%)	3.7	1.3–1.0
Males	4/115 (3.5%)	4/17 (23.5%)	8.5	1.9–38.3

Question A

NOTE: Each question is worth 10 marks. There are a total of 100 marks for the whole paper, 70 marks for Question A and 30 marks for Question B.

Question A1

In this paper, it is assumed that the GHQ−12 is a valid means of identifying depression and anxiety. Define what is meant by the validity of a measure.   [2 marks]

....
....
....
....

Briefly describe *two* types of validity of such instruments.   [6 marks]

....
....
....
....
....
....

When validating the GHQ (or any other instrument to measure an illness) what is the main requirement of subject samples used in such investigations?   [2 marks]

....
....
....
....

Question A2

The authors use a threshold score of 3 on the GHQ−12 for defining psychiatric disorder, because this was the optimal cut-off for defining 'caseness' when the GHQ−12 was compared with more detailed psychiatric assessment in a different study. Define the optimal threshold for any diagnostic test.   [3 marks]

....
....
....
....

Give *two* reasons why it may be difficult to set the optimal threshold score of the GHQ and psychiatric assessment in this study. [4 marks]

....
....
....
....

How might a Receiver Operator Curve (ROC) assist in this exercise? [3 marks]

....
....
....
....
....

Question A3

The results include the reported sensitivity and specificity of the general practitioners' diagnoses. Define sensitivity and specificity. [2+2 marks]

....
....
....
....

Calculate the sensitivity and specificity of the diagnostic categories given by the general practitioners from the data described in Table I. [2+2 marks]

....
....
....
....

Calculate the negative predictive value of diagnosis of a non-case by the GP. [2 marks]

....
....
....
....

Question A4

What is the positive predictive value of a test? [3 marks]

....
....
....
....

Use the data in Table 1 to calculate the positive predictive value of a general practitioner diagnosis of depression or anxiety in identifying GHQ-defined cases. [3 marks]

....
....
....
....
....

Explain whether or not you expect the positive predictive value to change, and in what direction, if the same study was carried out using patients in a general medical ward. [4 marks]

....
....
....
....

Question A5

Table 2 shows the relation between scores on the symptom attribution questionnaire, the rate of GHQ caseness, and the rate of non-detection of GHQ cases by the general practitioner. Give *five* main findings from the results shown in the table, with reference to differences between the three attributional style groups. [10 marks]

....
....
....
....
....
....
....
....

Question A6

The last rows of Table 2 present data showing the proportion of GHQ cases which were not detected by general practitioners. Associated with each rate is a 95% confidence interval. Define the 95% confidence interval. [3 marks]

....
....
....
....

Explain what it means. [4 marks]

....
....
....
....

Why is the confidence interval for the non-detection of patients with somatising attribution style wider than for the patients with a normalising style when the percentage of patients in each group is almost identical? [3 marks]

....
....
....
....

Question A7

Your general practitioner colleague's original question was about patients who finally are referred to a psychiatrist, querying whether initial presentation with physical symptoms might lead to the general practitioners initially missing a diagnosis of depression. How far does this paper assist her in proving or disproving her hypothesis that some depressed patients are not diagnosed because they present with physical symptoms? [I mark]

....
....
....

Explain your reasoning. [2 marks]

....
....
....
....

Does the paper help her in determining which patients she should refer to the psychiatrists?

[I mark]

....
....

Explain your conclusions.

[3 marks]

....
....
....
....

How accurate is the diagnosis of depression and anxiety made according to the threshold score of $\geqslant 3$ on the GHQ?

[I mark]

....
....

Indicate your reasoning.

[2 marks]

....
....
....
....

Question B

Question BI

The rate for major depression is expressed as a one-year prevalence. What type of prevalence is this called?

[3 marks]

....
....
....
....

What other type of prevalence is there? [1 mark]

....
....
....
....

Define this. [2 marks]

....
....
....
....

Indicate whether this alternative method of describing prevalence is likely to lead to a smaller or greater number of cases of depression. Explain your reasoning. [4 marks]

....
....
....
....
....

Question B2

If the *odds* of an event happening are 1 in 9, what would be the *rate* or *frequency* of that event? [3 marks]

....
....
....
....

Table 3 expresses the difference between the two groups as an odds ratio. Explain exactly what is meant by the odds ratio of 5.1 in Table 3? [4 marks]

....
....
....
....
....

If the odds ratio was 1.0 in any group of the sample population what would this mean? [3 marks]

....
....
....
....

Question B3

Give *four* main findings shown in Table 3 with particular relevance to the meaning of the odds ratios and their confidence intervals. Include in these the differences between men and women shown in the table, indicating whether these are likely to be significant. [10 marks]

....
....
....
....
....
....
....
....

Appendix 2
Critical Review Paper for the MRCPsych Part II Examination Information Pack[1]

1. General information

There will be a change to the papers that will be examined in the MRCPsych Part II Examination in the near future. The last sitting of the Short Answer Question (SAQ) paper will take place during the Autumn 1998 examination session. The Critical Review paper will be introduced at the spring 1999 examination session.

Reasons for introducing the Critical Review paper

(i) *The importance of developing critical appraisal skills and evidence-based practice*
Good clinical practice in psychiatry, as in other medical specialities, relies on the combination of sound clinical judgement and the appropriate application of research-based evidence. Increasingly, in their clinical work and as advocates for their services and patients, psychiatrists need to acquire new skills and confidence in critical appraisal of research evidence, and how this can be applied to their clinical work. Senior doctors must be able to determine the value of individual published scientific articles, not only in terms of the scientific validity of their results and conclusions, but in their applicability to clinical practice. The skills involved are of permanent value to the practising psychiatrist.

(ii) *Limitations of the current MRCPsych Examination*
The MRCPsych Part II Examination at present consists of six parts. There are two multiple choice question (MCQ) papers concerned with Basic Sciences and Clinical Topics, an Essay Paper, a SAQ paper and the Clinical Examination, comprising an Individual Patient Assessment (IPA) and Patient Management Problems (PMP). In addition, there has for many years been a Research Option in the Examination to encourage trainees to undertake and develop research. However, this option has rarely been exercised and has now been withdrawn owing to lack of interest.

An important requirement of the examination is that its different components should as far as possible measure different qualities and attributes of the candidates. This can be tested by measuring the extent of the correlation between the mark of the candidates in the different parts of the examination. On this basis, the MCQ exams, the Essay and the Clinical Examination test different aspects of candidates' knowledge and experience. However, the SAQ paper marks are closely correlated with the MCQ (Clinical Topics paper) marks and the paper does not introduce any extra dimension in the assessment.

The Court of Electors, on the advice of the Examinations Sub-Committee, has discontinued the Research Option. An alternative is needed to test the skills necessary to evaluate research and supplement the present examination curriculum. The SAQ paper will, therefore, be replaced by a Critical Review paper.

---

1. This information Pack was published by the Royal College of Psychiatrists in 1998.

Pilot examination paper

An examination paper was piloted in December 1997. The results of this pilot and of a paper that was piloted in 1995 will guide the development of the final paper for the examination. The pilot paper can be found on page 164. Comments from the examiners and from the candidates who sat this paper will be carefully considered before the final papers are produced. Additionally, a sample paper was produced in June 1997 and this can be found on page 183.

The intention of both papers is to move towards the testing of the principles and methodology of evidence-based medicine (EBM). The Examinations Sub-Committee is aware of the need for a 'gentle' introduction to EBM and initially the Critical Review paper examination will aim to test candidates' critical ability in a more traditional way, although the techniques and terminology of EBM will be introduced gradually. We are sensitive to the fact that many tutors and trainees will be unaware of the terms used in EBM, although most will know about the basic aims of this way of analysing research data. Tutors and trainees are strongly encouraged to learn more about EBM by looking at the material on the reading list (see page 160).

2. Aims of the Critical Review paper

The Critical Review paper is intended to assess skills and expertise that are not assessed in other parts of the MRCPsych Part II Examination. These include:

Knowledge

(a) Understanding the most appropriate design and methodology to examine the hypothesis proposed in a research investigation.

(b) Recognition of the key features, and common sources of problems or bias, of different types of research methodology, including randomised controlled trials, cohort studies, case–control studies, single case studies, studies involving economic analysis and qualitative studies.

(c) Understanding of basic statistical concepts (confidence intervals and probability) with sufficient knowledge to be able to interpret the results from common statistical tests used for parametric data (t-tests, ANOVA, multiple regression) and non-parametric data (chi-squared test, logistic regression).

(d) Understanding of the definition and meaning of measures important in critical appraisal (including relative and absolute risk reduction, sensitivity, specificity, likelihood ratio, odds ratio, and number needed-to-treat).

(e) Knowledge of the methodology of systematic reviews, including meta-analysis and the potential sources of bias in the interpretation of such analyses and overviews.

Skills

(a) The ability to determine the reliability and validity of information and results presented in a scientific paper.

(b) The ability to determine the clinical importance and relevance of results from the information given in a paper.

(c) The ability to detect errors in design and methodology that render the stated conclusions invalid or affect their impact.

(d)   The ability to understand and assess logically the process and results of critical appraisal of such a paper.

(e)   The capacity to suggest further experiments which would confirm or expand understanding in the field under investigation.

(f)   The ability to place the results of the paper in clinical context and assess how far clinical practice may be altered as a consequence.

3. Reading list

To guide tutors and trainees in preparing for the Critical Review paper, the Working Party has produced the following reference list of books on EBM.

Introductory textbooks

Author	Title	Publisher
Crombie, I. (1996)	*The Pocket Guide to Critical Appraisal*	BMJ Publishing
Dixon, R., Munro, J. & Silcocks, P. (1997)	*The Evidence-Based Medicine Workbook: Critical Appraisal for Clinical Problem Solving*	Butterworth-Heinemann
Greenhalgh, T. (1997)	*How to Read a Paper: The Basics of Evidence-Based Medicine*	BMJ Publishing
Sackett, D., Haynes, R., Guyatt, G., et al (1991)	*Clinical Epidemiology: A Basic Science for Clinical Medicine*	Little, Brown & Co
Sackett, D., Richardson, W., Rosenberg, W., et al (1996)	*Evidence-Based Medicine: How to Practise and Teach EBM*	Churchill Livingstone

General principles

Author	Paper title	Journal
Guyatt, G. (1992)	Evidence-based medicine: A new approach to teaching the practice of medicine	*Journal of the American Medical Association,* **268**, 2420–2425
Sackett, D., Rosenberg, W. Haynes, R., et al (1996)	Evidence-based medicine: What it is and what it isn't	*British Medical Journal,* **312**, 71–72

Evidence-based psychiatry

Author	Paper title	Journal
Geddes, J., Game, D., Jenkins, N., et al (1996)	What proportion of primary psychiatric intervention are based on randomized evidence?	*Quality in Health Care,* **5**, 215
Geddes, J. & Harrison, P. (1997)	Evidence-based psychiatry. Closing the gap between research and practice	*British Journal of Psychiatry,* **171**, 220–225
Summers, A & Kehoe, R. (1996)	Is psychiatric treatment evidence-based?	*Lancet,* **347**, 409–410

Critical appraisal

Author	Paper title	Journal
Earle, C. & Hébert, P. (1996)	A reader's guide to the evaluation of screening studies	*Postgraduate Medical Journal,* **72,** 77–83
Guyatt, G., Sackett, D. & Cook, D. (1993)	Users' guides to the medical literature. II. How to use an article about therapy or prevention. A. Are the results of the study valid?	*Journal of the American Medical Association,* **270,** 2598–2601
Guyatt, G., Sackett, D. & Cook, D. (1994)	Users' guides to the medical literature. II. How to use an article about therapy or prevention. B. What were the results and will they help me in caring for my patients?	*Journal of the American Medical Association,* **271,** 59–63
Guyatt, G., Sackett, D., Sinclair, J., et al (1995)	Users' guides to the medical literature. IX. A method for grading health care recommendations. Evidence-Based Medicine Working Group	*Journal of the American Medical Association,* **274,** 1800–1804
Jaeschke, R., Guyatt, G. & Sackett, D. (1994)	Users' guides to the medical literature. III. How to use an article about a diagnostic test. A. Are the results valid?	*Journal of the American Medical Association,* **271,** 389–391
Jaeschke, R., Guyatt, G. & Sackett, D. (1994)	Users' guides to the medical literature. III. How to use an article about a diagnostic test. B. What are the results and will they help me in caring for my patients?	*Journal of the American Medical Association,* **271,** 703–707
Laupacis, A., Wells, G., Richardson, W. et al (1994)	Users' guides to the medical literature. V. How to use an article about prognosis	*Journal of the American Medical Association,* **272,** 234–237
Levine, M., Walter, S. & Lee, H. (1994)	Users' guides to the medical literature. IV. How to use an article about harm	*Journal of the American Medical Association,* **271,** 1615–1619
Naylor, C. & Guyatt, G. (1996)	Users' guides to the medical literature. XI. How to use an article about a clinical utilization review	*Journal of the American Medical Association,* **275,** 1435–1439
Oxman, A., Cook, D. & Guyatt, G. (1994)	Users' guides to the medical literature. VI. How to use an overview	*Journal of the American Medical Association,* **272,** 1367–1371
Richardson, W. & Detsky A. (1995*a*)	Users' guides to the medical literature. VII. How to use a clinical decision analysis. B. What are the results and will they help me in caring for my patients? Evidence-Based Medicine Working Group	*Journal of the American Medical Association,* **273,** 1610–1613
Richardson, W. & Detsky A. (1995*b*)	Users' guides to the medical literature. VII. How to use a clinical decision analysis. A. Are the results of the study valid? Evidence-Based Medicine Working Group	*Journal of the American Medical Association,* **273,** 1292–1295
Richardson, W., Wilson, M., Nishikawa, J., et al (1995)	The well-built clinical question: A key to evidence-based decisions	*ACP Journal Club,* **123,** A12–13

Other methodology

Author	Paper title	Journal
Adams, C., Power, A., Frederic, K., *et al* (1994)	An investigation of the inadequacy of MEDLINE searches for randomized controlled trials (RCTs) of the effects of mental health care	*Psychological Medicine,* **24**, 741–748
Altman, D. (1996)	Better reporting of randomized controlled trials: the CONSORT statement	*British Medical Journal,* **313**, 570–571
Antman, E., Lau, J., Kupelnick, B., *et al* (1992)	A comparison of results of meta-analyses of randomized controlled trials and recommendations of clinical experts	*Journal of the American Medical Association,* **268**, 240–248
Bulpitt, C. (1988)	Subgroup analysis	*Lancet,* **ii**, 31–34
Charlton, B. (1994)	Understanding RCTs: Explanatory or pragmatic?	*Family Practice,* **11**, 243–244
Cook, R. & Sackett, D. (1995)	The number needed to treat. A clinically useful measure of treatment effect	*British Medical Journal,* **310**, 452–454
D'Agostino, R. & Kwan, H. (1995)	Measuring effectiveness: What to expect without a randomized control group	*Medical Care,* **33**, AS95–AS105
Detsky, A. & Sackett, D. (1985)	When was a 'negative' clinical trial big enough? How many patients you needed depends on what you found	*Archives of Internal Medicine,* **145**, 709–712
Easterbrook, P., Berlin, J., Gopalan, R. *et al* (1991)	Publication bias in clinical research	*Lancet,* **337**, 867–872
Egger, M. & Smith, G. (1995)	Misleading meta-analysis	*British Medical Journal,* **310**, 752–754
Feinstein, A. (1983)	An additional basic science for clinical medicine. II. The limitations of randomized trials	*Annals of Internal Medicine,* **99**, 544–550
Glaziou, P. & Irwig, L. (1995)	An evidence-based approach to individualising treatment	*British Medical Journal,* **311**, 1356–1359
Greenhalgh, T. (1997)	*How to Read a Paper: The Basics of Evidence-Based Medicine*	BMJ Publishing
Hayden, G., Kramer, M. & Horowitz, M. (1981)	The case–control study: A practical guide for the clinician	*Journal of the American Medical Association,* **247**, 326–331
Huston, P. & Moher, D. (1996)	Redundancy, disaggression and the integrity of medical research	*Lancet,* **347**, 1024–1026
Lewis, G., Churchill, R. & Hotopf, M. (1997)	Systematic reviews and meta-analysis	*Psychological Medicine,* **27**, 3–7
Michels, K. & Rosner, B. (1996)	Data trawling: To fish or not to fish	*Lancet,* **348**, 1152–1153
Mulrow, C. (1987)	The medical review article: State of the art	*Annals of Internal Medicine,* **106**, 485–488
Oakes, M. (1993)	The logic and role of meta-analysis in clinical research	*Statistical Methods in Medical Research,* **2**, 147–160
Sackett, D. (1979)	Bias in analytical research	*Journal of Chronic Diseases,* **32**, 51–63
Sackett, D. (1996)	On some clinically useful measures of the effects of treatment	*Evidence-Based Medicine,* **1**, 37–38
Schulz, K., Chalmers, I., Hayes, R., *et al* (1995)	Empirical evidence of bias. Dimensions of methodological quality associated with estimates of treatment effects in controlled trials	*Journal of the American Medical Association,* **273**, 408–412
Schulz, K. (1996)	Randomized trials, human nature and reporting guidelines	*Lancet,* **348**, 596–598
Schwartz, D. & Lellouch, J. (1967)	Explanatory and pragmatic attitudes in therapeutic trials	*Journal of Chronic Diseases,* **20**, 637–648
Streiner, D. (1991)	Using meta-analysis in psychiatric research	*Canadian Journal of Psychiatry,* **36**, 357–362

Other useful sources of methodological and other information

Evidence-Based Medicine, published bi-monthly by the *British Medical Journal*, includes some articles on mental illness in the papers it reviews.

Evidence-Based Mental Health, started publication in late 1997, and has adopted a similar format to *Evidence-Based Medicine*, but will concentrate on mental health.

The Cochrane Review Methodology Database, part of the Cochrane library, includes much valuable information about methodology. The Cochrane Library should be available on CD-ROM in most medical libraries.

4. Notice regarding the pilot paper and the sample paper

On the following pages you will find the question paper that was examined in the December 1997 pilot examination and the first sample question paper which was issued in June 1997. In light of feedback received from tutors, trainees and examiners, the Critical Review Working Party agreed to amend the pilot paper and created a new sample paper. What follows, therefore, is only an indication of what the paper will be like.

Critical Review Pilot Question Paper – 1–5 December 1997 (1 hour)

Read the following abridged paper carefully and then answer questions one to eight at the end of the paper. You may find it easier to read the questions first.

This paper studies the clinical relevance of subjective memory impairment in older people. It is based on an article in *Psychological Medicine* (1995, 779–786).

Introduction

The significance of self-perceived, subjective memory impairment (SMI) is uncertain. SMI may or may not occur in the presence of demonstrable cognitive impairment. It may be associated with mild memory impairment, as demonstrated on objective testing, but is not necessarily progressive and so may be distinct from dementia. SMI may be associated with concurrent depression.

The aims of this study were:

(a) To determine whether the presence of SMI is associated with an increased risk of developing either depression or dementia.

(b) To estimate the usefulness of SMI as a screening test for dementia and depression.

Method

Screening interviews

A population register of elderly subjects in one Inner London electoral ward was established. Eighty-seven per cent of all elderly residents were studied. A total of 705 residents over the age of 65 years and living in their own home were screened for the presence of objective memory disorder, depression, activity limitation and SMI in 1988. Of these, 524 were screened again in 1990.

The screening instrument used, the short-CARE, is the shortened version of the Comprehensive Assessment and Referral Evaluation (CARE; Gurland *et al*, 1994). This is a semi-structured interview containing indicator scales that suggest likely depression, dementia, subjective memory complaint, activity limitation, sleep disorder and somatic symptoms. The reliability and validity of the interview and its six indicator scales have been established. The indicator scales for depression and organic brain syndrome have been further refined to become depression and dementia diagnostic scales which detect cases of pervasive depression or dementia, at a severity at which a clinician would intervene.

For the SMI scale, items were derived by factor analysis of data derived from a large community sample in a separate study from the one described in this paper. The cut-off point of the SMI scale was validated in a community sample with the criterion of clinicians' judgement that subject's concern about memory constituted a significant problem for the person.

The SMI consists of the following nine items relating to the subjective perception of memory difficulty, following an initial probe as to whether or not the subject has experienced in this sphere:

(a)   Claims difficulty with memory.

(b)   Forgets what he or she has read or heard.

(c)   Forgets names of family or close friends.

(d)   Forgets where he/she has placed things.

(e)   Forgets safety precautions.

(f)   Cannot recall the right words.

(g)   Says impaired memory is a problem for him/her.

(h)   Is embarrassed by memory problem.

(i)   Has to make a greater effort to remember things.

Each positive response is given a score of one point. Previous work has shown that a score of three and above indicates the presence of SMI for the purpose of this study.

Diagnostic follow-up

The assessments performed were:

(a)   The Geriatric Mental State–A (GMS–A).

(b)   The History and Aetiology schedule (HAS).

(c)   The Cognitive Assessment schedule of the Cambridge Mental Disorders of the Elderly Examination (the CAMCOG of the CAMDEX).

The GMS–A (Copeland et al, 1976) is a standardised, semi-structured interview that allows for the classification of patients by symptom profile. It has an additional computerised diagnostic system, the Automated Geriatric Examination for Computerised Assisted Taxonomy (AGECAT; Copeland et al, 1986), which enables various levels of confidence to be achieved for seven diagnostic categories, including depression and organic states. For the purposes of this study diagnoses were generated both by the GMS–AGECAT programme and by a clinical interview. The HAS is a semi-structured interview schedule which complements the GMS and is a standardised means of collecting relevant information which would normally be obtained by clinical history-taking. The CAMDEX (Roth et al, 1986) is a standardised instrument for the diagnosis of mental disorders in the elderly which has three subsections, one of which, the CAMCOG, consists of a range of objective cognitive tests which constitute a neuropsychological battery.

Procedure for study

Subjects were visited at home, where the short-CARE, including the SMI scale, was administered. The same interviewer saw the subjects for initial and follow-up interviews. Each set of initial interviews was conducted over a nine-month period. There was a six-to nine-month interval between screening and diagnostic follow-up. The GMS–A, HAS and CAMCOG interviews were conducted during one visit by a psychiatrist who had been trained in the use of the interview schedules.

Data analysis

Analysis was carried out using the Statistical Package for the Social Sciences. Between-group comparisons were carried out using t-tests for parametric data. χ^2 tests (with Yates' correction where appropriate) were used for non-parametric comparisons and Fisher's exact test for categorical data. Multivariate Logistic Regression was used to evaluate whether future depression or dementia after two years was predicted by individual SMI items and demographic variables and items from the short-CARE were also included as dependant variables in this regression analysis. All confidence intervals are 95% confidence intervals (CI).

Background results

Characteristics of population at screening in 1988 and 1990

In 1988, the age of the population ranged between 65 and 98 years. The mean age was 74.59 years (s.d.=6.55). Using standard diagnostic instruments, 4.9% were classed as having dementia and 15.9% as having depression.

In 1990, 524 (74%) of the 705 were re-interviewed: 199 (17%) had died and 62 (9%) had either moved or refused interview. The mean age of the re-screened population was 76.01 years (s.d.=6.22). Of the remaining population 6.1% were classed as having dementia and 16% had depression.

Results of the study

SMI in 1988 and 1990

Fig. 1 shows the classification of the population according to short-CARE scales in terms of dementia, depression and SMI. The prevalence rate of SMI was 25% in 1988 and 27% in 1990. On both occasions there was a positive association between SMI and dementia and depression. The increased risk was

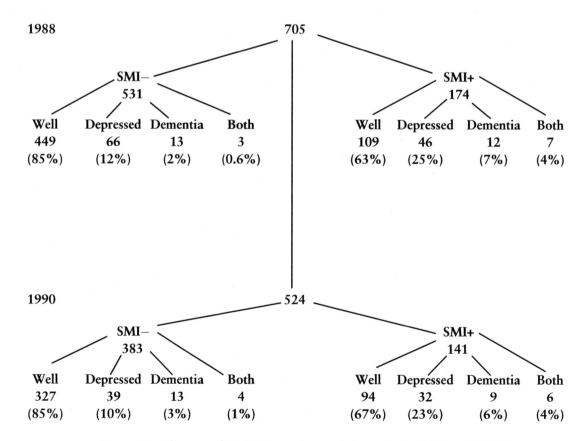

Fig. 1 Distribution of SMI, depression and dementia in 1988 and 1990

calculated using odds ratios as follows:

    (a)   Dementia: 1988, 3.95 (95% CI 1.09–8.28); 1990, 2.6 (95% CI 1.19–5.66).

    (b)   Depression: 1988, 2.85 (95% CI 1.85–4.36); 1990, 2.92 (95% CI 1.74–3.89).

On both occasions the majority of subjects with SMI, 63 and 67% respectively, received neither diagnosis.

Outcome of SMI

Fig. 2 shows the diagnostic status of those free of depression and dementia in 1988 subdivided according to SMI status, who were re-interviewed in 1990. There were 84 who reported SMI and 349 who did not. The majority (79%) of those with SMI in 1988 either had maintained similar complaints or had lost them. They were considered well. Eleven of those with SMI (13%) were diagnosed as depressed and six (7%) were diagnosed as suffering from dementia with one subject (1.2%) with both diagnoses. These figures compared with 21 (6%), three (0.9%) and three (0.9%) for dementia, depression and both disorders respectively, arising from those who were without SMI in 1988. Forty-two out of 349 (12%) of the population reported SMI for the first time in 1990. The odds ratios for developing dementia and depression on follow-up for subjects with SMI in 1988 compared with those without SMI were calculated as 4.26 (95% CI 1.63–13.20) and 2.16 (95% CI 0.97–4.74) respectively

SMI items as predictors of dementia and depression

The nine SMI items were analysed with univariate comparisons in order to assess whether any particular SMI question predicted dementia or depression in a population free of these conditions. A total of 433 subjects were included (the 524 followed up, less those with depression or dementia in 1988). Items 2 and 7 were strongly associated with developing future dementia: 'forgetting what they have read or heard' (odds ratio=5.33, 95% CI 1.15–49.7, $P<0.02$) and 'claiming that their memory posed a significant problem for them' (odds ratio=4.25, 98% CI 1.33–13.7, $P<0.001$). A second analysis, using multivariate

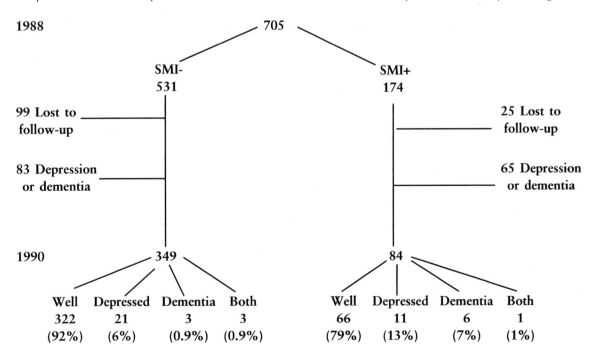

Fig. 2 Outcome of those screened for SMI

logistic regression in order to ascertain whether these effects were independent, was then carried out. The same items were found to have a significant effect for predicting dementia. The only item to predict depression at a significant level was Item 8 'being embarrassed by their perceived memory problem' (odds ratio = 4.06, 98% CI 1.70–9.72, $P < 0.01$).

The SMI scale was tested in this population for its efficacy as a screen for dementia at the cut-point 3/4. The sensitivity was 50% and specificity 84% but positive predictive value (PPV) was 17%. Optimal PPV was 25% at a cut-off point of 4/5, but with a loss of sensitivity (41%). Items 2 and 7 were tested alone as a screen and were shown to have a PPV of 40% with specificity of 97% but sensitivity of 28% if both items were given a positive response. As a screen for depression the SMI scale performed with optimal sensitivity and specificity to a cut-off point of 2/3–40% and 79% respectively, with a PPV of 26%. PPV could be increased to 40% at a cut-off point of 4/5, but with loss of sensitivity to 26%.

Please write your answers to questions I to VIII in the spaces provided.

SECTION I

Validity of the study

I.   (a) Selection

(i)   Was the duration of the symptoms of SMI well defined?   [3 marks]

....

....

....

(ii)   Were subjects assessed at a similar time with regard to their SMI symptoms?   [3 marks]

....

....

....

(iii)   Was the selection of patients taking part in the study a representative sample of the
        population?   [3 marks]

....

....

....

(b)   Follow-up

(i)   Not all the patients were seen for follow-up. How far do you believe this affects the validity
        of the results?   [3 marks]

....

....

....

(ii)   Were the outcome measures objective? Give two reasons to explain your
        reasoning.   [3 marks]

....

....

(iii)   Did the authors omit any potentially important prognostic factors?   [3 marks]

....

....

....

(c)   Statistical Analysis

(i)   What does a 95% confidence interval (CI) mean?   [4 marks]

....
....
....
....

(iii) If a 95% CI of an odds ratio contains the number 1.0, what does this mean?   [3 marks]

....
....
....

Importance of the study

2.   Are the results that are valid of the study of outcome of SMI clinically important?
     Judge, with particular reference to the statistics, the likely risk of future dementia
     or depression.   [10 marks]

....
....
....
....
....
....
....

Further questions

3.   If you were to use the SMI with a cut-off score of 3/4, what proportion
     of patients with dementia would you currently identify? Show how you arrive
     at your result.   [5 marks]

....
....
....
....

4.   What proportion of those without dementia test positive for it on the SMI at a cut-off score
     of 3/4? Show how you arrive at your result.   [5 marks]

....
....
....
....

5.   Define positive predictive value (PPV).   [5 marks]

....
....
....
....

6.   Is the PPV likely to be smaller or greater in patients in hospital?   [5 marks]

....
....
....
....

Summary of the study

7.   What do you consider to be the five main findings of this study?   [25 marks]

(i) ....
....
....
....
(ii) ....
....
....
....
(iii) ....
....
....
....
(iv) ....
....
....
....
(v) ....
....
....
....

Clinical implications

8. Are the results that are valid of the SMI scale of clinical value in its proposed use as a screening instrument? Indicate, from the results of this study, how far the SMI scale is likely to be of value in caring for your elderly patients. How would you use the SMI scale in practice? [10 marks]

....
....
....
....
....
....
....
....
....
....

[Total: 90 marks]

Please write your answers to questions I to IV in the spaces provided.

SECTION 2

Question I

Your surgical colleagues are trying to identify elderly patients with dementia who seem to do worse following operations and are more likely to develop acute confusional states. They ask you if there is a quick and easy way of identifying elderly patients who have dementia.

You agree to help them, and find a study which investigates the usefulness of the Mini-Mental State Examination (MMSE) in detecting dementia among elderly patients living in the community.

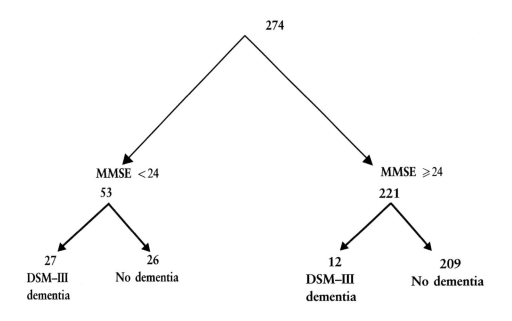

You decide that the paper is methodologically adequate and you decide to see if the MMSE would be a useful screening test for your surgical colleagues.

I.(a) What proportion of patients classed as cognitively impaired by the MMSE really have dementia?   [2 marks]

....
....
....
....

I.(b) What is this measure called?   [2 marks]

....
....
....
....

1.(c) What proportion of patients classed as cognitively unimpaired by the MMSE really do not have dementia? [2 marks]

....
....
....
....

1.(d) What is this measure called? [2 marks]

....
....
....
....

1.(e) How would you interpret these findings clinically? [4 marks]

....
....
....
....

Question 2

After a 'quick and dirty' survey of the surgical wards, you find that the prevalence of dementia among the over six-year-olds on the surgical wards is actually 40%.

2.(a) In the study, what is the prevalence of dementia? [2 marks]

....
....
....
....

2.(b) What difference does this make to the use of the test on the surgical ward? [3 marks]

....
....
....
....

Question 3

You know that there are two characteristics of the test which you can assume will be constant and would enable you to use the results of this study on the surgical ward. These are the sensitivity and the specificity of the test.

In this study, the sensitivity of the test is 27/39=69% and the specificity is 209/235=89%.

3.(a) How would you explain to the surgeons what the sensitivity represents?   [3 marks]

....
....
....
....

3.(b) What about the specificity?   [3 marks]

....
....
....
....

3.(c) What measure can be produced using these test characteristics to allow you to use the findings in a clinical setting where there was a different prevalence of dementia? [3 marks]

....
....
....
....

3.(d) Calculate this measure.   [3 marks]

....
....
....
....

3.(e) How would you use this measure to help the surgeons decide if someone was likely to have dementia?   [5 marks]

....
....
....
....

3.(f) The surgeons would find it difficult to begin to calculate pre-test odds at the bedside — is there anyway to avoid having to do this? [10 marks]

....
....
....
....

Question 4

The surgeons decide that they want a test which will detect more of the subjects with dementia.

4.(a) How might you achieve this using the MMSE? [3 marks]

....
....
....
....

4.(b) What would happen to the specificity? [3 marks]

....
....
....
....

[Total: 50 marks]

Validity of the study

1. (a) Selection

(i) Was the duration of the symptoms of SMI well defined?

There is no mention that the phase or duration of the SMI were assessed.

(ii) Were subjects assessed at a similar time with regard to their SMI symptoms?

We do not know if the phase of SMI was uniform — not assessed. The interval of 6–9 months between screening and further study reported here may have allowed some respondents to change their mental state.

(iii) Was the selection of patients taking part in the study a representative sample of the population?

The subjects were visited at home, thus avoiding the bias inherent in studies of SMI subjects in memory clinics or hospital populations. But only 87% of community sample was initially screened.

(b) Follow-up

(i) Not all the patients were seen for follow-up. How far do you believe this affects the validity of the result?

There was an attrition or response bias with 7% who had either moved or refused to be interviewed and 17% who had died at the second screening. This degree of drop-out is small and deaths in this population are likely. The follow-up period was only two years. A longer period may have revealed greater predictive value but greater attrition. As it is the attrition rate that largely affects the validity, and this was small, the result can be validly applied to a larger sample.

(ii) Were the outcome measures objective? Give the two reasons to explain your reasoning.

The main findings depend on the validity of the short-CARE classification for dementia and depression, and also on the independence of the SMI scale from the depression and dementia scales. The interview was standardised and psychometric testing served to minimise observer bias.

(iii) Did the authors omit any potentially important prognostic factors?

Additional prognostic factors were not discussed. Were some people with SMI treated with antidepressants?

(c) Statistical analysis

(i) What does a 95% confidence interval (CI) mean?

If a series of identical studies was carried out repeatedly on different samples from the same population and a 95% CI for the odds ratio calculated in each study, then, in the long run, 95% of these CIs would include the true population.

Alternatively, there is a one in 20 chance that a similar study carried out in a similar population would produce results within this range.

(ii) If a 95% CI of an odds ratio contains the number 1.0, what does this mean?

The odds ratio is not significant.

Importance of the study

2. Are the results that are valid of the study of outcome of SMI clinically important? Judge, with particular reference to the statistics, the likely risk of future dementia or depression.

SMI is not entirely benign. Twenty-one per cent of subjects with SMI alone identified at the first screen, went on to develop detectable psychopathology, either depression or dementia.

The prognostic estimates are not that precise, with wide CIs. Moreover the lower limit of the CI for depression falls below one, so the study does not show a definite association.

3. If you were to use the SMI with a cut-off score of 3/4, what proportion of patients with dementia would you currently identify?

Fifty per cent. This is because the sensitivity of the instrument at cut-off point 3/4 is 50%.

4. What proportion of those without dementia test positive for it on the SMI at a cut-off score of 3/4? Show how you arrive at your result.

16%, 1 — specificity. The specificity of the instrument at cut-off point 3/4 is 84%. (Therefore 100%–84% do not have dementia when this screening level is used).

5. Define positive predictive value (PPV).

PPV is the proportion of screening test positives who have the target disorder.

6. Is the PPV likely to be smaller or greater in patients in hospital?

Greater. It depends on the pre-test prevalence of the disorder which differs between community and hospital populations. Patients in hospitals are likely to have a higher prevalence of subclinical depression and dementia and so PPV will be greater.

Summary of the study

7. What do you consider to be the five main findings of this study?

The five main findings:

(a) SMI is common and occurs in one in four of people over the age of 65 years.
(b) Subjects with SMI are significantly more likely to be suffering from dementia or depression than those without the complaint.
(c) Nonetheless, 60% of subjects with SMI do not have evidence of these disorders.
(d) When followed up over two years, subjects with SMI were found to be at four-fold greater risk of developing future dementia, and two-fold greater risk of developing a depression compared with those without SMI.
(e) The SMI scale was not found to be useful as a population screen for dementia or depression, although two of the nine items might have value as screening questions in clinical circumstances to determine those with memory complaints at risk for dementia.
(f) Five per cent of elderly subjects had dementia and 16% depression on short-CARE assessment.

Clinical implications

8. Are the results that are valid of the SMI scale of clinical value in its proposed use as a screening instrument? Indicate, from the results of this study, how far the SMI scale is likely to be of value in caring for your elderly patients. How would you use the SMI scale in practice?

The SMI scale is not particularly useful because the predictive values both for dementia and depression are low. Optimising them to 25% for dementia or to 40% for depression caused loss of sensitivity in each case. Two items on the short-CARE Assessment were strongly associated with a diagnosis of dementia, and if both these items were positive it was highly likely that the person with these complaints had a dementing illness. Likewise, one item on the short-CARE assessment was strongly associated with a diagnosis of depression. These three items may therefore be clinically useful, and should be re-tested in a new population to establish their predictive validity.

Although 60% of subjects with SMI do not have evidence of dementia or depression at two year follow-up, there is a four-fold greater risk of developing dementia and a 2.5 times greater risk of developing depression, compared with those without SMI. Therefore, clinical assessment for dementia and depression is important in patients with SMI.

If the whole scale is used, the specificity of 84% at the cut-point 3/4 is high enough to rule in the diagnoses of depression or dementia, but the sensitivity of 50% is too low to rule these diagnoses out with confidence. Therefore, consider further assessment — questionnaires or clinical or both.

Question 1

Your surgical colleagues are trying to identify elderly patients with dementia who seem to do worse following operations and are more likely to develop acute confusional states. They ask you if there is a quick and easy way of identifying elderly patients who have dementia.

You agree to help them and find a study which investigates the usefulness of the Mini-Mental State Examination (MMSE) in detecting dementia among elderly patients living in the community.

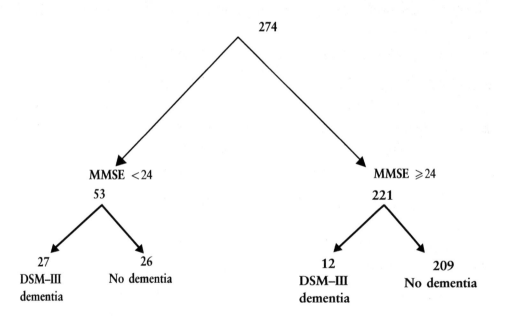

You decide that the paper is methodologically adequate and you decide to see if the MMSE would be a useful screening test for your surgical colleagues.

1.(a) What proportion of patients classed as cognitively impaired by the MMSE really have dementia?

27/53=51%.

1.(b) What is this measure called?

Positive predictive value.

1.(c) What proportion of patients classed as cognitively unimpaired by the MMSE really do not have dementia?

209/221=95%.

1.(d) What is this measure called?

Negative predictive value.

1.(e) How would you interpret these findings clinically?

If a patient scores less than 24 on the MMSE, they have about a 50% chance of having dementia. If a patient scores 24 or more on the MMSE, they have a 95% chance of not having dementia. The test is better at excluding dementia than it is at confirming it.

Question 2

After a 'quick and dirty' survey of the surgical wards, you find that the prevalence of dementia among the over 65-year olds on the surgical ward is actually 40%.

2.(a) In the study, what is the prevalence of dementia?

(27+12)/274=14%

2.(b) What difference does this make to the use of the test on the surgical ward?

It means that, when used on the surgical ward, the positive predictive value will be higher and the negative predictive value will be lower than those found in the study.

Question 3

You know that there are two characteristics of the test which you can assume will be constant and would enable you to use the results of this study on the surgical ward. These are the sensitivity and the specificity of the test.

In this study, the sensitivity of the test is 27/39=69% and the specificity is 209/235=89%.

3.(a) How would you explain to the surgeons what the sensitivity represents?

The sensitivity is the proportion of patients who really are cognitively impaired who score positive on the MMSE.

3.(b) *What about the specificity?*

The specificity is the proportion of patients who really do not have cognitive impairment who score negative on the test.

3.(c) *What measure can be produced using these test characteristics to allow you to use the findings in a clinical setting where there was a different prevalence of dementia?*

The likelihood ratio – this is the likelihood that a positive test result will be observed in a patient with, as opposed to one without, the disorder.

3.(d) *Calculate this measure*

Sensitivity/(1 – specificity) = 6.3

3.(e) *How would you use this measure to help the surgeons decide if someone was likely to have dementia?*

The likelihood ratio can be multiplied by the pre-test odds to produce the post-test odds, and hence the post-test probability of having dementia.

6.3 × 0.7 = 4.4

4.4/5.4 = 81%

3.(f) *The surgeons would find it difficult to begin to calculate pre-test odds at the bedside – is there anyway to avoid having to do this?*

A nomogram can be used. Anchor a straight line on the left hand axis of the nomogram at the appropriate pre-test probability. Continue the line through the central line at the value of the likelihood ratio (about six). The appropriate post-test probability can then be read directly off the right hand axis:

Question 4

The surgeons decide that they want a test which will detect more of the subjects with dementia.

4.(a) *How might you achieve this using the MMSE?*

Using a higher cut-point on the MMSE (i.e. 25 or 26) would detect more of the patients who had dementia.

4. (b) *What would happen to the specificity?*

The specificity would fall – that is there would be more false positives. The sensitivity and specificity work against each other – as one gets better, the other gets worse.

Critical Review paper – Sample paper (45 minutes)

Read the following abridged paper carefully and then answer questions I to V at the end of the paper.

Dr Kurt Schneider, the pioneering German psychiatrist, stated that certain psychotic symptoms were found in schizophrenia. He categorised these symptoms in order of importance and listed eleven of these symptoms as 'first-rank'. In the absence of an organic psychosis he believed that these first-rank symptoms were characteristic of schizophrenia and their presence made other diagnoses unlikely, although he added that they were in no way fundamental to that disorder and that schizophrenia could be diagnosed in their absence.

In a study of Schneiderian first-rank symptoms (O'Grady, 1990) a symptom questionnaire was devised specifically for the study to elicit first-rank symptoms at interview. Research Diagnostic Criteria (RDC) were used as the 'gold standard' for diagnosis. The sample was representative of people admitted to an acute general psychiatry admission unit at Newcastle, and comprised 59 women and 40 men. Of 105 patients eligible for inclusion, three refused to be interviewed and three interviews were unsuitable for research purposes. In these six cases there was no evidence of first-rank symptoms from interview or scrutiny of case notes.

The definition of first-rank symptoms has given rise to controversy. Koehler in 1979 showed that first-rank symptoms were described differently by different authors. He believed that each first-rank symptom could be viewed as a continuum according to whether it was defined in a narrow or wide fashion. Mellor *et al* (1981) have shown that when narrow definitions of such symptoms were employed the diagnosis of schizophrenia remained stable in 88% of subjects with these symptoms over an 11-year period.

O'Grady therefore believed it would be useful to examine the relationship between the presence or absence of first-rank symptoms defined according to narrowly described stringent criteria compared to wider-ranging definitions. Thus, for the symptom of third-person auditory hallucinations the narrow definition is confined to voices heard outside the head whereas the wider definition also includes voices heard inside the subject's head or mind. All core Schneiderian first-rank symptoms were similarly defined according to narrow and wide criteria employed by Koehler.

The most common first-rank symptom found in the investigation was third-person auditory hallucinations, found in eight of the patients. No subject was found who had a delusional perception. Passivity experiences were rare.

The table below shows the relationship between RDC diagnosis and first-rank symptoms (FRS).

References

Koehler, K. (1979) First-rank symptoms of schizophrenia: questions concerning clinical boundaries. *British Journal of Psychiatry*, **134**, 236–248.

Mellor, C. S., Sims, A. C. P. & Cope, R. V. (1981) Changes of diagnosis in schizophrenia and first-rank symptoms: an eight year follow-up. *Comprehensive Psychiatry*, **22**, 184–188.

O'Grady, J. C. (1990) The prevalence and diagnostic significance of Schneiderian first-rank symptoms in a random sample of acute psychiatric in-patients. *British Journal of Psychiatry*, **156**, 496–500.

Critical Reviews in Psychiatry

Number of patients in different Research Diagnostic Criteria categories with Schneiderian first-rank symptoms (FRS)

RDC diagnosis	Number of patients		
	Total	With narrow FRS	With only wide FRS
Schizophrenia	15	11	0
Schizo-affective depressed	5	2	1
Schizo-affected manic	1	0	0
Mania	12	0	0
Depressive disorder	46	0	2
Other	20	0	0
Total	99	13	3

The following questions all deal with the possible diagnostic importance of first-rank symptoms for schizophrenia as opposed to other diagnoses. Unless otherwise indicated, answer the questions according to the narrow definition of first-rank symptoms.

1.(a) Define sensitivity, specificity and positive predictive value. [5% of marks]
  (b) What are the sensitivity, specificity and positive predictive value of first-rank symptoms for schizophrenia in this sample? [10% of marks]
  (c) In this sample of acute admissions who received the symptom questionnaire, what is the prevalence of schizophrenia? [5% of marks]

2.(a) What is the likelihood in this sample of:
    (i) a patient who has schizophrenia having a first-rank symptom (i.e. what proportion of those with schizophrenia have a first rank symptom)?;
    (ii) a patient who does not have schizophrenia having a first-rank symptom? [10% of marks]
  (b) (i) Define the likelihood ratio. What is it for the present data? [10% of marks]
    (ii) How can this result be interpreted in diagnosing schizophrenia in this sample? [10% of marks]

3(a) How far would you expect the results indicated above to differ if the sample was taken from the community rather than from in-patient admissions? In particular, indicate how far the different prevalence of schizophrenia within a community sample would affect the value of the presence or absence of first-rank symptoms as a diagnostic pointer towards schizophrenia [15% of marks]
  (b) What would be the approximate positive predictive value of the presence of first-rank symptoms in such a community sample? [5% of marks]

4. If you were designing a similar study to examine the value of first-rank symptoms in the diagnosis of schizophrenia, what modifications would you make to this study? [20% of marks]

5. From the data presented in this paper, indicate how far the presence of first-rank symptoms helps us in determining the relationship of schizo-affective disorder to schizophrenia or to affective disorders. [20% of marks]

Marking scheme for sample paper

The table can be represented in a simple 2 × 2 fashion.

First-rank symptoms	Schizophrenia		
	Present	Absent	Total
Present	11	2	13
Absent	4	82	86
Total	15	84	99

1.(a) Define sensitivity, specificity and positive predictive value.

The sensitivity of a test is the ability of that test to identify a disease when it really is present, that is the proportion identified by the test who actually have the disease.

The specificity of a test is the ability of that test to identify the absence of a disease when the disease really is not present i.e. the proportion identified by the test as not having the disease.

The positive predictive value of a test is the proportion of subjects with positive test results who actually have the disease.

1.(b) What are the sensitivity, specificity and positive predictive value of first-rank symptoms schizophrenia in this sample?

For the study in question – sensitivity is the proportion of the sample with schizophrenia who have first-rank symptoms (11/15=0.73), often expressed as a percentage (73%).

Specificity is the proportion of the sample without schizophrenia who do not have first-rank symptoms (82/84=0.98 or 98%).

Positive predictive value is the proportion of patients with first-rank symptoms who have schizophrenia (11/13=0.85 or 85%).

1.(c) In this sample of acute admissions who received the symptom questionnaire, what is the prevalence of schizophrenia?

The prevalence of schizophrenia is the proportion of the total sample diagnosed as having schizophrenia (15/99=15%).

2.(a)(i) What is the likelihood in this sample of a patient who has schizophrenia having a first-rank symptom (i.e. what proportion of those with schizophrenia have a first rank symptom)?

The likelihood of a subject with schizophrenia having a first-rank symptom is 11/15 or 73% (i.e. the sensitivity).

2.(a)(ii) A patient who does not have schizophrenia having a first-rank symptom?

The likelihood of a subject without schizophrenia having a first-rank symptom is $2 \div 84$ (i.e. $1 -$ specificity).

2.(b)(i) Define the likelihood ratio. What is it for the present data?

The likelihood ratio is the ratio of the likelihood of first-rank symptoms being present given the diagnosis of schizophrenia to the likelihood of first-rank symptoms given the diagnosis is not schizophrenia. Using the table, this is $(11/15)/(2/84) = 30.8$ (using sensitivity and specificity as integer percentages as above, the result comes to 36.5).

(ii) How can this result be interpreted in diagnosing schizophrenia in this sample?

The magnitude of this likelihood ratio is high, mainly because of the results showing that only two patients had first-rank symptoms in the absence of schizophrenia. The test is therefore highly specific, indicating that a positive result rules in the diagnosis (sometimes termed SpPin).

3.(a) How far would you expect the results indicated above to differ if the sample was taken from the community rather than from in-patient admissions? In particular, indicate how far the different prevalence of schizophrenia within a community sample would affect the value of the presence or absence of first-rank symptoms as a diagnostic pointer towards schizophrenia.

It is usually assumed that the sensitivity and specificity of a diagnostic test (as this is) are independent of the prevalence of the underlying disorder. The likelihood ratio depends only on these, and will therefore also remain constant. However, the positive predictive value of the test depends on the prevalence of the disorder. In this case, the prevalence of schizophrenia in the sample was 15%. In the community the prevalence of schizophrenia would be much lower and so the predictive value of first-rank symptoms would be lower.

3.(b) What would be the approximate positive predictive value of the presence of first-rank symptoms in such a community sample?

In the community, the point prevalence of schizophrenia is expected to be between 0.1 and 0.5%. In a sample of 1000 people in the community with a prevalence of schizophrenia of 0.5%, the equivalent figures in the above table become the following.

First-risk symptoms	Schizophrenia		
	Present	Absent	Total
Present	4	20	24
Absent	1	975	976
Total	5	995	1000

This gives a positive predictive value of only 0.16 or 16%. This indicates that the presence of first-rank symptoms in the community is of little value in diagnosing schizophrenia, but their presence in an acute admission is closely linked with schizophrenia.

(This is not the only correct answer to the problem posed. A good candidate could point out that it is unrewarding to search for a rare diagnosis of schizophrenia in a completely random community sample. For instance, a sample of patients attending a general practitioner's surgery is likely to have a much greater proportion of people with schizophrenia than a random community sample and yet could quite justifiably be considered a community sample. Answers that estimate the prevalence of schizophrenia as between 0.5% and 5%, depending on how the community sample is defined, would give a positive predictive value of between 16 and 62%. Marks should be awarded based on the calculation indicated above, not just on the absolute figure given.)

4. If you were designing a similar study to examine the value of first-rank symptoms in the diagnosis of schizophrenia, what modifications would you make to this study?

The value of examining the presence or absence of first-rank symptoms in the diagnosis of schizophrenia depends on the population studied. A study would be most valuable in a newly-admitted group of patients with psychosis. Ideally, a larger number of subjects should be used. It would also be helpful to find out which first-rank symptoms were most predictive of schizophrenia. Diagnostic ratings should be made by a separate investigator than the one examining for the presence or absence of first-rank symptoms. The study should also follow patients up long enough to confirm the diagnosis of schizophrenia (remember that DSM–IV, for example, requires some symptoms to have been present for at least six months to make a confident diagnosis of schizophrenia).

5. From the data presented in this paper, indicate how far the presence of first-rank symptoms helps us in determining the relationship of schizo-affective disorder to schizophrenia or to affective disorders.

The figures indicated in this study, although small (which should be mentioned) suggest that schizo-affective depressive disorder is closer to the diagnostic entity of schizophrenia than to bipolar affective disorder. The presence of first-rank symptoms in schizo-affective illness may be a pointer to a course and prognosis that is similar to that in schizophrenia and this is suggested by outcome studies and what we know of the genetics of schizo-depressive disorder. Nevertheless, the value of first-rank symptoms in schizo-affective disorder cannot be categorically stated from the information presented here as the numbers are so small.

Appendix 3 – Original papers

Health of the Nation Outcome Scales (HoNOS)

Research and development

J. K. WING, A. S. BEEVOR, R. H. CURTIS, S. B. G. PARK, S. HADDEN and A. BURNS

Background An instrument was required to quantify and thus potentially measure progress towards a Health of the Nation target, set by the Department of Health, "to improve significantly the health and social functioning of mentally ill people".

Method A first draft was created in consultation with experts and on the basis of literature review. This version was improved during four stages of testing: two preliminary stages, a large field trial involving 2706 patients (rated by 492 clinicians) and tests of the final Health of the Nation Outcome Scales (HoNOS), which included an independent study (*n*=197) of reliability and relationship to other instruments.

Results The resulting 12-item instrument is simple to use, covers clinical problems and social functioning with reasonable adequacy, has been generally acceptable to clinicians who have used it, is sensitive to change or the lack of it, showed good reliability in independent trials and compared reasonably well with equivalent items in the Brief Psychiatric Rating Scales and Role Functioning Scales.

Conclusions The key test for HoNOS is that clinicians should want to use it for their own purposes. In general, it has passed that test. A further possibility, that HoNOS data collected routinely as part of a minimum data set, for example for the Care Programme Approach, could also be useful in anonymised and aggregated form for public health purposes, is therefore testable but has not yet been tested.

The Government White Paper *Health of the Nation* (Department of Health, 1992, 1993) identified five key areas, one of which was mental health, where priority should be given to the development of local strategies for reducing mortality and morbidity. One of the mental health targets was "to improve significantly the health and social functioning of mentally ill people". This could be expressed either in terms of clinical and social improvement or by maintenance of an optimal functional state by preventing, slowing and/or mitigating deterioration. In an optimal functional state people with disabilities are able to function, if they wish to do so, reasonably close to the peak of their intact abilities. This is also close to the concept of 'optimal functional autonomy'. In order to set a quantified target and to measure how far it was being met, a dedicated instrument would be needed that could be used routinely, within the context of other necessary information, in the National Health Service (NHS).

PLAN OF DEVELOPMENT

To be useful to clinicians, the instrument would need to be brief enough for routine use by keyworkers, cover common clinical problems and social functioning, be sensitive to change or lack of it and have known reliability and relationship to more established scales. If successful, Health of the Nation Outcome Scales (HoNOS) data could be used as part of a minimum data set containing information on diagnosis, treatment, settings and background population, within which the indicators could be properly interpreted, comparing like with like. The creation of this essential context was not, however, part of the remit of this study.

Reviews of the literature revealed a huge number of scales but none met the chief criterion, which was that they must be brief enough for routine use across the country while also covering the clinical and social range required. A first mock-up was therefore created, with the help of consultants, and tested and modified during four phases of development (Table 1).

TWO PILOT PHASES

HoNOS-1 was a 20-item instrument, drafted with the help of consultants and covering four key areas of functioning: behaviour, impairment, symptoms and social functioning. Item 20 was a global (0–100) disability score. This version was tested during a first pilot study (*n*=152) to discover how it performed in terms of clinical acceptability, simple structure and sensitivity to change. The results were satisfactory. In the light of comments from users it was shortened to 12 items, each rated on a 0–4 scale of severity. HoNOS-2 was then tested again (*n*=100) with results closely similar to those of the first pilot. HoNOS-3 (see Table 2), used in the main field trials, reflected the lessons learned. A glossary based on this experience was provided containing a definition at each rating point on each of the 12 items. A set of answers to common questions raised by raters and a description of the basic rationale and methods of using the system was included.

FIELD TRIALS – HoNOS-3

Large-scale trials were needed in order thoroughly to test feasibility and clinical acceptability and establish a substantial base of data from ratings made by clinicians as part of their everyday work. The community teams taking part were recruited partly from those already involved in the first two stages, partly by contacts through the Royal College of Psychiatrists' Research Unit (CRU), which holds a list of district audit convenors, and partly from volunteers who had heard of the HoNOS projects. A choice was made on the basis of contrasting service and staffing patterns, geography and socio-demographic indices. District rankings on the Jarman index of social deprivation (Jarman & Hirsch, 1992), for example, ranged from 8 to 188 out of the total 192 districts.

The task in each area was routinely to collect HoNOS data on a consecutive series of up to 200 patients (T1), and to follow as many as possible for at least three months

Table I HoNOS project: phases of development

Phase of work (Dates)	1. Start-up (Sep. 92–Mar. 93)	2. Pilot tests (Apr. 93–Dec. 93)		3. Field trials (Jan. 94–Mar. 95)	4. Reliability/comparisons (Apr. 95–Sep. 95)
Version of HoNOS	–	HoNOS-1	HoNOS-2	HoNOS-3	Final HoNOS
Sites (n)	–	9	7	25	2 (main)
					4 (supplementary)
Patients (n)	–	152	100	2706	Reliability 293+188
					Comparisons 166+107
Nature of work	Literature search	Acceptability		Acceptability	Acceptability
	Consultation	Structure		Structure	Structure
	Design of trials	Sensitivity		Sensitivity	Sensitivity
				Reliability	Reliability
				Profiles	Comparisons
					Profiles

or to the end of the episode of contact, if earlier (T2). Local supervisors and coordinators were trained on-site. Completed score sheets were returned to the CRU for checking and recording before being forwarded in batches for data entry.

The statistical analyses were based on data from the charts and score sheets of 2706 patients from 25 sites. Of these, 1678 were rated on a second occasion (872 by the same rater on both occasions and 806 by a different rater on the second occasion), making 4380 sets of data in all. The same issues (clinical acceptability, simple structure and sensitivity to change) were studied as in the pilots but the larger numbers allowed more complexity in analysis. Checks were made on the proportions of missing item values. For example, of the 872 same-rater pairs, 6.4% contained missing data in at least one item. There was little effect on the histograms of distributions or on the means. The analysis for different-rater pairs gave similar results.

Analysis of HoNOS-3 structure

It was intended that, in a 12-item instrument covering a broad socio-clinical area, each item should be informative. High internal consistency was not sought. The 12×12 item matrix was satisfactory in this respect in that it showed only three correlations with values of 0.30 or higher. The four sub-scores (A–D) were no more intercorrelated (0.08–0.25) than the individual items. The correlations between A–D sub-scores and the total score were 0.62, 0.45, 0.63 and 0.72. The equivalents for the global score were 0.06, 0.37, 0.33 and 0.28. Principal components analysis of

data at T1 with varimax rotation gave five factors accounting for 63% of the variance. These were fairly close to the grouping into sections A–D adopted on clinical grounds.

The relationship between ratings of severity on individual items and the total score (ratings on items 1–11 summed) is important if a single indicator of severity is to be derived. Table 3 shows data derived

from HoNOS-3 and also provides results from a subsequent check using the final HoNOS. The index is based on the fact that each item rating represents a clinical judgement of severity: the more zeros there are, the less the severity; the more fours the greater the severity; and *pro rata* in between. The threshold for the highest level in the hierarchy shown in Table 3 is defined by four or more ratings of four (very severe),

Table 2 HoNOS-3 and the final HoNOS compared (all items scored 0–4)

HoNOS-3 items	Final HoNOS items
Sub-score A: max. 12	Sub-score A: max. 12
1. Aggression	1. Aggression & overactivity
2. Self-harm	2. Self-harm
3. Substance use	3. Substance use
Sub-score B: max. 8	Sub-score B: max. 8
4. Cognition	4. Cognition
5. Physical health	5. Physical health
Sub-score C: max. 12	Sub-score C: max. 12
6. Affective disorders	6. Hallucinations & delusions
7. Psychotic disorders	7. Depression
8. Other symptoms	8. Other symptoms
Sub-score D: max. 12	Sub-score D: max. 16
9. Social relations	9. Social relations
10. Housing	10. General functioning
11. Activities	11. Housing
12. —	12. Activities
Total score: max. 44	Total score 1–12: max. 48
Global score (0–100)	Total score 1–10: max. 40[1]

1. If relevant social information is not available, items 11 and 12 should be omitted from the total score and Total 1–10 used instead.

Table 3 Item severity ratings at Time I by total scores: HoNOS-3 and final HoNOS

Minimal value	HoNOS-3		Final HoNOS	
	Mean=9.86	n=2612	Mean=9.98	n=641
4 or more 4s	24.2	41	22.5	6
3 × 4s	19.5	44	20.4	16
2 × 4s	16.2	148	16.6	47
I × 4	12.4	487	13.8	99
4 or more 3s	17.9	57	17.7	27
3 × 3s	14.7	103	13.7	24
2 × 3s	11.8	263	10.9	71
I × 3s	8.8	573	8.1	134
4 or more 2s	10.8	66	10.3	25
3 × 2s	8.4	112	7.9	38
2 × 2s	6.4	205	5.3	55
I × 2	4.7	264	3.5	67
4 or more Is	4.9	54	4.7	3
3 × Is	3.0	51	3.0	6
2 × Is	2.0	63	2.0	6
I × I	1.0	44	1.0	9
only 0s	0.0	37	0.0	9

that is, a score of 16. In fact, other items are rated as well, giving a mean of 24.2. Because of this, there is an acceptable overlap in some of the means shown. Thus, four or more ratings at level three suggest higher total severity than two ratings at level four,

three ratings at level three suggest more severity than one at level four, and so on.

Sensitivity to change

The main field trials provide evidence of change between first and second ratings (T1

and T2) and how far this is supported by the clinical judgement of the rater at T2. Change in individual item scores is indicated by the profiles of means at T1 and T2, shown in Figure 1 for the same and different pairs of raters. Items six, eight and nine have the highest mean ratings on both occasions. The overall pattern of improvement on the second occasion of rating is evident.

Table 4 shows the means for sub-scores A–D, the total score derived from items 1–11 (0–44) and the global item 12 (0–100), at T1 and T2. All means show a substantial and highly significant improvement, whether derived from same- or different-rater pairs. The largest mean change per item is found in the symptom sub-score, followed by behaviour, social functioning, and impairment, in that order. The sub-scores thus provide a degree of prediction about likely change.

Table 4 also shows, what is clear from inspection of Figure 1, that the means from different-rater pairs were all higher at T1 than those from same-rater pairs. A possible reason for the interactions is that, because of the shift system, different-rater pairs constitute 65% of those in acute wards compared with 12% in non-ward settings. This is illustrated in Table 5, which also shows that the higher severity in different-rater pairs at T1 occurs, though to a lesser extent, in non-acute settings as well. A confirmatory factor analysis, carried out separately for short-stay in-patients and others, showed that the underlying latent variable for same-rater pairs remained consistent over the two occasions in both kinds of setting. Changes in sub-scores between T1 and T2 correlated well with changes in total score, whether calculated using same-rater or different-rater pairs. Correlations with the global score were generally low.

To provide a check on the changes in score over time, raters on the second occasion were asked to make a clinical estimate of change during the period between ratings using a scale of 'much better', 'better', 'no change', 'worse' and 'much worse'. Table 6 shows the mean change between total HoNOS scores at T1 and T2 for each of these intervals. A one-way analysis of variance for each type of pair showed a very highly significant relationship for both between the overall outcome estimated by retrospective clinical judgement and the change in total score. Apart from the interval between 'much better' and 'better' for same-rater pairs, all

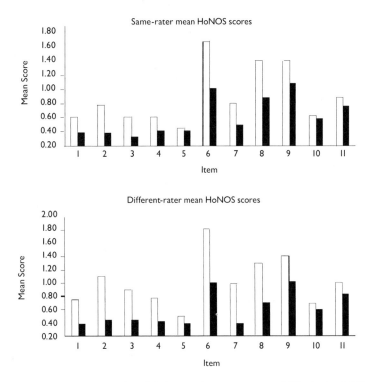

Fig. I Mean scores on items I–II at TI and T2, by type of rater-pair. □, time I (TI); ■, time 2 (T2).

Table 4 HoNOS-3 sub-scores and summary scores at Time 1 and Time 2: by type of rater pairs

Type of score	Same raters[1] (n=871)		Different raters[1] (n=798)	
	T1	T2	T1	T2
A (0–12) Behaviour	1.97	1.08	2.62	1.35
B (0–8) Impairment	1.03	0.83	1.22	0.85
C (0–12) Symptoms	3.92	2.41	4.13	2.23
D (0–12) Social	2.91	2.43	3.04	2.45
Total (0–44)	9.77	6.67	10.96	6.86
Global (0–100)	43.37	33.65	44.37	34.10

1. Numbers vary because of missing data.
All T1-T2 differences are significant (P < 0.001). Difference between same-rater pairs and different-rater pairs: A P < 0.001; total P < 0.001; Interaction: A P < 0.001; B P < 0.013; C P < 0.002; total P < 0.001.

Table 5 Mean total scores at Time 1 and Time 2: by setting and type of rater pair

Time when rated	In-patient less than 3 months		All other patients	
	SRP (n=329)	DRP (n=611)	SRP (n=295)	DRP (n=39)
Time 1	10.93	11.05	8.59	10.28
Time 2	6.88	5.54	6.15	7.49
Improvement T1–T2	4.05	5.51	2.44	2.79

SRP, same-rater pairs; DRP, different-rater pairs.

Table 6 Changes in total score T1–T2, by retrospective judgement

Estimated outcome	Same-rater pairs		Different-rater pairs	
	Mean change	n	Mean change	n
Much better	5.69	156	6.13	193
Better	4.48	327	4.37	331
No change	0.66	194	2.22	155
Worse or much worse	−1.11	45	−2.2	25
Total	3.37	722	4.15	704

mean score changes between the raters' categories are individually significant. Although the second rater was not always blind to the earlier HoNOS ratings, this does lend extra clinical support (particularly in the case of different-rater pairs) for the suggestion that the scales measure change.

Test–retest reliability

Tests of reliability were deferred to the fourth phase of the project since it was necessary to ensure that the information was available for the final version of HoNOS. However, an opportunity to consider test–retest reliability is provided by a comparison of the 212 pairs of ratings made by the same rater on two occasions for which the clinical estimate at T2 was zero (no change). This avoids the usual problems arising from marked changes in patients' item-profiles over time or the rater at T2 being different from the rater at T1. The mean interval for this group was 35.3 days and the gender and diagnostic spread was much the same as for the total series. The intraclass correlation coefficients for items, the total score (sum of items 1–11) and the global score were all between 0.74 and 0.88, except for aggression (0.61).

Rating styles

Nearly all raters were nurses (n=399) or doctors (n=60) and the statistical analysis is

heavily weighted by their data. There were 19 social workers and seven each of psychologists and occupational therapists. It is important to know whether, as separate professions, they have different rating styles and, if so, what the consequences are for the measurement of outcomes. Table 7 shows the mean total HoNOS score for short-stay in-patients and for those in other settings (generally in longer-term contact and the majority not in-patients), according to the profession of the rater.

The difference in mean total score between nurses and doctors rating short-stay in-patients is significant but relatively small (1.8) for acute wards and not significant for longer-term settings. Selective factors, such as duties connected with the Mental Health Act, could be part or all of the explanation. This may also explain part of the high mean total by the few social workers in the acute ward setting. But the comparatively high mean score of social workers in other settings (mostly day centres) is more remarkable. The effect is seen in all four sub-scores (i.e. both clinical and social items) and in both psychotic and affective disorders.

Clinical profiles

If profiles of HoNOS-3 ratings and/or scores did not illustrate associations that have already been clearly demonstrated by other research, the instrument would lose clinical validity. For example, items with the highest mean score should differ predictably between diagnostic groups. Thus, among the ICD–10 disorders, F0 (mainly dementias) should score highest on cognitive problems and physical disability; F1 (substance use) should be associated with item three; F2 (affective disorders) with depression, and so on. This holds true. Age category is found to be associated with different items in predictable ways. There is a gradient of aggression, highest under age 25, lowest over 65. Cognition, as expected, has the opposite pattern. Patients in hospital for less than three months have high mean scores on almost every item compared with people not in hospital care; the only exception is item eight, mostly representing anxiety and phobic conditions, the mean for which is slightly higher in those who are not in-patients. Items on aggression and substance use are higher in males than in females. Pre-onset social and role performance shows a clear gradient, from above average to markedly below

Table 7 Mean total scores by profession and setting

Staff category	In-patient < 3 months		Other settings		All settings	
	Mean	n patients	Mean	n patients	Mean	n patients
Nurse	10.46	1094	8.28	696	9.61	1790
Doctor	12.26	360	7.94	345	10.15	705
Social worker	17.30	10	13.81	73	14.43	83
Occupational therapist			11.56	25	11.56	25
Clinical psychologist			7.28	40	7.28	40

average, in association with five items: aggression, cognition, psychotic symptoms, housing and activities.

Amendments to HoNOS-3 resulting from the phase three field trials

Comments made during follow-up visits to 14 sites, responses to a request in the regular HoNOS newsletter, and returns of a questionnaire sent to all raters, yielded few suggestions for further change and most amendments were small. One concerned the conjunction of manic (rare) and depressive (common) symptoms in one item; a practice that was in any case against the spirit of the rule that the scales deal with symptoms and dysfunctions, not diagnoses. Overactivity was therefore included at item one, while manic and depressive delusions, hallucinations and bizarre behaviour were included with other psychotic symptoms placed at item six, with depression following as item seven. The global rating and its change score were not closely associated with items, sub-scores or total score. Raters found it difficult to switch from the 0–4 scales to the 0–100. They tended to avoid the lowest and highest sectors and to cluster ratings round the remaining anchor points, resulting in a more normal distribution. Since it was not entirely clear how the global scale was being used, it was dropped and a more specific definition of disability provided, in terms of activities of daily living rated on the usual 0–4 scale, with glossary definitions for each severity point. This was placed at item 10, followed by the social environment item split into two for residential and daytime environments, with clarified glossary definitions in terms of autonomy. These changes were incorporated in the final version of HoNOS (see

Table 2). Although the 0–48 score range appears to give less scope for measuring change than one of 0–100, the top and bottom sections of the global score were hardly used and the quality of the information conveyed is unknown. If a global scale is required, it can be used independently.

RELIABILITY AND RELATIONSHIP TO OTHER SCALES

Studies in Nottingham and Manchester

The fourth phase consisted of tests to show whether the final form of the instrument remained acceptable to clinicians, had comparable characteristics to its predecessor, performed well when subjected to independent tests of reliability, and had reasonable compatibility with larger instruments with a long track record. The studies were carried out in academic departments in Nottingham and Manchester, in consultation with the CRU team.

Design of the reliability trials

In each city, a preliminary pilot was carried out to assess training and conditions of testing, followed by a main reliability trial. The Biometrics Department at the Institute of Psychiatry advised that, for most reasonable target coefficient requirements, 200 pairs would be appropriate. Altogether, 293 patients were rated during the two phases of testing, 96 during the pilots, 197 during the main study. The main difference from the group of patients in the field trials was that more patients in Manchester were elderly, many suffering from dementia.

In Nottingham, the trainer and central rater was a psychiatrist, in Manchester an experienced mental health nurse. This

arrangement was adopted in order to study the performance of HoNOS under a broad range of training and working conditions and to represent the expertise of the professions principally involved.

Reliability

In a first rapid assessment in order to discover any major problems, nine patients were rated by the Nottingham trainer and 13 other clinicians, eight of whom were the patients' keyworkers. Comparing the score sheets of each rater against those of each of the other 12 provided 78 sets of ratings for one patient, resulting in 702 sets of ratings (351 rater-pairs) for all nine. A few nurses had to leave early and, with some missing data, the actual number of rater-pairs analysed is 325. The exercise was intended to be used to provide initial feedback on the way the 12 items were being rated. In fact, only three were unsatisfactory and were dealt with by clarification of the wording of the related anchor points in the glossary. Subsequent work proceeded on the basis of these revisions, which were also fed back to the Manchester trainer in time for the main study there.

In the Nottingham main trial, 100 patients were rated by the trainer, and by each patient's keyworker or the person most knowledgeable about the patient's clinical condition. The first data column of Table 8 shows the intraclass correlation coefficients (ICC) attained, the coefficients of which are good to very good,[11] apart from item 12 which is moderate. There was also good equivalence between results examined when numbers reached 60 and 100, indicating good structural stability. The ICC data for four sub-scores and two total scores are all very satisfactory.

In Manchester, having first secured the collaboration of local hospital and community teams, the nurse trainer attended routine ward rounds and team meetings in order to ensure the inclusion of a spread of disorders and settings. Nine consultants conducted interviews with their patients following a general introduction. Further discussion ensued after the patient had left. The nurse trainer observed, but did not take part in, these proceedings. HoNOS was then rated by the trainer and relevant consultant.

1. Agreement categories (Landis & Koch, 1977): 0.41–0.60, moderate; 0.61–0.80, good; 0.81+, very good.

Table 8 Intraclass correlation coefficients (ICC) for HoNOS-4. Tests of reliability: Nottingham and Manchester

HoNOS item	Main study in Nottingham n=100	Main study in Manchester n=97
1. Aggression	0.97	0.80
2. Self-harm	0.88	0.92
3. Drug & alcohol use	0.99	0.61
4. Cognitive problems	0.81	0.92
5. Physical illness & disability	0.88	0.89
6. Hallucinations & delusions	0.87	0.92
7. Depression	0.84	0.89
8. Other symptoms	0.95	0.52
9. Relationships	0.74	0.78
10. Activities of daily living	0.71	0.90
11. Residential environment	0.83	0.72
12. Day-time activities	0.49	0.51
HoNOS subscores		
A: 1–3 Behaviour	0.89	0.74
B: 4–5 Impairment	0.87	0.95
C: 6–8 Symptoms	0.88	0.81
D: 9–12 Social	0.82	0.68
HoNOS total scores		
E: 1–12	0.86	0.77
F: 1–10	0.86	0.86

As in Nottingham, data collection was divided into a pilot and a main phase. In the pilot, ratings were provided from 87 trainer–doctor pairs. After minor adjustments on the basis of these results and suggestions from the Nottingham pilot, the trainer in Manchester rated a further 97 patients, each also rated by the relevant consultant. The second data column of Table 8 shows that the ICC coefficients are good to very good for all items but two (items 8 and 12), which are moderately good and acceptable.

Comparisons

An update of the earlier search, and reference to a similar survey by Andrews & Morris-Yates (1994), found no instrument of reasonable length that covered both the clinical and the social items in HoNOS. Two sets of scales, the 24-item Brief Psychiatric Rating Scale (BPRS-24) (Overall & Gorham, 1962; Ventura *et al*, 1993) and the Role Functioning Scale (RFS; Goodman *et al*, 1993), were selected because of a long track record and because, between them, they cover most of the content of the final HoNOS. However,

both instruments have a much wider range and the BPRS is intended to be completed at an interview with the patient, which is only an option for HoNOS. See Wing *et al* (1996) for papers describing the properties of each instrument.

In Nottingham, the trainer completed the comparison instruments for 33 of the patients in the reliability study. The product–moment correlation between the total HoNOS and total RFS scores was 0.65. That between the four social HoNOS items (9–12) and RFS 1–4 was 0.75. The correlation between total HoNOS and total BPRS scores was 0.84 and that between the clinical items HoNOS 1–8 and BPRS 1–15 (omitting the behavioural items 16–24) was 0.85.

The exercise in Manchester was more complicated and less appropriate for comparisons, since nine consultants rated a total of 97 patients. Five contributed too few BPRS and RFS forms for separate analysis; a total of 20. The other four between them provided a total of 77 score sheets. Of these, 37 (22 with a diagnosis of dementia) were contributed by one rater. The correlations between total HoNOS and total RFS scores, in order of magnitude, were 0.52, 0.64,

0.67 and 0.73. The equivalents for total HoNOS and total BPRS scores were 0.49, 0.57, 0.71 and 0.71.

Detailed information on individual items is provided for both samples in Table 9, which shows the symptomatic BPRS-24 items that are correlated at a level of 0.50 or higher with HoNOS items. Data from the four Manchester raters are combined. Bearing in mind the different diagnostic mix of the two patient groups, and the fact that there were four raters in Manchester, the results show reasonably good equivalence.

DISCUSSION

Meeting the remit

The first five necessary (though not sufficient) requirements for an instrument capable of routinely measuring changes in mental health outcomes have been met as well as they reasonably could be during the stages of construction. HoNOS is simple to use and generally clinically acceptable; it covers a broad range of clinical problems and social dysfunctions; it is sensitive to change or the lack of it over time; it has acceptable reliability and is compatible with longer and well-established instruments. It is now in the public domain and released for more widespread use and experiment.

Training users is simple. Most clinicians need and already collect and record such information, albeit not in standard format. Apart from the numbers participating in the trials (see Table 1), on average 15 clinicians at each of 40 sites have since been trained to use the final HoNOS and 55 have received the full trainers' course at the CRU. The scales and glossary are in the public domain. A software application (HoNOSoft) can be used to enter data rapidly, make simple analyses and print results or export them to statistical packages. Materials and manuals, and a full report on the research, can be obtained from the CRU.

Clinical use of HoNOS

The most obvious use for HoNOS is as a simple record of a patient's progress. It takes only a few minutes to complete a small 'peel-off' rating form, which can be stuck at once into the case file and updated as needed. If the instrument continues to be found useful in this way by individual clinicians, the quality of information

Table 9 Correlations between final HoNOS and BPRS-24 items, Nottingham and Manchester

HoNOS item	BPRS-24 item		Nottingham	Manchester
1. Aggression	B5	Hostility	0.87	0.60
	B10	Disorientation	0.52	–
2. Self-harm	B19[1]	Suicidality	0.97	0.72
	B5	Hostility	–	0.60
	B3	Depression	0.59	–
	B4	Guilt	–	0.50
4. Cognition	B10	Disorientation	0.74	0.84
	B11	Conceptual disorganisation	0.61	–
	B14	Blunted affect	0.61	–
	B16[1]	Mannerisms	0.55	–
	B18[1]	Emotional withdrawal	0.51	–
	B7	Hallucinations	0.78	0.88
6. Hallucinations & delusions	B7	Unusual thought content	0.81	0.58
	B6	Suspiciousness	0.75	0.59
	B24[1]	Distractability	0.66	–
	B21[1]	Bizarreness	0.57	–
7. Depression	B3	Depression	0.91	0.87
	B4	Guilt	0.81	–
	B2	Anxiety	–	0.61
	B19[1]	Suicidality	0.60	–
	B15	Tension	–	0.59
	B18[1]	Emotional withdrawal	–	0.50
8. Other symptoms	B1	Somatic concern	0.54	–
	B15	Tension	0.51	–
	B2	Anxiety	0.49	–

NB: HoNOS items 3 (drug misuse), 5 (physical problems) and 9–12 (social functioning) are not represented in BPRS-24.
1. BPRS items 16–24 are behavioural.

recorded is likely to be acceptable and many other ways of using HoNOS data become feasible.

The key to these would be incorporation into a structured clinical data set, for example serving a clinical team's need to implement the Care Programme Approach. There would be opportunities to compare specific problems or interventions or settings, and to audit outcomes in the context of care plans, case mix and case load (Lelliot, 1994, 1995). Rationally derived episodes could be substituted for the current method based on artificial divisions between periods of in-patient and other forms of care (Glover, 1995a,b).

Possible administrative uses of HoNOS

Whether the total HoNOS score would prove suitable as a single indicator for administrative purposes (such as monitor-

ing the attainment of a quantified target) can only be assessed in a realistic context such as a sector or district register. The total has proved robust throughout the four stages of the trials and the four sub-scores may also be found useful. Profiles of items provide the most detailed information but much will depend on the nature of the comparisons to be made. The most important criterion, whatever the question being asked, is that like should be compared with like. The more detailed the database, the easier that will be.

The incorporation of clinical information, following aggregation and anonymisation, into sector or district registers used for administrative as well as clinical and epidemiological purposes, requires assurance not only of the confidentiality, quality and security of clinical data, but also of the integrity of its use (Andrews & Morris-Yates, 1994). A discussion of the issues raised for

HoNOS, and for computerised health records more generally, by comparisons that have been made involving the work of institutions and practitioners in various fields of professional work will be the subject of another paper.

CONCLUSION

HoNOS performs to specification for clinical purposes. It has an official entry in the NHS Data Dictionary and is recommended for further testing within the secondary mental health services. It is being tested in Australia, Denmark, Italy and Spain.

A version for children and adolescents has been completed, others for old age psychiatry and learning disability are under test, and one for mentally disordered offenders is being developed. If a comparable primary care HoNOS were devised, tested and widely used, the age-old problem of relating data collected from secondary health and social agencies to a relevant population base would be much simplified.

ACKNOWLEDGEMENTS

The research on which this report is based was supported by the Department of Health. This study could not have been mounted without the hard work and cooperation of site coordinators who organised start-up, training and feedback meetings, supervised the running of projects and data collection, disseminated information during the project and were in many cases HoNOS raters themselves. We are indebted to Professor Brian Everitt, Dr Graham Dunn and Mr Charlie Sharp for their advice and help with analysis and interpretation of data.

APPENDIX

HoNOS scales, HoNOSoft software and further details are available from the College Research Unit, 11 Grosvenor Crescent, London SW1X 7EE.

REFERENCES

Andrews G. & Morris-Yates, A. (1994) Ethical implications of the electronic storage of medical records. In *Computers in Mental Health*, Vol. 1 (eds G. Andrews, T. B. Ustun, H. Dilling, *et al*), pp. 129–135. St Andrews: Churchill Livingstone/WHO.

Department of Health (1992) *Health of the Nation*. White Paper. London: HMSO.

__ **(1993)** *Key Area Handbook. Mental Health*. London: Department of Health.

Glover, G. (1995a) The public health perspective. In *Measurement for Mental Health*, Chapter 6 (ed Wing, J. K.). London: College Research Unit.

___ **(1995b)** Mental health informatics and the rhythm of community care. *British Medical Journal*, **311**, 1038–1039.

Goodman, S. H., Sewell, D. R., Cooley, E. L., et al (1993) Assessing levels of adaptive functioning: the Role Functioning Scale. *Community Mental Health Journal*, **29**, 119–131.

Jarman, B. & Hirsch, S. (1992) Statistical models to predict district psychiatric morbidity. In *Measuring Mental Health Needs* (eds G. Thornicroft, C. R. Brewin & J. K. Wing), pp. 62–80. London: Gaskell.

Landis, J. R. & Koch, G. G. (1977) The measurement of observer agreement for categorical data. *Biometrics*, **33**, 159–174.

Lelliot, P. (1994) Making clinical informatics work. Don't forget the doctor is the customer. *British Medical Journal*, **308**, 802–803.

___ **(1995)** Mental health information systems. *Measurement for Mental Health. Contributions from the College Research Unit*, chapter 8, (ed. Wing, J. K.). London: College Research Unit.

Overall, J. E. & Gorham, D. R. (1962) The Brief Psychiatric Rating Scale. *Psychological Reports*, **10**, 799–812.

Ventura, J., Green, M. F., Shaner, A., et al (1993) Training and quality assurance with the BPRS. 'The drift busters'. *International Journal of Methods in Psychiatric Research*, **3**, 221–244.

Wing, J. K., Curtis, R. H. & Beevor, A. S. (1996) HoNOS. Health of the Nation Outcome Scales. Report on research and development. London: College Research Unit.

CLINICAL IMPLICATIONS

■ HoNOS is suitable for routine use by nurses and psychiatrists because of its simplicity, broad clinical and social coverage and adequate psychometrics.

■ Item profiles, subscores and totals can be used to measure progress.

■ It would be suitable for incorporation into a data set for CPA monitoring.

LIMITATIONS

■ The use of HoNOS by other keyworker groups has not been tested.

■ The instrument is not intended to explain why the outcomes it measures have occurred.

■ The research has provided an instrument that could be used within a broader data set to monitor progress towards local, regional and national targets. Further study is needed to test this proposition.

J. K. WING, FRCPsych, A. S. BEEVOR, R. H. CURTIS, College Research Unit, 11 Grosvenor Crescent, London SWIX 7EE; S. G. B. PARK, MRCPsych, University of Nottingham, Duncan Macmillan House, Porchester Road, Nottingham; J. HADDEN, A. BURNS, FRCPsych, University of South Manchester, Withington, Manchester M20 9BX

Correspondence: Professor J. K. Wing, College Research Unit, 11 Grosvenor Crescent, London SWIX 7EE

(First received 23 January 1997, final revision 12 August 1997, accepted 26 August 1997)

Auditing electroconvulsive therapy

The third cycle

RICHARD DUFFETT and PAUL LELLIOTT

Background   This is the third large-scale audit in the past 20 years and compares the practice of electroconvulsive therapy (ECT) in England and Wales with the standards derived from the Royal College of Psychiatrists' 2nd ECT handbook.

Method   Facilities, equipment, practice, personnel and training were systematically evaluated during visits to all ECT clinics in the former North East Thames and East Anglia regions and Wales. All other English ECT clinics were surveyed with a postal questionnaire. Information was obtained for 184 (84%) of the 220 ECT clinics identified.

Results   Although some aspects of ECT administration had improved since the last audit in 1991, overall only one-third of clinics were rated as meeting College standards. Only 16% of responsible consultants attended their ECT clinic weekly and only 6% had sessional time for ECT duties. Fifty-nine per cent of all clinics had machines of the type recommended by the College and 7% were still using machines considered outdated in 1989. Only about one-third of clinics had clear policies to help guide junior doctors to administer ECT effectively.

Conclusions   Twenty years of activity by the Royal College of Psychiatrists and three large-scale audits have been associated with only modest improvement in local practice.

This paper reports the findings of a third audit of electroconvulsive therapy (ECT), which was conducted between September 1995 and July 1996.

PREVIOUS AUDITS OF ECT IN BRITAIN

The College first set standards for the administration of ECT in 1977 (Royal College of Psychiatrists, 1977). Pippard & Ellam (1981) subsequently conducted a review of practice by visiting 180 ECT clinics in the UK – about one-half of the total number. The audit revealed that some centres were using obsolete machines and that training of junior doctors in the administration of ECT was generally poor. In response to these findings the College produced its first ECT handbook in 1989 (Royal College of Psychiatrists, 1989).

In a second audit, Pippard (1992) evaluated the administration of ECT against standards contained in the 1989 handbook during visits to 35 National Health Service (NHS) and five private ECT clinics in the old North East Thames and East Anglia Regions. Although he reported an improvement since 1981 in the standard of ECT facilities and some aspects of practice, many clinics were still failing to meet the 1989 recommendations, particularly with regard to the training of junior doctors and the use of modern machines.

After his second evaluation, Pippard (1992) made a number of further recommendations. These focused on the role of the College and its members in ensuring that ECT clinics meet certain standards. These included the allocation of consultant sessions to administer and supervise ECT, accreditation of consultants in charge of ECT clinics, external inspection visits and better training of junior doctors.

The College established a working group to consider Pippard's suggestions and recent research findings. The revised College recommendations related both to structures (including the quality of ECT suites and equipment for administering ECT and monitoring seizures) and to processes (the administration of the electrical current, management of anaesthesia and recovery, the training and supervision of personnel). These revised guidelines were disseminated in the 2nd ECT handbook (Royal College of Psychiatrists, 1995), a video for psychiatrists involved in administering ECT (400 had been sold by the autumn of 1996), two articles in a journal supporting continuing medical education of psychiatrists (Lock, 1994; Robertson & Fergusson, 1996) and a series of training courses organised by the College (about 300 psychiatrists had attended these by the autumn of 1996). Pippard's recommendations about external audit and accreditation were not, however, implemented.

THE THIRD AUDIT

Method

Two hundred and fifteen ECT clinics, and the consultant responsible for ECT, were identified by phoning all NHS mental health trusts in England and Wales. Private clinics in North Thames and East Anglia were also identified. There were two components to the audit:

(a) Visits by R.D. to all ECT clinics in the old North East Thames and East Anglia regions (the area covered by Pippard's second audit) and to all clinics in Wales;

(b) A postal questionnaire sent to consultant psychiatrists responsible for ECT in all other English NHS mental health services.

Component 1: visits to ECT clinics

All 33 NHS clinics in the North East Thames and East Anglia regions and 17 in Wales were visited by R.D. between September 1995 and July 1996. In addition, visits were made to the two private clinics in the North East Thames and East Anglia regions and to three private clinics in north-west London. Whenever possible, visits were made on a day when ECT was due to be given. Clinics were rated using a schedule of standards derived from the 1995 ECT handbook. Some standards, such as presence of adequate equipment could be rated simply as present or absent. The standards of rooms, personnel and training were given a summary rating of poor, average or good and each clinic was also assigned a global rating using a similar scale. Each of these ratings took account of a number of factors (see Results). Similar methods were used to those employed by Pippard, who was consulted both on the design of the rating methods and on assigning ratings to individual clinics.

A total of 130 ECT treatments were observed in 40 (80%) of the NHS clinics and five treatments in three of the private clinics. During the sessions, observations were made about the testing of equipment, preparation of the patient, nursing care, stimulus used and the adequacy of medical records.

Component 2: the postal questionnaire

An eight-page postal questionnaire was sent to the consultant responsible for the 165 ECT clinics in England which were not visited as part of Component 1. The questionnaires were posted at the end of 1995 with a second mailing made to non-responders in spring 1996. The questionnaire was also completed by 10 of the consultants whose units were visited.

RESULTS

Returns were received from 129 of the 165 clinics in Component 2. Thus, data were available from 184 of the 220 clinics identified (response rate of 84%). Comparison of information from the 10 clinics which completed both the postal questionnaire and received a visit suggested that the two approaches yielded results which were sufficiently similar for the data from both methods to be combined; this is done in the Results, where possible. The relevant standards (derived from Royal College of Psychiatrists (1995)) are displayed at the beginning of each Results sub-section.

The ECT suite

ECT suites should consist of separate waiting room, treatment room and recovery room, and be warm, clean and of an adequate size. Clinics should provide a separate office for staff and a further recovery area for patients when they no longer need to be on the treatment trolley

An overview of the results is presented in Table 1. None of the NHS clinics wheeled the ECT machine from cubicle to cubicle, as had been found previously, and a further recovery area was provided by 46% of services. Four of the private clinics administered ECT in patient rooms and as such

did not have a separate waiting and recovery room. Despite the improvements, the quality of the environment in which ECT was administered varied widely; while some services had neglected the fabric of their ECT suite for many years, others provided a very well-maintained facility.

Equipment

ECT machines should be capable of a wide range of current settings (machines from four manufacturers are recommended in the 1995 handbook).

Recent research has shown that the minimum current required to induce a seizure may vary up to 40-fold between patients (although a narrower range is often found in ordinary clinical practice; Lock, 1994). The latest College handbook therefore recommends machines which deliver at least a 14-fold range of currents. By 1996, 108 clinics (59%) had installed these 'state of the art' machines (see Table 2). About one-third of clinics were using the Ectron 5 which can deliver a less than three-fold range of current and so limits the ability to titrate the current delivered. Twelve clinics (7%) were still using machines that were no longer recommended in the 1989 handbook. These older machines are underpowered, deliver a very restricted range of current and do not record the current actually delivered.

Anaesthetic equipment should include tilt trolleys, suction facilities, a supply of oxygen in the recovery and treatment rooms, electrocardiograms, pulse oximeters and capnographs.

Only two services visited provided capnographs and nine did not have tilt trolleys, otherwise these standards were generally well met; 21 clinics (41%) had pulse oximiters in both the treatment and recovery room.

Personnel, supervision and training

The consultant psychiatrist responsible for ECT should attend the clinic regularly and be acquainted with College recommendations on ECT practice.

In all services a named consultant psychiatrist was identified as being responsible for

the ECT clinic. Of the clinics visited only three consultants (6%) had sessional time allocated specifically for ECT. For the remainder, the times at which ECT was given often conflicted with other fixed commitments such as ward rounds and out-patient clinics. Twenty (36%) had read the 1995 ECT handbook and 23 consultants in the clinics visited (42%) had personally attended the ECT training course run by the College. In five (9%) of the clinics visited the consultants never attended ECT sessions; in 18 (33%) the consultant attended on average every 2–6 months; in 23 (42%) once a month and in nine (16%) once a week. In only three clinics did the consultant or another senior doctor, administer treatment routinely, and junior doctors attend principally for training purposes. The respondents to the postal survey reported spending on average three hours a month devoted to ECT (range 0–20). Sixty-six per cent of respondents to the postal questionnaire (n=85) claimed to have read the College handbook.

Junior doctors should observe ECT being given before they administer it themselves and should be supervised for the first few treatments they administer by a psychiatrist who has passed the Membership examination.

The issue of junior doctor involvement in ECT, their training and supervision is reported more fully elsewhere (Duffett & Lelliott, 1997). In brief, junior psychiatrists usually give ECT; all but four of the 184 clinics included senior house officers and registrars in psychiatry on the roster to give ECT and 140 (76%) included general practice vocational trainees. The College does not encourage the latter practice.

Anaesthetists should be sufficiently trained and experienced to manage any complication likely to arise during ECT administration (particularly if ECT is given at a site without an anaesthetic department). Rosters should include a consultant anaesthetist and be arranged to provide some continuity of care for patients over their course of treatment.

Standards relating to anaesthetic practice were derived from the College's ECT handbook and measures agreed with a

Table I Standards of rooms in the ECT suite

	Visited sites (%) n=55	Rest of England (%) n=129	Total (%) n=184
Good	14 (25)	47 (36)	61 (33)
Deficient in some areas	27 (49)	73 (57)	100 (54)
Poor	14 (25)	9 (7)	23 (13)

Table 2 ECT machines in use

ECT machines in use	Visited sites (%) n=55	Rest of England (%) n=129	Total (%) n=184
Thymatron[1]	9 (16)	24 (18)	33 (18)
Mecta[1]	3 (5)	18 (12)	21 (11)
Neurotronics[1]	1 (2)	8 (6)	9 (5)
Ectron 5 a/b[1]	12 (22)	33 (24)	45 (24)
Ectron 5	27 (49)	37 (26)	64 (34)
Older Ectrons	3 (5)	9 (7)	12 (7)

1. Currently recommended by the Royal College of Psychiatrists.

Council representative from the Royal College of Anaesthetists. In only four services visited (7%) was anaesthetic input rated as poor, either due to the inexperience of staff or to a failure to provide regular cover. Eight clinics (15%), however, reported experiencing difficulty in obtaining anaesthetic cover at least once a month resulting in cancelled clinics or the need to transport patients between hospitals.

Visited clinics located in district general hospitals and teaching hospitals ($n=23$) more frequently included junior anaesthetists (senior house officers and registrars) on the ECT roster than those located elsewhere ($n=32$), 65% $v.$ 9% $\chi^2=16$, $P<0.001$. For 68% of all clinics ($n=126$) anaesthesia was administered by a consultant anaesthetist for at least one session a week. No senior house officers administered anaesthesia for ECT in a setting outside of a district general or teaching hospital unsupervised. An operating department assistant was available in 88 (48%).

Nursing staff should be familiar with ECT procedures and trained in recovery techniques. There should be at least one senior nurse with special responsibility for ECT who is supported during the clinic by additional appropriately trained staff.

The quality of nursing input to the clinic varied greatly. When staff had sessional time allocated for ECT, nurses were keen to ensure high standards and in some services routinely met patients prior to them starting a course of ECT. In 23 clinics visited (42%) the senior nurse was dual trained (Registered Mental Nurse and State Registered Nurse), although many others had gained experience recovering patients in the theatre recovery area of general hospitals. However, many of the other nursing staff accompanying patients, and involved in patient recovery, were not as highly trained.

Policies and procedures

There must be policies giving guidance on what settings to use to stimulate patients, what to do in the absence of a seizure and when to terminate a prolonged seizure.

ECT is a relatively simple and circumscribed medical procedure, and is a good subject for locally developed structured protocols for its administration. Despite this, 36 of the clinics visited (67%) lacked any clear written stimulation policy, 35 (65%) gave no written guidance on restimulating patients with short seizures and 48 (89%) gave no guidance on terminating prolonged seizures. Of the clinics visited, 13 (24%) had ECT recording forms which were judged to be inadequate.

Observed treatment sessions

Patient preparation and delivery of treatment

Consistent with College recommendations, only nine (7%) of the 130 patients (47 men, 83 women) observed being treated received unilateral ECT. Twenty-one patients ($n=21$, 16%) were detained under Sections of the 1983 Mental Health Act, with 17 (13%) being given ECT against their will under the provisions of Sections 62 or 58.

Propofol was used as the induction agent for 22 patients (17%) (while there is no clear evidence that this compound impedes the efficacy of ECT, its use is not recommended either by the manufacturers or the 1995 ECT handbook). In response to the first stimulus, 21 patients (16%) had a seizure duration of 14 seconds or less, 11 of whom (8%) appeared to have no seizure. All but one of the 13 patients with a seizure duration below 10 seconds were re-stimulated, although not always on a high enough setting. No patient was stimulated more than twice during the same session. Seizures were generally timed appropriately with 21% ($n=27$) monitored using an electroencephalogram (EEG), 8% ($n=10$)

using the Hamilton cuff technique and 71% ($n=93$) relying on naked eye observation of the modified seizure. The recorded mean length of seizure activity when EEG monitoring was used was longer than when it was not (37 $v.$ 29 seconds; Mann–Whitney, $P<0.05$).

Only 14 clinics (36%) followed the recommendation that someone other than the doctor holding the electrodes should trigger the stimulus. In two clinics the administering doctor removed live electrodes early from the patient's head.

The College recommends that patients receiving ECT should be subject to regular review. However, no information had been recorded on mental state in the preceeding week for 32 patients (25%) and for only 67 (52%) had an entry in the case notes been made since the last ECT treatment (or the last week, if this was shorter). Stimulus settings and duration of seizure were adequately recorded.

Punctuality and staffing

In the services visited all patients were either accompanied to the ECT clinic or treated by a staff member who knew them. The level of support patients received while in the treatment room was generally high, with nursing staff in particular endeavouring to minimise the distress associated with the procedure. However, in two clinics the level of reassurance and support patients received was poor, with patients left lying on a trolley unattended while staff members busied themselves with 'other duties'. Although the majority of clinics started on time, 10 (23%) started more than 20 minutes late. The most common cause of a delay in starting was late arrival of medical staff.

Overall performance of clinics

Table 3 shows summary ratings of the quality of aspects of facilities and staffing. The global rating took account of facilities, personnel and how smoothly the clinic ran and were influenced by the level of patient care and the effectiveness of the observed ECT session. It was therefore a better rating of the quality of clinics where treatment was actually observed. R.D.'s view was that, had he required it, he would have been reluctant to receive ECT in 13 of the clinics visited (24%).

Impact of the College initiative

Consultants responsible for 147 (80%) of all clinics surveyed reported that they had seen the College video. In the clinics visited, 17 of the 23 consultants (74%) who had attended the one-day training course run by the College had also read the 1995 handbook compared with only three (9%) in the 32 clinics where the consultant had not attended the course ($\chi^2=24$, $P<0.001$). The overall performance of clinics whose consultants had attended the course was rated better than those where the consultant had not and none of the former received a poor rating; this association was statistically significant ($P<0.05$).

Although some of its recommendations related to nursing practice, in only 21 of the clinics visited (38%) had any nursing staff heard of the handbook.

DISCUSSION

Problems of multi-centre audits

This project illustrates some of the problems of conducting a multi-centre clinical audit. Whenever possible the standards, which were derived from the lengthy handbook, were converted into a format which facilitated measurement. Some, however, such as those relating to the adequacy of rooms, required subjective judgement to be made. The use of a single rater means that ratings were likely to have been made in a consistent way in all the clinics visited, and the involvement of Dr Pippard means that some comparisons can be made with his findings from 1991.

Changes since the previous audit

There has been improvement between 1991 and 1996 in some aspects of ECT administration. ECT machines are no longer wheeled from patient to patient (evident

Table 3 Summary ratings of the 55 clinics visited

	Poor (%)	Average (%)	Good (%)
ECT suite	14 (25.5)	27 (49)	14 (25.5)
ECT/anaesthetic equipment	5 (9)	31 (56)	19 (34)
Psychiatric staff	10 (18)	34 (62)	11 (20)
Anaesthetic staff	4 (7)	30 (56)	20 (37)
Nursing staff	11 (20)	23 (42)	21 (38)

in three clinics in the 1991 audit), operating department assistants have been introduced and further recovery areas made available for patients prior to them returning to their ward. ECT machines pre-dating the Ectron 5 (used by 46% of clinics in 1991) have been largely phased out. Fewer of the consultants responsible for ECT had never visited the clinic during its operation (9% v. 40% in 1991) and the number of services where anaesthetic practice was rated as poor has fallen from 28% to 7%.

Problems of implementation of ECT guidelines

The extent to which the slow improvement in ECT practice can be attributed to the College's actions could only have been gauged by a prospective, controlled study which, even if methodologically possible, would have been prohibitively expensive. There is, however, circumstantial evidence that the activities of the College over the years have had some impact. Consultants who had attended the College course had better clinics (although consultants keen to raise standards are probably also more likely to attend the College course). Also, staff in good clinics often attributed their high standards to following the College recommendations and reported using the results of the 1991 audit to argue for resources to improve facilities.

Although the 1996 audit was conducted only a few months after the publication of the ECT handbook, it is disappointing that only one-third of the consultants in the clinics visited had actually read it, most of whom had also attended the College course. Dissemination of the College recommendations across professional boundaries was also poor, with two-thirds of senior nurses in ECT clinics not even aware of the handbook's existence (despite liaison with the Royal College of Nursing at the time the standards were set). The College video had been more widely circulated, having been seen by more than one-half of junior doctors administering ECT (Duffett & Lelliott, 1997) and about 80% of consultants.

It is known that even after well-planned dissemination, guidelines frequently reach only a small proportion of their target audience (Grol, 1992; Lomas, 1993). The College ECT initiative is consistent with what is known about effective dissemination of guidelines in that it included presentation through a variety of media

(video, workshops, a handbook, papers in peer review journals and journals of continuing professional development), interventions targeted at the key audience (the ECT course for responsible consultants) and the involvement of respected colleagues (in teaching and promoting good practice; Lomas, 1993).

However, even if the handbook were to reach all of its intended audience it would not necessarily lead to change of practice. Its weakness, common to other national initiatives, is that it was developed 'top-down' and so may not be 'owned' by those to whose practice it relates (Grimshaw & Russell, 1993).

Options for accreditation

Given the number of clinics which do not meet standards the question has to be asked as to when sanctions should replace exhortation and education. In the USA, the American Psychiatric Association requires a psychiatrist to receive special training and accreditation before giving ECT unsupervised (American Psychiatric Association, 1990). If applied in the UK, this would end the practice of junior doctors, who might be in their first psychiatric post, being assigned to ECT rosters simply on the basis of their availability for this duty.

Alternatively, accreditation could apply to the whole process of ECT administration including facilities, equipment, practice, personnel, supervision and training. Although ECT facilities are inspected at College visits to accredit training schemes, this has not assured uniformly high standards to date. It is likely that the detailed inspection required for accreditation of ECT clinics would have to be conducted as a separate activity. There is a precedent; Clinical Pathology Accreditation (UK) Ltd started by the Royal College of Pathologists has been accrediting departments of clinical pathology since 1992. Although accreditation is not statutory, increasingly health authorities will only commission services from accredited departments.

CURRENT STANDARDS IN ECT

Many aspects of the organisation and administration of ECT improved between 1991 and 1996. Very old ECT machines have largely been replaced, senior psychiatrists are more actively involved and anaesthetic input is better. However, two-thirds of ECT clinics fall short of the most recent College standards, particularly in relation to the frequency of consultant attendance and the training of junior doctors. These problems have not been fully resolved by 20 years of audit and College activity. There should be a continuing debate as to what further interventions might be considered.

ACKNOWLEDGEMENTS

We thank the staff of the sites visited and those who completed the questionnaire and Dr John Pippard for assistance in designing the protocol and for commenting on the draft paper. The work was funded by an NHS Executive Clinical Audit Grant.

REFERENCES

American Psychiatric Association (1990) *The Practice of Electroconvulsive Therapy: Recommendations for Treatment, Training and Privileging.* Washington, DC: APA.

Duffett, R. & Lelliott, P. (1997) Junior doctors training in the theory and practice of electroconvulsive therapy. *Psychiatric Bulletin,* **21**, 563–565.

Grimshaw, J. M. & Russell, I. T. (1993) Effect of clinical guidelines on medical practice: a systematic review of rigorous evaluations. *Lancet,* **342**, 1317–1322.

Grol, R. (1992) Implementing guidelines in general practice care. *Quality Health,* **I**, 184–191.

Lock, T. (1994) Advances in the practice of electroconvulsive therapy. *Advances in Psychiatric Treatment,* **I**, 47–56.

Lomas, J. (1993) Diffusion, dissemination, and implementation; who should do what? *Annals of New York Academy of Science,* **703**, 226–235.

Pippard, J. (1992) Audit of electroconvulsive treatment in two national health service regions. *British Journal of Psychiatry,* **160**, 621–637.

___ **& Ellam, L. (1981)** Electroconvulsive treatment in Great Britain: a report to the college. *British Journal of Psychiatry,* **139**, 563–568.

Robertson, C. & Ferguson, G. (1996) Electroconvulsive therapy machines. *Advances in Psychiatric Treatment,* **2**, 24–31.

Royal College of Psychiatrists (1977) The Royal College of Psychiatrists' memorandum on the use of electroconvulsive therapy. *British Journal of Psychiatry,* **131**, 261–272.

___ **(1989)** *The Practical Administration of Electroconvulsive Therapy.* London: Gaskell.

___ **(1995)** *The ECT Handbook: The 2nd Report of the Royal College of Psychiatrists' Special Committee on ECT.* Council Report CR39. London: Royal College of Psychiatrists.

CLINICAL IMPLICATIONS

- Only one-third of ECT clinics in England and Wales can be regarded as good. Local clinicians should work with managers to improve the quality of clinics and instigate regular local audit.

- Many consultants responsible for ECT devote less time to this activity than is recommended by the Royal College of Psychiatrists.

- After more than 20 years of College activity to improve standards, including three large-scale audits, consideration might be given to a system of accreditation.

LIMITATIONS

- The audit began only a few months after publication of the standards on which it was based.

- A postal questionnaire supplemented data collected on site visits; the national picture is based on a combination of the two data sets.

- Many ratings relied on the subjective view of the author who visited the clinics.

RICHARD DUFFET, MRCPsych, PAUL LELLIOTT, MRCPsych, Royal College of Psychiatrists' Research Unit, London

Correspondence: Richard Duffett, Royal College of Psychiatrists' Research Unit, 11 Grosvenor Crescent, London SW1X 7EE

(First received 25 August 1997, final revision 20 January 1998, accepted 21 January 1998)

Trends in deliberate self-harm in Oxford, 1985–1995

Implications for clinical services and the prevention of suicide

KEITH HAWTON, JOAN FAGG, SUE SIMKIN, ELIZABETH BALE
and ALISON BOND

Background   Deliberate self-harm (DSH) has been a major health problem in the UK for nearly three decades. Any changes in rates of DSH or the demographic characteristics of the patient population are likely to have important implications for clinical services and suicide prevention.

Method   Data collected by the Oxford Monitoring System for Attempted Suicide were used to review trends in DSH between 1985–1995.

Results   There was a substantial increase in DSH rates during the 11-year study period, with a 62.1% increase in males and a 42.2% increase in females. The largest rise was in 15–24-year-old males (+194.1%). Changes in DSH rates correlated with changes in national suicide rates in both males and females in this age group. Rates of repetition of DSH increased in both genders during the study period. Paracetamol self-poisoning has continued to increase, half of all overdoses in 1995 involving paracetamol, and antidepressant overdoses have become more common.

Conclusions   The increase in DSH, especially in young males, has important implications for general hospital DSH and medical services. It may herald a reversal of recent progress towards achievement of national suicide targets.

Rates of deliberate self-harm (DSH) (self-poisoning and self-injury) in the UK escalated during the late 1960s and early 1970s to such an extent that it became a major health problem (Bancroft *et al*, 1975; Holding *et al*, 1977). This problem was particularly marked in adolescents and young adults (Kreitman & Schreiber, 1979; Hawton & Goldacre, 1982). Following a decline in rates during the late 1970s and early 1980s, notably in older teenage girls (Platt *et al*, 1988; Sellar *et al*, 1990*a*), we subsequently reported that rates in Oxford had begun to rise again in the late 1980s (Hawton & Fagg, 1992*a*), especially in older adolescent females (Hawton & Fagg, 1992*b*). Subsequently, it became clear that the rates of DSH in the UK are among the highest in Europe (Schmidtke *et al*, 1996). Because of the size of the problem of DSH and its associated significant risk of suicide (Hawton & Fagg, 1988), any changes in its prevalence can have important clinical implications both for general medical and psychiatric services and for suicide prevention. The aims of this study were to review trends in DSH which are relevant to the prevention of self-harm and service provision for this population. In this paper we have utilised data collected through the Oxford Monitoring System for Attempted Suicide (Hawton & Fagg, 1992*a*) to review trends in DSH in Oxford during the 11 years 1985 to 1995.

METHOD

The study population consisted of all persons referred to the general hospital in Oxford between 1985 and 1995 following self-poisoning or self-injury. The general hospital receives all hospital-referred cases from Oxford City and the surrounding area. Patients referred to the hospital following self-poisoning or self-injury are identified by the Monitoring System maintained by the University Department of Psychiatry (Hawton &

Fagg, 1992*a*). Most attempted suicide patients are routinely referred to the emergency psychiatric service in the hospital. All patients referred to the service receive a detailed psychosocial assessment by a specially trained psychiatrist, psychiatric nurse, or social worker. Most assessments are discussed in detail with a senior psychiatrist. A range of patient characteristics and clinical items are recorded by the assessors on data sheets which are then coded and the data entered into a computerised data file. Through scrutiny of the records of the accident and emergency department a limited amount of information is also available on patients presenting to the hospital but not seen by the psychiatric service. We have previously demonstrated the reliability of our method of data collection (Sellar *et al*, 1990*b*).

Self-poisoning is defined as the intentional self-administration of more than the prescribed dose of any drug whether or not there is evidence that the act was intended to cause self-harm. This category also includes overdoses of 'drugs for kicks' and poisoning by non-ingestible substances and gas, provided the hospital staff consider that these are cases of deliberate self-harm. Alcohol intoxication is not included unless accompanied by other types of self-poisoning or self-injury. Self-injury is defined as any injury recognised by hospital staff as having been deliberately self-inflicted.

Calculation of rates

For those findings which are based on rates, the data have been analysed for referrals from Oxford City only. This is because the rest of the hospital catchment area is somewhat ill-defined; therefore rates can only be calculated for the City referrals. The population figures for Oxford City are mid-year estimates and were provided by the Office for National Statistics (formerly the Office of Population Censuses and Surveys). Age- and sex-specific rates per 100 000 population were calculated, using appropriate mid-year population estimates as the denominators.

In the calculation of annual rates and examination of trends in rates, each individual could only contribute to the data once in any one year. However, they were included in the calculations of rates for other years if they made further attempts in those years. Where findings for the whole study period are averaged this is either on the basis of persons, in which case each individual could only contribute to the data once (i.e. 'true' persons), or episodes.

Clinical variables

Findings with regard to demographic variables, methods of self-harm, and repetition of attempts, are based on the total population of patients referred to the hospital. Most of the other clinical information was only available for patients assessed by the clinical service. We have reported on the problems patients referred in 1995 were facing, these problems being indicated by the clinical assessors on a standard checklist. A problem was defined as 'a factor which was causing current distress for the patient and/or contributed to the attempt'.

Repetition of attempts has been studied according to (a) previous attempts leading to hospital referral before the first referral during the study period, and (b) repeat attempts resulting in re-referral to the general hospital in Oxford during the year following the first referral in any one year (1985–1994 only).

Suicide rates

Data on annual suicide rates for England and Wales were obtained from the Office for National Statistics. Rates of suicide in the category 'suicide' (E950–E959) and 'undetermined cause' (E980–E989) were combined to provide a more valid estimate of the overall rates of suicide (Charlton *et al*, 1992).

Statistical analysis

The data were analysed with the SPSSX statistical package (SPSS, 1993) using χ^2 and Spearman's rho (two-tailed) tests where appropriate. In testing for trends the χ^2 test for trend was used where trends were approximately linear and χ^2 for proportions in grouped years where the trends were clearly non-linear.

RESULTS

Referrals to the general hospital

During the 11 years 1985 to 1995, 7437 persons presented to the hospital following 10 631 episodes of DSH (Table 1). There was an increase in both the annual number of persons (mean annual increase +4.6% per year) and episodes (+7.2% per year) during the study period. This was more marked for males (persons +5.8% per year; episodes +7.9% per year) than females (persons +3.8% per year; episodes +5.6% per year). The gender ratio for episodes steadily

Table I Numbers of persons and episodes referred to the general hospital following deliberate self-harm, by gender, 1985–1995

Year	Males		Females		Both genders	
	Persons	Episodes	Persons	Episodes	Persons	Episodes
1985	278	326	400	463	678	789
1986	290	339	451	494	741	833
1987	292	332	466	514	758	846
1988	279	329	425	490	704	819
1989	298	350	465	548	763	898
1990	331	409	479	553	810	962
1991	323	368	445	504	768	872
1992	303	359	498	586	801	945
1993	344	450	497	590	841	1040
1994	419	540	565	727	984	1267
1995	452	611	568	749	1020	1360
1985–1995[1]	3042	4413	4395	6218	7437	10 631

1. 'True' persons.

declined, from 1.43 (F:M) in 1985 to 1.35 in 1990 and 1.23 in 1995.

Rate of DSH

Person-based rates for Oxford City reflected these changes (Fig. 1). The overall rate rose between 1985 and 1995 by 50.9% (χ^2 for trend=26.18, 1 d.f., $P<0.0001$), the rates in males by 62.1% (χ^2 for trend=19.59, 1 d.f. $P<0.0001$) and the rate in females by 42.2% (χ^2 for trend=8.42, 1 d.f., $P<0.01$). The gender ratio for rates decreased from 1.40 (F:M) in 1985 to 1.33 in 1990 and 1.23 in 1995.

When the trends were examined according to gender and age groups it was apparent that the increase in male rates (Fig. 2) was especially marked in 15–24-year-olds. The annual rates per 100 000 in 15–24-year-old males increased from 162.2 in 1985 to 477.1 in 1995, an increase of 194.1% (χ^2 for trend based on raw data=27.72, 1 d.f., $P<0.0001$). Rates also increased in females aged 25–34 years, with a 35.6% increase during the study period (χ^2 for trend=3.98, 1 d.f., $P<0.05$), and 35–54 years, with a 67.7% increase during the study period (χ^2 for trend=4.56, 1 d.f., $P<0.05$). Rates in other age groups did not change significantly.

Associations with rates of suicide

In males aged 15–24 years, annual rates of DSH in Oxford correlated positively with the combined annual rates of suicide (ICD codes E950–E959) and undetermined cause

Fig. I Rates of deliberate self-harm in Oxford City in persons aged 15 years and over, by gender, 1985–1995

of death (E980–E989) in England and Wales between 1985 and 1995 (Spearman's rho=0.60, $P=0.053$). When the association was examined in 15–24-year-old females, it was also close to statistical significance (rho=0.58, $P=0.06$). The correlations in other age groups for both males and females were much smaller, although all were positive apart from those for females aged 35–54 years and 55 years and over.

Repetition of DSH

Repetition of DSH also increased, as reflected in an increase in the episodes : persons ratio from an annual average of 1.15 in 1985–1990 to 1.24 in 1991–1995. The repetition rate within a year of an episode in each calendar year also increased, averaging 13.1% in 1985–1989 and 16.1% in 1990–1994 (χ^2=13.81, $P<0.001$). While the repetition rate within a year of a first episode in each year was generally higher in males (mean=15.8%) than females (mean=

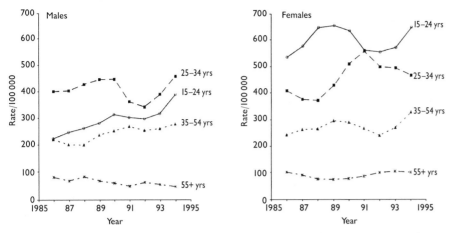

Fig. 2 Age group specific rates of deliberate self-harm in Oxford City, 1985–1995 (rates are shown as three-year moving averages).

14.0%), the increase in annual repetition rates was more marked in females (11.9% in 1985–1989 to 15.8% in 1990–1994; $\chi^2=15.05$, $P<0.01$) than males (15.0% to 16.5%, NS).

There was some indication of a diminution in the percentage of individuals (who received a psychiatric assessment) carrying out their first episodes of DSH (hospital referred or otherwise) during the study period. This proportion declined from 58.7% in 1985–1990 to 51.3% in 1991–1995. However, the mean annual numbers of 'first-timers' were very similar in the two time periods, being 353 in 1985–1990 and 350 in 1991–1995.

Methods used

During the period of the study, 87.9% ($n=9345$) of episodes of DSH involved self-poisoning, 8.3% ($n=887$) involved self-injury, and 3.8% ($n=399$) both self-poisoning and self-injury. There were major changes in the substances used for self-poisoning (Fig. 3). There was a steady increase in the use of non-opiate analgesics (χ^2 for trend$=38.14$, $P<0.0001$), this increase being entirely accounted for by the massive increase in the use of paracetamol (including paracetamol-containing compounds). Thus whereas in 1985 31.3% of overdoses involved paracetamol, by 1995 this figure had risen to 49.6% (χ^2 for trend$=98.14$, $P<0.0001$). This increase was most marked in females, in whom paracetamol overdoses increased from 29.6% in 1985 to 52.6% in 1995. The comparable increase in males was from 34.1 to 45.9%.

There was also an increase in antidepressant overdoses, from 11.6% in 1985 to 18.2% in 1995 (χ^2 for trend$=55.46$, $P<0.0001$). This increase was somewhat more marked in males (from 8.0% in 1985 to 18.1% in 1995) than in females (from 13.9% in 1985 to 18.3% in 1995). Of those who took antidepressant overdoses in 1995, 58.9% used tricyclics and 29.5% used selective serotonin reuptake inhibitors (SSRIs). The previously noted decline in overdoses of minor tranquillisers and sedatives continued between 1985 and 1995, with a drop from 25.5 to 15.6% (χ^2 for trend$=49.19$, $P<0.0001$).

Problems preceding self-harm

The most frequent problems identified as being present at the time of self-harm in the patients who presented in 1995 and were assessed by a member of the hospital psychiatric service showed some marked sex differences (Table 2). Problems concerning a partner, employment or studies, alcohol, drugs and finances were all more common in the males and problems with family members other than a partner were more common in the females.

In terms of living circumstances, an annual mean of 3.2% of individuals (6.4% of males and 1.0% of females) were of no fixed abode. This figure increased between 1985–1990 and 1991–1995, from 2.4 to 3.9% ($\chi^2=16.61$, $P<0.001$).

Admissions to the general hospital, psychiatric assessment and in-patient psychiatric admission

In spite of the considerable increase in the numbers of patients presenting to the general

hospital following DSH the proportion admitted to an in-patient bed varied little during the study period, averaging 86.5% per year. However, the proportion who received a psychiatric assessment declined, averaging 82.4% in 1985–1990 and 77.4% in 1991–1995 ($\chi^2=41.65$, $P<0.0001$). This decline was particularly marked in the last three years of the study period when the numbers of referrals to the hospital increased substantially (Table 1), with only 73.2% receiving a psychiatric assessment in 1993–1995. In part this reflected the fact that male patients took their own discharge from hospital more than females (10.6% $v.$ 7.5%; $\chi^2=20.14$, 1 d.f., $P<0.001$).

An average of 10.2% of all patients each year were admitted to in-patient psychiatric care from the general hospital, approximately half of whom were already in current psychiatric care and a third were current in-patients. This proportion increased from a mean of 7.9% in 1985–1987 to 12.5% in 1993–1995 ($\chi^2=30.78$, $P<0.001$). This change was more marked in females (from 7.7 to 13.5%; $\chi^2=27.82$, $P<0.001$) than males (from 8.2 to 11.2%; $\chi^2=5.33$, $P<0.05$).

DISCUSSION

Increased rates of DSH and implications for suicide prevention

The rising trends in DSH identified in Oxford appear to reflect what is happening

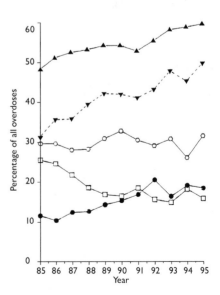

Fig. 3 Trends in substances used for self-poisoning, 1985–1995. ▲—▲, non-opiate analgesics; ▼- - -▼, paracetamol; ○—○, other; ●—●, antidepressants; □—□, tranquillisers and sedatives

Critical Reviews in Psychiatry

Table 2 The 10 most frequent types of problems identified at assessment in patients presenting in 1995

Problem	Both genders (n=738)%	Males (n=316)%	Females (n=422)%	P
Partner	55.8	60.1	52.5	<0.05
Other family member	41.2	31.0	48.8	<0.0001
Employment/studies	35.8	46.8	27.5	<0.0001
Alcohol	21.3	30.7	14.2	<0.0001
Financial	20.1	26.6	15.2	<0.001
Social isolation	17.1	16.8	17.3	NS
Housing	16.1	18.7	14.2	NS
Friends	13.4	12.0	14.5	NS
Physical health	12.6	11.4	13.5	NS
Drugs	8.1	13.0	4.5	<0.0001

elsewhere in the UK. Thus our results are in keeping with recent findings based on admissions to general hospitals in Scotland (McLoone & Crombie, 1996) and to a district poisons treatment unit in Wales (Bialas et al, 1996). We previously estimated on the basis of Oxford rates that the mean annual number of people presenting to hospitals following DSH in 1989 and 1990 in England and Wales would have been 120 000 (Hawton & Fagg, 1992a). On the basis of the 1995 rate the figure would be 142 000, a substantially increased proportion of whom are males. The rise in the numbers of DSH patients is putting considerable pressure on hospital services, and especially on in-patient beds, and must be an important factor in the worsening bed crisis affecting many general hospitals in the UK. Although there was no reduction in the proportion of DSH patients admitted to a bed in the general hospital in Oxford during the study period, this is probably not true elsewhere. There has certainly been a trend towards more rapid discharge from the general hospital, and a consequent decrease in the proportion who receive a psychosocial assessment.

The increase in DSH has been most marked in young males. This trend has clearly paralleled the recent trend in deaths from suicide and probable suicide. In view of the association between DSH and subsequent suicide in all age groups (Hawton & Fagg, 1988), but especially in young males, the current trend raises serious concerns about whether the recently reported decrease in suicide rates in England and Wales toward The Health of the Nation targets (Department of Health, 1995) will be sustained.

One factor contributing to the recent rise in DSH appears to have been an increase

in frequency of repetition, particularly in females. The reasons for this are unclear, but in addition to placing greater demands on clinical services it may have important implications in view of the known link between repetition and risk of suicide (Hawton & Fagg, 1988). On the other hand, over the duration of our study there was an encouraging reduction in the proportion of patients engaging in their first episode of DSH, but not, unfortunately, in the overall number of 'first-timers', thus providing no evidence of effective primary prevention of DSH.

Implications for clinical services

The great increase in male DSH patients presents considerable problems for service provision. Not only do males, as we have shown, take their own discharge from hospital more often than females, a recent review of outcome of treatment studies following DSH has shown that they are less easy to engage in treatment and that currently available methods of treatment appear to be less efficacious in males (Hawton, 1997). The recent trends will therefore place increasing pressure on clinical services to develop more effective treatments for males, especially those in the younger age groups. It may well be that current therapy strategies need to be reviewed for this growing population of DSH patients, perhaps utilising a more practical approach (e.g. an open-house workshop format) combined with aggressive outreach in order to try to keep patients in the programme (Van Heeringen et al, 1995). Given the clear evidence that continuity of care is important in sustaining compliance of many DSH patients with treatment

(Möller, 1989) and the risk that transfer of care from general hospital services to community mental health teams can interfere with this, attention needs to be paid to how continuity can be maintained for those patients not already in treatment at the time they self-harm.

Changes in substances used in overdoses

The increasing rise in the use of paracetamol for self-poisoning and the concomitant rise in paracetamol-related deaths (Gunnell et al, 1997) clearly necessitates urgent preventive strategies, with reduction in paracetamol pack size seeming the best approach (Hawton et al, 1996). The rise in antidepressant overdoses in recent years presumably reflects more widespread prescribing, including greater use of SSRIs and other less toxic preparations in patients thought to be at risk of overdose.

Problems preceding DSH

The pattern of problems facing DSH patients showed an interesting change from that found in earlier studies in that whereas problems with partners used to be far more common in female DSH patients (e.g. Bancroft et al, 1977), the reverse was true in our study. This finding, which probably reflects the large increase in the number of younger male DSH patients, may have implications for the content of therapeutic interventions. The considerable excess of substance misuse in males, with its well-recognised association with greater risk of subsequent suicide, especially in young males (Hawton et al, 1993), necessitates that there must be close collaboration between general hospital DSH services and services for alcohol and drug misusers.

ACKNOWLEDGEMENTS

We thank members of the Barnes Unit, Department of Psychological Medicine, Oxford Radcliffe Hospital (John Radcliffe), Oxford, for their continuing support of the Monitoring System. Data from the system are contributed to the WHO:EURO Study on Parasuicide by means of which trends in DSH are being monitored throughout Europe. The Monitoring System is funded by a grant from the Department of Health.

REFERENCES

Bancroft, J., Skrimshire, A., Reynolds, F., et al (1975) Self-poisoning and self-injury in the Oxford area: epidemiological aspects 1969–1973. *British Journal of Preventive and Social Medicine,* **29,** 170–177.

—, —, **Casson, J., et al (1977)** People who deliberately poison or injure themselves: their problems and their contacts with helping agencies. *Psychological Medicine*, **7**, 289–303.

Bialas, M. C., Reid, P. G., Beck, J. H., et al (1996) Changing patterns of self-poisoning in a UK health district. *Quarterly Journal of Medicine*, **89**, 893–901.

Charlton, J., Kelly, S., Dunnell, K., et al (1992) Trends in suicide deaths in England and Wales. *Population Trends*, **69**, 10–16.

Department of Health (1995) *Fit for the Future. Second Progress Report on the Health of the Nation.* London: Department of Health.

Gunnell, D., Hawton, K., Murray, V., et al (1997) Use of paracetamol for suicide and non-fatal poisoning in the UK and France: Are restrictions on availability justified? *Journal of Epidemiology and Community Health*, **51**, 175–179.

Hawton, K. (1997) Attempted suicide. In *Science and Practice of Cognitive Behaviour Therapy* (eds D. M. Clark & C. G. Fairburn), pp. 285–312. Oxford: Oxford University Press.

__ **& Goldacre, M. (1982)** Hospital admissions for adverse effects of medicinal agents (mainly self-poisoning) among adolescents in the Oxford Region. *British Journal of Psychiatry*, **141**, 166–170.

__ **& Fagg, J. (1988)** Suicide, and other causes of death, following attempted suicide. *British Journal of Psychiatry*, **152**, 359–366.

__ **& __ (1992a)** Trends in deliberate self-poisoning and self-injury in Oxford, 1976–90. *British Medical Journal*, **304**, 1409–1411.

__ **& __ (1992b)** Deliberate self-poisoning and self-injury in adolescents: a study of characteristics and trends in Oxford, 1976–89. *British Journal of Psychiatry*, **161**, 816–823.

—, —, **Platt, S., et al (1993)** Factors associated with suicide after parasuicide in young people. *British Medical Journal*, **130**, 1641–1644.

—, **Ware, C., Mistry, H., et al (1996)** Paracetamol self-poisoning: characteristics, prevention and harm reduction. *British Journal of Psychiatry*, **168**, 43–48.

Holding, T., Buglass, D., Duffy, J. C., et al (1977) Parasuicide in Edinburgh – a seven year review 1968–74. *British Journal of Psychiatry*, **130**, 534–543.

Kreitman, N. & Schreiber, M. (1979) Parasuicide in young Edinburgh women, 1968–75. *Psychological Medicine*, **141**, 37–44.

McLoone, P. & Crombie, I. K. (1996) Hospitalisation for deliberate self-poisoning in Scotland from 1981 to 1993: trends in rates and types of drugs used. *British Journal of Psychiatry*, **169**, 81–86.

Möller, H. J. (1989) Efficacy of different strategies of aftercare for patients who have attempted suicide. *Journal of the Royal Society of Medicine*, **82**, 643–647.

Platt, S., Hawton, K., Kreitman, N., et al (1988) Recent clinical and epidemiological trends in parasuicide in Edinburgh and Oxford: a tale of two cities. *Psychological Medicine*, **18**, 405–418.

Schmidtke, A., Bille-Brahe, U., Deleo, D., et al (1996) Attempted suicide in Europe: rates, trends, and sociodemographic characteristics of suicide attempters during the period 1989–1992. Results of the WHO/EURO Multicentre Study on Parasuicide. *Acta Psychiatrica Scandinavica*, **93**, 327–338.

Sellar, C., Hawton, K. & Goldacre, M. J. (1990a) Self-poisoning in adolescents: hospital admissions and deaths in the Oxford Region 1980–1985. *British Journal of Psychiatry*, **56**, 866–870.

—, **Goldacre, M. J. & Hawton, K. (1990b)** Reliability of routine hospital data on poisoning as measures of deliberate self-poisoning in adolescents. *Journal of Epidemiology and Community Health*, **44**, 313–315.

SPSS (1993) *SPSSX for Unix: Base System User's Guide, Release 5.0.* Chicago, IL: SPSS Inc.

Van Heeringen, C., Jannes, S., Buylaert, W., et al (1995) The management of non-compliance with referral to out-patient after-care among attempted suicide patients: a controlled intervention study. *Psychological Medicine*, **25**, 963–970.

CLINICAL IMPLICATIONS

■ Rising rates of DSH are placing increasing demands on general hospital medical and psychiatric services.

■ Reduction in the dangers of paracetamol overdoses is becoming increasingly necessary.

■ Increased rates of DSH in young males have implications for treatment provision and prevention of suicide.

LIMITATIONS

■ The data are limited to that which can reasonably be collected in routine monitoring.

■ The findings regarding repetition take no account of treatment effects.

■ No data are available on completed suicide in the study population.

KEITH HAWTON, DM, JOAN FAGG, SUE SIMKIN, BA, ELIZABETH BALE, ALISON BOND, BA, University Department of Psychiatry, Warneford Hospital, Oxford

Correspondence: Professor Keith Hawton, University Department of Psychiatry, Warneford Hospital, Oxford OX3 7JX

(First received 11 March 1997, final revision 17 June 1997, accepted 30 June 1997)

The psychiatric status of patients with the chronic fatigue syndrome

IAN HICKIE, ANDREW LLOYD, DENIS WAKEFIELD and GORDON PARKER

The prevalence of psychiatric disorder in 48 patients with chronic fatigue syndrome (CFS) was determined. Twenty-two had had a major depressive (non-endogenous) episode during the course of their illness, while seven had a current major (non-endogenous) depression. The pre-morbid prevalence of major depression (12.5%) and of total psychiatric disorder (24.5%) was no higher than general community estimates. The pattern of psychiatric symptoms in the CFS patients was significantly different to that of 48 patients with non-endogenous depression, but was comparable with that observed in other medical disorders. Patients with CFS were not excessively hypochondriacal. We conclude that psychological disturbance is likely to be a consequence of, rather than an antecedent risk factor to the syndrome.

"Acquired neurasthenia is characterised by a diminished power of attention, distractibility, defective mental application, difficulty of thinking, an increased susceptibility to fatigue, increased emotional irritability, and a greater variety of physical symptoms, mostly subjective, including hypochondriasis." (Emil Kraepelin, 1981, first published 1907).

The chronic fatigue syndrome (also termed 'myalgic encephalomyelitis', 'Royal Free disease', 'post-viral fatigue syndrome'), recently defined by the Centers for Disease Control in Atlanta, Georgia (Holmes *et al*, 1988), has been subject to ongoing controversy (Dawson, 1987; David *et al*, 1988; Swartz, 1988). Psychological features have often been noted (David *et al*, 1988), leading some physicians to regard DFS as a psychiatric disorder (McEvedy & Beard, 1973). The demonstration of persistent infection (Yousef *et al*, 1988) and immunological abnormalities (Behan *et al*, 1985; Straus *et al*, 1985; Caliguiri *et al*, 1987; Lloyd *et al*, 1989), however, have supported alternative hypotheses (e.g. that of Wakefield & Lloyd, 1987) that highlight the role of biological factors in the condition.

Straus (1988) stated that "ultimately, any hypothesis regarding the cause of the chronic fatigue syndrome must incorporate the psychopathology that accompanies and, in some cases, precedes it," emphasising the importance of assessing psychopathology both pre-morbidly and during the illness.

The frequency of neuropsychiatric and depressive symptoms in these patients (David *et al*, 1988; Straus, 1988) suggested the specific hypothesis that CFS occurs in individuals with a pre-morbid vulnerability to depression. A case–control study of 24 subjects by Taerk *et al* (1987) supported this notion but may be challenged as controls were healthy hospital personnel, and no attempt was made to validate prevalence estimates. Similarly, Kruesi *et al* (1989) have reported an increased life-time prevalence of depressive and anxiety disorders in patients with CFS.

In this paper we record the prevalence of psychiatric morbidity in patients with CFS both during and before the illness episode to determine whether the syndrome is associated with an increase in psychological disturbance, and whether subjects had a higher pre-morbid rate of psychiatric disturbance. We included a control group of patients with non-endogenous depression to assess whether CFS patients resembled patients with depression, either during the illness episode or on pre-morbid measures.

The non-specific nature of the key symptom of fatigue has necessitated the development of strict criteria for CFS (Holmes *et al*, 1988; Lloyd *et al*, 1988*a*,*b*). The Centers for Disease Control (CDC) criteria (Holmes *et al*, 1988) specifically exclude patients with a number of psychiatric disorders and those taking psychotropic medication, effectively preventing accurate quantification of psychological symptoms in patients with CFS. The difficulty created by those criteria is exemplified by the study of Manu *et al* (1988), who reported that 95% of 135 consecutive patients who had attended a fatigue clinic in a university hospital, with at least a six-month history of debilitating fatigue, failed to meet CDC criteria. The overwhelming reason for exclusion was current psychiatric disorder (91/135) and the most prevalent psychiatric diagnosis was "major depression" (67/91). Such concurrent psychiatric morbidity was assumed to be "a *major cause* of these patients' fatigue" (italics added). The criteria used in the present study, however, do not make this assumption, and thereby avoid the limitation of excluding subjects on the basis of psychological symptoms.

METHOD

We studied 48 subjects with marked and persistent fatigue who met the following operational criteria for CFS (Lloyd *et al*, 1988*a*):

To fulfil the criteria a patient must have chronic, persistent or relapsing fatigue of a generalised nature, causing major disruption of usual daily activities, present for more than six months, plus two major *or* one major and three minor criteria (symptoms, signs, or assessments):

(a) Symptoms: persisting at least six months continuously, or relapsing on three or more occasions with a similar pattern over six months or more:

    (i) Major: concentration/memory impairment

    (ii) Minor: myalgia, arthralgia, depression, tinnitus, paraesthesia, headaches.

(b) Signs: present on at least one occasion subsequent to the initial illness:

    (i) Major: lymphadenopathy

    (ii) Minor: pharyngitis, muscle tenderness.

(c) Immunological assessment:

    (i) Major: cutaneous anergy, T4 or T8 lymphopenia

    (ii) Minor: hypoergy

The criteria that we have recommended since are a simplification of those original criteria (Lloyd et al, 1988b). Both of our sets of criteria emphasise the importance of a characteristic pattern of physical and neuropsychological impairment and the demonstration of impaired cell-mediated immunity.

All patients had been referred by their general practitioner to the immunology or infectious diseases' department of a university teaching hospital for evaluation of their chronic fatigue. Patients referred to this service typically had been extensively investigated by their own practitioners and/or other consultant physicians. Additionally, many had been assessed previously by a psychiatrist. The patients in this report were drawn from a previously described sample of 200 patients (Lloyd et al, 1988b) who had been assessed rigorously to exclude other possible physical causes of fatigue (infectious diseases or thyroid, neurological, haematological, hepatic, renal, or autoimmune dysfunction). Although the CDC criteria were not established at the time our patients were enrolled, the process of physical evaluation and investigation we used was as extensive as that recommended by Holmes et al (1988).

Twenty-nine of the 48 patients had developed their persistent fatigue immediately after an acute infectious illness. Five of these illnesses had been documented serologically (four Epstein–Barr virus infections, one toxoplasmosis). Patients were approached to progress to a treatment trial on the basis of the persistence of their symptoms and their willingness to give informed consent to participate in a double-blind, placebo-controlled, treatment trial of intravenous immunoglobulin therapy (to be reported elsewhere). The extensive process of physical evaluation within a tertiary referral service, the application of strict clinical and laboratory criteria, and the delay between initial contact with the clinic and inclusion in the treatment trial, all limited the clinical heterogeneity that one might expect within such a sample.

Initially, each subject was asked by the psychiatrist (I.H.) to describe their 'key symptoms'. The interviewer recorded the frequency with which psychological and neuropsychological symptoms were reported spontaneously before administering a standardised psychiatric interview schedule (SCID–P; Spitzer & Williams, 1985) which generated DSM–III–R (American Psychiatric Association, 1987) diagnostic data. A relative of each patient was interviewed independently to corroborate the patient's report. Because of a delay in the commencement of the psychiatrist's involvement in the trial, 33 patients were interviewed before treatment, and the remaining 15 patients after completion of immunoglobulin infusions.

All subjects completed a number of psychometric measures, including the 30-item General Health Questionnaire (GHQ; Goldberg, 1979), the Zung Self-Rating Depression Scale (Zung, 1965), the Eysenck Personality Inventory (Eysenck & Eysenck, 1964), and the Illness Behaviour Questionnaire (Pilowsky & Spence, 1983). The latter scale generates scores on seven dimensions which indicate the subject's attitudes towards the illness. The 17-item Hamilton Rating Scale for Depression (Hamilton, 1960), and the Newcastle Depression Scale (Carney et al, 1965), used to identify patients with endogenous depression, were administered by the psychiatrist.

Forty-eight patients with non-endogenous depression (Newcastle Depression Scale score less than five) were selected from the in-patient and out-patient psychiatric services of the same hospital for comparison with the patients with CFS.

RESULTS

The mean age of the patients was 36 (range 15–63) years, and there were equal numbers of men and women. The mean duration of illness was 56 (median 46, range 12–156) months. The sample therefore contained patients with chronic illness with little prospect of spontaneous remission.

The control subjects suffering from non-endogenous depression were matched exactly for sex, and similarly for age (36.1 v. 37.8 years, $t=1.56$, NS) and social class (mean Congalton (1969) score: 3.69 v. 3.89, $t=1.01$, NS). Of the 48 control patients, 28 met DSM–III–R criteria for major depression, while the remaining 20 had minor depressive disorders. None of these control patients had been depressed continuously for two years, so that there were no cases of dysthymic disorder. Nineteen were in-patients of a general hospital psychiatry unit, while 29 were from out-patient and liaison psychiatry clinics.

Table I Frequency of spontaneous reports of neuropsychological or psychological symptoms as 'key' features by patients with CFS ($n=48$)

Spontaneous symptoms	No. of patients	Percentage of patients
Neuropsychological impairments		
concentration/attention	25	52%
short-term memory	13	27%
dysphasia	4	8%
planning tasks	2	4%
Total	29	60%
Psychological symptoms		
depression	18	38%
irritability	8	17%
anxiety/worry/tension	4	8%
Total	19	40%
Total (neuropsychological and/or psychological)	38	80%

Of the 48 patients with CFS, 19 spontaneously reported psychological and 29 reported neuropsychological complaints among their key symptoms (Table 1).

Twenty-four warranted a psychiatric diagnosis during the course of their illness. The commonest disorder was major (non-endogenous) depression (8 men, 14 women). Six of these 22 depressed patients with CFS also experienced panic attacks, although these were frequent enough in only one case to justify an additional diagnosis of panic disorder. In addition, three non-depressed patients had experienced at least one panic attack, and two of these subjects met criteria for panic disorder. Only one patient, who also met criteria for major depression, fulfilled criteria for somatisation disorder (Briquet's hysteria). There were no cases of generalised anxiety disorder and, although a number of patients reported simple phobias, none was associated with avoidant behaviour leading to significant impairment of daily functioning.

The overall concordance of subject/witness reports was very high (kappa= 0.87), with relatives reporting a psychiatric diagnosis in 23 of the patients, strongly supporting the accuracy of our estimate. In the 33 patients assessed before treatment, the prevalence rate of psychiatric disorder in the preceding month was 21% (7/33), all having major (non-endogenous) depression.

The GHQ scores of the 33 subjects assessed immediately before treatment established that 15 had a score of five or above, generally suggestive of psychiatric morbidity (Goldberg, 1979). In patients with known medical disorders, however, significant physical symptoms inevitably lead to positive responses on more of the GHQ items. Zung depression scores for the 33 subjects assessed before treatment showed that 19 scores above the recommended cut-off point of 40 (Zung, 1972) for identifying mild depression in community settings. As with the GHQ, the raw Zung score is known to be significantly elevated in medical patients (Zung et al, 1983). It is possible to overcome this effect, in part, by comparing the number of patients and depressive controls assigned to at least the moderately depressed range (48 or above) on the Zung scale. Using this higher cut-off point, a highly significant difference ($\chi^2=22.06$, $P<0.001$) remained between the number of patients with CFS (8/33) in comparison to the number of

Table 2 Mean scores from the Zung Self-Rating Depression Scale (n=33)

Item no.	Mean
Most frequently reported Zung items	
12 Not easy to do things	3.5
10 Tiredness	3.4
2 Worse in a.m.	2.8
11 Mind not clear	2.8
16 Indecisive	2.4
Least frequently reported Zung items	
19 Suicidal	1.1
7 Weight loss	1.2
3 Tearful	1.4
13 Restless	1.5
9 Palpitations	1.5

depressive controls (37/48). This established that depressive disorders of clinical severity were rare in the CFS sample. Table 2 shows patients' mean scores on the Zung items.

This distinction was supported by the significant differences between the mean scores of the CFS patients and depressive controls on the Hamilton (10.6 v. 19.0, $t=8.92$, $P<0.001$) and Zung (40.7 v. 55.2, $t=7.67$, $P<0.001$) scales. Importantly, patients with CFS also reported significantly lower levels of neuroticism (7.3 v. 15.8, $t=7.71$, $P<0.001$). This suggested that any psychiatric morbidity in the CFS sample was less severe, in addition to being less prevalent, than in depressed patients.

Table 3 records the patients', their relatives', and the depressives' estimates of prior psychological morbidity. Again there was substantial agreement between the patients' and relatives' estimates of overall pre-morbid psychiatric morbidity in the CFS group (kappa=0.81). Thirty of the 48

depressive controls had had a previous episode that met DSM–III–R criteria for major depression, compared with 6 of the 48 CFS patients ($\chi^2=25.6$, $P<0.001$).

The scores of the patients with CFS on the seven dimensions of the Illness Behaviour Questionnare are shown in Table 4. Comparison of these data with previously reported Australian general practice samples (Pilowsky & Spence, 1983) and patients with Briquet's hysteria (Singer et al, 1988) suggests that the illness behaviour of patients with CFS is characterised by the strong conviction that they are physically ill (i.e. high scores on 'disease conviction': "an attitude of determined certainty as to the presence of disease, and a resistance to reassurance" (Pilowsky, 1988) and low scores on 'psychological v. somatic concern', which is said to be indicative of "somatic focusing" (Pilowsky, 1988)).

In contrast to patients with Briquet's hysteria, who typically present their psychological concerns in a somatic form, patients with CFS are not hypochondriacal and are not inhibited in their expression of affectively laden topics. (A high score on 'affective inhibition' is said to indicate "a reluctance to communicate inner feelings to others, particularly those of hostility" and is felt to be related to the notions of "introspection and . . . alexithymia" (Pilowsky, 1988)). Patients with CFS do differ from general practice patients, however, principally in terms of their reluctance to accept psychological interpretations of their somatic symptoms. Further, they have somewhat higher scores on the 'denial' subscale, which purports to measure "the tendency to regard illness as the sole problem, whose resolution would result in a circumstance devoid of difficulties" and "the tendency to displace attention from psychosocial stressors onto physical problems" (Pilowsky, 1988).

Table 3 Numbers of patients and relatives reporting psychiatric morbidity before onset of CFS (n=48), and controls (n=48) before onset of depression

DSM–III–R	Patients		Depressive controls
	Self-report	Relatives' report	
Major depression	6 (12.5%)	6 (12.5%)	30 (62%)
Panic disorder	1 (2%)	1 (2%)	3 (6%)
Alcohol dependence	4 (8%)	4 (8%)	18 (38%)
Benzodiazepine dependence	–	–	5 (10%)
Psychotic episode	1 (2%)	1 (2%)	–
Total previous morbidity	12 (24.5%)	12 (24.5%)	43 (90%)

Table 4 Mean scores on dimensions of illness behaviour of patients with CFS as measured by the Illness Behaviour Questionnaire (IBQ)

IBQ subscale	CFS patients (n=44) mean (s.d.)	General practice[1] (n=147) mean	Briquet's syndrome[2] (n=17) mean
General hypochondriasis (range=0–9)	1.96 (1.9)	1.44	4.0
Disease conviction (range=0–6)	4.25 (1.2)	1.59	4.0
Psychological v. somatic focusing (range=0–5)	0.45 (0.8)	1.99	1.0
Affective inhibition (range=0–5)	1.98 (1.7)	2.46	4.0
Dysphoria (range=0–5)	2.00 (1.7)	2.31	5.0
Denial (range=0–5)	3.43 (1.6)	2.93	2.0
Irritability (range=0–6)	2.93 (1.8)	2.45	3.0

1. Pilowsky & Spence (1983).
2. Singer et al (1988).

DISCUSSION

Eighty per cent of patients with CFS spontaneously reported that neuropsychological and/or psychological difficulties were among their key complaints, confirming that such symptoms are common components of the CFS syndrome. Half had a psychiatric diagnosis (usually major depression) during the course of the illness, and 21% met criteria for major (non-endogenous) depression at the start of treatment.

The existence of significant psychological morbidity during the illness raises the question as to whether CFS is a mislabelled depressive disorder or a depressive equivalent. As early as 1907 Kraepelin noted that "acquired neurasthenia" needed to be carefully differentiated from melancholia. If CFS is a form of depressive disorder, a similar pattern of current symptoms and past psychiatric disorder might be expected in CFS patients to that observed in depressed psychiatric patients. Our findings do not support that proposition.

The estimated prevalence of pre-morbid lifetime psychiatric disorder in our CFS subjects (24%) is comparable with that reported in three sites of the Epidemiological Catchment Area Survey (ECA), where the lifetime prevalences of psychiatric disorder (excluding phobic disorders) were 24.9%, 23.9%, and 26.2% respectively (Robins et al, 1984). Previous large epidemiological studies have indicated a lifetime prevalence rate for major depression of 18–25% (Weissman et al, 1978; Reich et al, 1980; Bromet et al, 1986), larger than our estimate of a 12.5% pre-morbid prevalence rate of depression in CFS patients. Corroborative data from relatives were highly consistent with reports by the subjects and offer strong support for the validity of our data.

When compared with non-endogenously depressed controls, our CFS patients did not have a similar high pre-morbid rate of psychiatric disorder, were significantly less neurotic, and, when unwell, neither clinically resembled nor had the psychometric profile of non-endogenous depressive patients seen in psychiatric settings. The percentage of subjects with non-specific psychiatric symptoms as determined by the GHQ in our sample is consistent with previous findings in general medical (Goldberg & Blackwell, 1970; Maguire et al, 1974) and neurological settings (Bridges & Goldberg, 1984).

The interviewing psychiatrist was not blind to the clinical diagnosis of the patients with CFS or depressive disorders, and so it is important to consider whether a systematic bias may have been introduced in the evaluation of prevalence rates of pre-morbid psychiatric disorder. Given the important differences in the type of symptoms reported by patients with CFS as compared with patients with depressive disorders, it is doubtful that a truly 'blind' investigation is possible. We sought, however, to avoid any potential bias by using a highly structured interviewing technique. Further, we corroborated our data in the CFS patients with prevalence results reported by relatives, and we established high levels of agreement. Neither the interviewees nor the relatives were reluctant to report recent psychiatric morbidity. It is unlikely, therefore, that the low pre-morbid rates of disorder can be attributed to

systematic under-recording of psychiatric morbidity. It is possible, however, that a recall bias may have been operating, such that past psychiatric morbidity was not remembered by either patients or their relatives as readily as that morbidity associated with their current protracted illness.

Our findings do not confirm those of Taerk et al (1987), who suggested a much higher pre-morbid risk of depressive disorder in patients with CFS. The patients in that study were not as extensively evaluated as the patients in this study or that of Kruesi et al (1989), so that it is likely that their sample was less homogeneous. In their study, however, if one compares the pre-morbid prevalence rate of major depression in the patients (12/24), rather than the total lifetime prevalence rates (67%, which includes the period of the current illness), with the lifetime prevalence rate in the 'healthy' controls (7/24), then there is only a non-significant trend ($\chi^2=2.2$, NS) towards higher affective disorder in the patient group. Further, the use of the criteria from the Diagnostic Interview Schedule (DIS) and DSM–III in that study produced high prevalence rates of all psychiatric disorders in both the patients and the 'healthy controls', suggesting that the actual threshold for psychiatric diagnosis was low.

Although Taerk et al (1987) did not suggest that depression alone was the cause of their subjects' illnesses, they did suggest that "sporadic neuromyasthenia may be the result of an organic illness in psychologically susceptible (i.e. premorbidly depressed) individuals". By contrast, our results suggest that CFS patients are no more psychologically disturbed before the onset of their illness than members of the general population. Taerk et al used DSM–III criteria for major depression, whereas we used the more strict criteria of DSM–III–R, and so we would expect lower prevalence rates for this disorder in our study.

Kruesi et al (1989) studied 28 patients who were said to have met CDC criteria for CFS. The patients were interviewed with the DIS to assess lifetime prevalence rates of psychiatric disorder. Patients in that study had been ill for a mean of 6.8 years and had been extensively investigated to exclude other possible disorders, thereby creating a sample quite similar to our own. Contrary to the actual CDC criteria, however, the presence of a current or past psychiatric diagnosis did not exclude those patients from participation in a treatment trial of acyclovir, an antiviral therapy. Lifetime depressive disorders were identified in 54% (15/28) of their patients (13 cases of major depression), while 21% (6/28) were currently depressed. These depressive diagnoses, however, were closely related in time to the onset or course of the fatigue syndrome. Simple phobia was reported as clinically significant in eight patients (29%), a remarkably high proportion. Only two of their patients met criteria for somatisation disorder, while other significant anxiety disorders were rare (one case of panic disorder and no cases of generalised anxiety disorder).

Examination of the pre-morbid prevalence rates suggested that eight of their patients had simple phobia, one had panic disorder/agoraphobia, and only two had a major depressive disorder. Attaching surprising importance, however, to the pre-morbid diagnoses of simple phobia, the authors concluded that "psychiatric disorders more often preceded the chronic fatigue than followed it". Robins *et al* (1984) have noted the high inter-site variation in the prevalence of the diagnosis of simple phobia using the DIS and DSM–III criteria, and reported their lifetime prevalence data for all disorders both with and without this diagnostic category. The high rate of simple phobia reported by Kruesi *et al* (1989) is therefore likely to be a result of the interview method and is unlikely to be of psychopathological significance in patients with CFS.

If one limits evaluation of their cases to those with axis I diagnoses, but excludes simple phobia, then there are important similarities between their findings and ours. The pre-morbid rate of psychiatric disorder was low, 18% (5/28) (one patient with agoraphobia, two with major depression, and two cases of alcohol abuse, allowing that each diagnosis was actually for a different individual), comparable with our premorbid rate of 25%. Depressive disorders were common in association with the fatigue syndrome (54% as compared with our rate of 46%), with a currently depressed case rate of 21%, which is identical to our figure.

Our method of case selection involved the enrolment of individuals who had been extensively evaluated within a tertiary referral service and who had often experienced considerable delay between confirmation of the diagnosis and participation in the treatment trial. This process may have decreased the rate of current psychiatric symptoms. No active psychiatric screening was undertaken by the hospital medical staff before inclusion in the trial, but our patients cannot be considered comparable with patients presenting for the first time complaining of fatigue in general medical settings. Establishing the pattern of pre-morbid and current psychopathology in a group of patients who clearly meet strict clinical and immunological criteria for the disorder is essential, however, before progressing to the evaluation of patients who may share only the symptom of fatigue in common.

The pattern of illness behaviour recorded in our patients was not similar to that previously described in patients with defined Briquet's hysteria (Singer *et al*, 1988), as patients with CFS were not particularly hypochondriacal, affectively inhibited, or dysphoric. If patients with CFS were dealing principally with psychological distress by the process of somatisation, one might have expected higher scores on those relevant subscales.

Our patients differed from those in Australian general practice, principally in terms of their conviction that they were physically ill. Given the controversy surrounding this disorder, the referral of these patients to a tertiary assessment service and their participation in a pharmacological treatment trial, the firmness with which they held this belief and rejected psychological interpretations of the cause of their illness is not surprising. It may be of considerable clinical importance, however, as conflict may quickly arise between such patients and medical practitioners who are openly sceptical about the disorder.

In conclusion, we have demonstrated that while depression and anxiety are common symptoms in patients suffering from CFS, there is no evidence from our well-defined sample to support the hypothesis that CFS is a somatic presentation of an underlying psychological disorder. In particular, there is no evidence that CFS is a variant or expression of a depressive disorder. Instead, our study supports the hypothesis that the current psychological symptoms of patients with CFS are a consequence of the disorder, rather than evidence of antecedent vulnerability. We are unable to say whether the psychological symptoms occur purely as a result of the fatigue, or as an integral symptom of the disease process. Comparisons between pa-

tients with CFS and patients who have fatigue on a peripheral basis (e.g. myasthenia gravis) or on a central basis (e.g. multiple sclerosis (Krupp *et al*, 1988)) will be undertaken to clarify this issue further.

It is possible that the chronic production of cytokines, such as interferon, which is released by lymphocytes in response to viral infections, may account for the morbidity reported by these patients. These soluble products of lymphocytes may precipitate fatigue and neuropsychiatric syndromes in humans (Denicoff *et al*, 1987; McDonald *et al*, 1987) and, therefore, ongoing localised production of these substances within the central nervous system of patients with CFS constitutes a possible explanation for the diverse physical, neuropsychiatric, and psychological symptoms encountered in this syndrome (Wakefield & Lloyd, 1987).

ACKNOWLEDGEMENTS

Dr Hickie is funded by the NSW Institute of Psychiatry, and Dr Lloyd by the National Health and Medical Research Council of Australia.

REFERENCES

American Psychiatric Association (1987) *Diagnostic and Statistical Manual of Mental Disorders* (3rd edn, revised). Washington, DC: APA.

Behan, P. O., Behan, W. M. H. & Bell, E. J. (1985) The postviral fatigue syndrome – analysis of the findings in 50 cases. *Journal of Infection*, **10**, 211–222.

Bridges, K. W. & Goldberg, D. P. (1984) Psychiatric illness in inpatients with neurological disorders: patients' views on discussion of emotional problems with neurologists. *British Medical Journal*, **289**, 656–658.

Bromet, E. J., Dunn, L. O., Connell, M. M., et al (1986) Long-term reliability of diagnosing lifetime major depression in a community sample. *Archives of General Psychiatry*, **43**, 435–440.

Caliguiri, M., Murray, C., Buchwald, D., et al (1987) Phenotypic and functional deficiency of natural killer cells in patients with chronic fatigue syndrome. *Journal of Immunology*, **139**, 3306–3313.

Carney, M. W. P., Roth, M. & Garside, R. F. (1965) The diagnosis of depressive symptoms and the prediction of ECT response. *British Journal of Psychiatry*, **111**, 659–674.

Congalton, A. A. (1969) *Status and Prestige in Australia*. Melbourne: F. W. Cheshire Publishing Pty Ltd.

David, A. S., Wessely, S. & Pelosi, A. J. (1988) Postviral fatigue syndrome: time for a new approach. *British Medical Journal*, **296**, 696–699.

Dawson, J. (1987) Royal Free disease: perplexity continues (editorial). *British Medical Journal*, **294**, 327–328.

Denicoff, K. D., Rubinow, D. R., Papa, M. Z., et al (1987) The neuropsychiatric effects of treatment with interleukin-2 and lymphokine-activated killer cells. *Annals of Internal Medicine*, **107**, 293–300.

Eysenck, H. J. & Eysenck, S. B. (1964) *Manual of the Eysenck Personality Inventory.* London: Hodder & Stoughton.

Goldberg, D. P. (1979) *Manual of the General Health Questionnaire.* Windsor: NFER Publishing Co.

__ & Blackwell, B. (1970) Psychiatric illness in general medical practice. *British Medical Journal,* ii, 439–443.

Hamilton, M. (1960) A rating scale for depression. *Journal of Neurology, Neurosurgery and Psychiatry,* 23, 56–62.

Holmes, G. P., Kaplan, J. E., Gantz, N. M., et al (1988) Chronic fatigue syndrome: a working case definition. *Annals of Internal Medicine,* 108, 387–389.

Kraepelin, E. (1981) *Clinical Psychiatry* (ed. R. I. Watson). New York: Scholars' Facsimiles & Reprints.

Kruesi, M. J. P., Dale, J. & Straus, S. E. (1989) Psychiatric diagnoses in patients who have chronic fatigue syndrome. *Journal of Clinical Psychiatry,* 50, 53–56.

Krupp, L. B., Alvarez, L. A., LaRocca, N. G., et al (1988) Fatigue in multiple sclerosis. *Archives of Neurology,* 45, 435–437.

Lloyd, A. R., Hales, J. P. & Gandevia, S. C. (1988a) Muscle strength, endurance and recovery in the post-infection fatigue syndrome. *Journal of Neurology, Neurosurgery and Psychiatry,* 51, 1316–1322.

__ , Wakefield, D., Boughton, C., et al (1988b) What is myalgic encephalomyelitis? *Lancet,* i, 1286–1287.

__ , __ , __ , et al (1989) Immunological abnormalities in the chronic fatigue syndrome. *Medical Journal of Australia,* 151, 122–124.

Maguire, G. P., Julier, D. L., Hawton, K. E., et al (1974) Psychiatric morbidity and referral on two general medical wards. *British Medical Journal,* i, 268–270.

Manu, P., Lane, T. J. & Matthews, D. A. (1988) The frequency of the chronic fatigue syndrome in patients with symptoms of persistent fatigue. *Annals of Internal Medicine,* 109, 554–556.

McDonald, E. M., Mann, A. H. & Thomas, H. C. (1987) Interferons as mediators of psychiatric morbidity. An investigation in a trial of recombinant α-interferon in hepatitis-B carriers. *Lancet,* ii, 1175–1177.

McEvedy, C. P. & Beard, A. W. (1973) A controlled follow-up of cases involved in an epidemic of benign myalgic encephalomyelitis. *British Journal of Psychiatry,* 122, 141–150.

Pilowsky, I. (1988) Abnormal illness behaviour. In *Handbook of Social Psychiatry* (eds A. S. Henderson & G. Burrows). Amsterdam: Elsevier Science publishers.

__ & Spence, N. D. (1983) *Manual for the Illness Behaviour Questionnaire (IBQ)* (2nd edn). Adelaide: University of Adelaide.

Reich, T., Rice, J., Andreasen, N., et al (1980) A preliminary analysis of the segregation distribution of primary major depressive disorder. *Psychological Bulletin,* 16, 34–36.

Robins, L. N., Helzer, J. E., Weissman, M. M., et al (1984) Lifetime prevalence of specific psychiatric disorders in three sites. *Archives of General Psychiatry,* 41, 949–958.

Singer, A., Thompson, S., Kraiuhin, C., et al (1988) An investigation of patients presenting with multiple physical complaints using the Illness Behaviour Questionnaire. *Psychotherapy and Psychosomatics,* 47, 181–189.

Spitzer, R. L. & Williams, J. B. W. (1985) *Structured Clinical Interview for DSM–III–R, Patient Version (SCID–P, 7/1/85).* New York: Biometrics Research Dept, Psychiatric Institute.

Straus, S. E. (1988) The chronic mononucleosis syndrome. *Journal of Infectious Diseases,* 157, 405–412.

__ , Tosato, G., Armstrong, G., et al (1985) Persisting fatigue and illness in adults with evidence of persisting Epstein–Barr virus infection. *Annals of Internal Medicine,* 102, 7–16.

Swartz, M. N. (1988) The chronic fatigue syndrome – one entity or many (editorial)? *New England Journal of Medicine,* 319, 1726–1728.

Taerk, G. S., Toner, B. B., Salit, I. E., et al (1987) Depression in patients with neuromyasthenia (benign myalgic encephalomyelitis). *International Journal of Psychiatry in Medicine,* 17, 49–56.

Wakefield, D. & Lloyd, A. (1987) Pathophysiology of myalgic encephalomyelitis. *Lancet,* ii, 918–919.

Weissman, M. M., Myers, J. K. & Harding, P. S. (1978) Psychiatric disorders in a US urban community: 1975–76. *American Journal of Psychiatry,* 135, 459–462.

Yousef, G. E., Bell, E. J., Mann, G. F., et al (1988) Chronic enterovirus infection in patients with postviral fatigue syndrome. *Lancet,* i, 146–149.

Zung, W. W. K. (1965) A self-rating depression scale. *Archives of General Psychiatry,* 12, 63–70.

__ (1972) How normal is depression? *Psychosomatics,* 12, 174–178.

__ , Magill, M., Moore, J. T., et al (1983) Recognition and treatment of depression in a family medicine practice. *Journal of Clinical Psychiatry,* 44, 3–6.

IAN HICKIE, FRANZCP, Staff Specialist in Psychiatry, Mood Disorders Unit, Prince Henry Hospital, Sydney, Australia; ANDREW LLOYD, FRACP, NH & MRC Research Fellow, School of Pathology, University of New South Wales, Kensington NSW, Australia; DENIS WAKEFIELD, MD, FRACP, Associate Professor of Pathology, School of Pathology, University of New South Wales, Kensington NSW, Australia; GORDON PARKER, MD, PhD, FRANZCP, Professor of Psychiatry, School of Psychiatry (University of New South Wales), Prince Henry Hospital, Sydney, Australia

Correspondence: Ian Hickie, Mood Disorders Unit, Division of Psychiatry, Prince Henry Hospital, Sydney, 2036 Australia

Cognitive deficits in patients suffering from chronic fatigue syndrome, acute infective illness or depression

UTE VOLLMER-CONNA, DENIS WAKEFIELD, ANDREW LLOYD, IAN HICKIE, JIM LEMON, KEVIN D. BIRD and REGINALD F. WESTBROOK

Background Patients with chronic fatigue syndrome (CFS) report neuro-psychological symptoms as a characteristic feature. We sought to assess cognitive performance in patients with CFS, and compare cognitive performance and subjective workload experience of these patients with that of two disease comparison groups (non-melanchonic depression and acute infection) and healthy controls.

Method A computerised performance battery employed to assess cognitive functioning included tests of continuous attention, response speed, performance accuracy and memory. Severity of mood disturbance and subjective fatigue were assessed by questionnaire.

Results All patient groups demonstrated increased errors and slower reaction times, and gave higher workload ratings than healthy controls. Patients with CFS and non-melancholic depression had more severe deficits than patients with acute infection. All patient groups reported more severe mood disturbance and fatigue than healthy controls, but patients with CFS and those with acute infection reported less severe mood disturbance than patients with depression.

Conclusions As all patients demonstrated similar deficits in attention and response speed, it is possible that common pathophysiological processes are involved. The differences in severity of mood disturbance, however, suggest that the pathophysiological processes in patients with CFS and acute infection are not simply secondary to depressed mood.

The formal assessment of cognitive functioning in patients with CFS has produced inconsistent results (see Moss-Morris et al, 1996, for review). While some studies have failed to detect cognitive impairments (Grafman et al, 1993), others have found that patients with CFS demonstrate a variety of deficits including poor memory, slowed response execution, poor detection of target stimuli, and a heightened vulnerability to interference (Prasher et al, 1990; Scheffers et al, 1992; Sandman et al, 1993; Smith et al, 1993; DeLuca et al, 1993, 1995; Wearden & Appleby, 1997). The main aims of this study were: (a) to provide a detailed assessment of cognitive performance in patients suffering from CFS; and (b) to compare the performance and the reports of workload of patients suffering from CFS with that of two relevant positive control groups (patients with major, non-melancholic depression and patients suffering from an acute infective illness), as well as healthy control subjects. We also studied the relationship between mental activity and fatigue, by examining changes in performance and mental workload ratings as a function of time or task difficulty.

METHOD

Subjects

Patients who met our modified diagnostic criteria for CFS, which require six months or more of unexplained disabling fatigue and constitutional symptoms, but do not require demonstration of abnormal cell-mediated immunity (Lloyd et al, 1990) were selected from those referred to the Department of Immunology at the Prince Henry and Prince of Wales Hospitals, Sydney, for evaluation of chronic fatigue. Their mean duration of illness was five years (range eight months to 10 years). Twenty of the 21 patients reported developing CFS subsequent to an acute infectious illness. In 10 cases the illness had been documented serologically (eight

Epstein–Barr virus infections, two Ross River fever). Patients with acute infective illness were recruited through the Casualty and the Infectious Disease Departments at the Prince Henry Hospital, general practitioners, and public notices in local newspapers and on radio. Five patients had documented acute Epstein–Barr virus infections, the remaining patients suffered from influenza-like illnesses. Patients with depression were recruited from in- and out-patient services at the Mood Disorders Unit, Prince Henry Hospital, and met DSM–III–R (American Psychiatric Association, 1987) criteria for major depressive episode (non-melancholic type). These control subjects were specifically chosen as they exhibit comparable socio-demographic characteristics to patients with CFS, including female predominance and age at onset of symptoms between 20–40 years of age. Healthy control subjects were recruited from hospital staff and the general community.

Subjects were excluded if on drugs known to impair cell-mediated immunity (in particular, corticosteroids and non-steroidal anti-inflammatory drugs). However, seven of the depressed patients and two patients with CFS remained on low-dose antidepressant therapy. Potential subjects were excluded if: they had a history of physical illness associated with abnormal immunity (particularly, auto-immune diseases, diabetes or malignancy); and if there was a history of viral infection within the previous two weeks (with the exception of those belonging to the group with an acute infective illness). Subjects in the four groups were matched for gender, age, education, and scores on two standardised tests of general intelligence (the National Adult Reading Test, NART (Nelson, 1982) and an abbreviated version of Raven's Advanced Progressive Matrices (Raven, 1962)). The study was approved by the institutional ethics committee and informed consent was obtained from all subjects.

Procedure

Subjects attended a 3–4 hour testing session. A structured interview was used to obtain relevant demographic information and medical history. Subjects completed the self-report Profile of Mood States (POMS) questionnaire (McNair et al, 1981) to obtain data from the tension/anxiety, depression, confusion, and fatigue subscales. A modified, computerised Rozelle Test Battery (Lemon, 1990) was used to assess cognitive performance. This battery consisted of six tests chosen to provide a relatively broad assessment of attention and concentration, while permitting an examination of specific difficulties previously described in patients with CFS, including a vulnerability to interference, slowed response execution, difficulties with sustained concentration, spatial orientation and short-term memory. The tests were: an auditory discrimination task; a pursuit-tracking task; a divided attention task, which involved the concurrent performance of the first two tests; a task-shifting task, consisting of a Sternberg-type, short-term memory task (Sternberg, 1966) and an arithmetical task; a left–right discrimination/spatial orientation task; and the Mackworth clock, vigilance task (Mackworth, 1948). The order of the tests was counterbalanced across subjects. After the completion of each of the tasks, task-related subjective workload experience was assessed by visual analogue scales (0–9) with end-point descriptions. Variables of interest were perceived mental demand, physical demand, time pressure, effort, fatigue, and frustration level (Hart & Staveland, 1988). Workload experience was assessed by a composite measure derived by summing a subject's scores on the separate workload variables.

Statistical analyses

ANOVAs were performed on each of the three sets of outcome measures (i.e. performance, workload and mood data). Between-group differences on each of the dependent measures and some planned linear combinations of these were analysed using the analysis of variance option available on the SYSTAT statistical package (Wilkinson, 1990). Logarithmic transformations were applied to normalise performance measures. Standardised coefficients were used when between-group differences on any linear combination of dependent measures were assessed.

Post-hoc orthogonal contrasts were written and the decision-wise error rate was controlled by the technique described by Rodger (1967) which yields F critical=5.58, with α=0.05 and d.f.=3, 80.

The data collected continuously (at five-second intervals) during the pursuit-tracking task were used for a detailed assessment of the stability of subjects' performance under conditions of sustained attention and effort. Fast Fourier transform algorithms (Quinn-Curtis, 1990) were used to determine the power in subjects' performance curves at frequencies above or equal to 0.016 Hz (see below). The power scores produced by these

analyses represent a measure of performance stability. High values indicate a more unstable performance.

Correlational analyses were performed to examine relationships between variables.

RESULTS

There were no significant between-group differences in age ($F(3, 80) < 1$), education ($F(3, 80) < 1$) or measures of general intelligence: NART ($F(3, 80)=1.5$) and Raven's Matrices ($F(3, 80) < 1$) (Table 1). Descriptive statistics only for group performance on the different tasks are shown in Table 2. Comparative analyses were performed on summed error and reaction time data for each group.

Performance measures

Levels of performance

Overall, subjects in the three patient groups made significantly more errors ($F=9.69$) and took considerably longer to make their

responses ($F=21.33$) than did healthy subjects on tests involving auditory discrimination, short-term memory, left–right discrimination and sustained attention. Patients with CFS and those with depression did not differ from each other ($Fs < 1.0$), but were significantly slower ($F=9.49$) and less accurate ($F=10.88$) than those with an acute infective illness. Subjects in all patient groups were also less able to control the tracking display than were healthy subjects, both when this task was easy (performed in isolation, $F=17.29$) and difficult (in combination with the auditory discrimination task, $F=11.52$). The tracking performances of patients with CFS and with depression did not differ from each other, but were significantly worse than those of patients with acute infections under both easy ($F=8.38$) and difficult ($F=10.78$) task conditions.

Effects of task difficulty

Most tests contained an easy and a more difficult component. This permitted an

Table 1 Characteristics of patients in the study

	Age mean (s.d.)	Gender F:M	School leaving age mean (s.d.)	Number with tertiary degree	NART mean (s.d.)	Raven's matrices mean (s.d.)
Patients with CFS ($n=21$)	35.0 (14)	12:9	16.9 (1.3)	10	14.3 (5.6)	8.9 (2.5)
Patients with infections ($n=21$)	32.4 (11)	12:9	17.1 (1.3)	11	11.2 (6.5)	9.4 (1.9)
Patients with depression ($n=21$)	35.9 (11)	12:9	16.6 (1.4)	10	11.9 (4.4)	8.9 (1.9)
Healthy subjects ($n=21$)	33.5 (12)	12:9	16.9 (1.2)	10	11.5 (3.9)	9.7 (2.1)

Table 2 Summary table of performance indices for five computerised tasks

	Beeps		STM		'Little Man'		Vigilance		Tracking
	Errors	RT	Errors	RT	Errors	RT	Errors	RT	
Patients with CFS ($n=21$)	2.23	0.69	2.53	1.09	1.62	1.54	3.66	0.74	7.14
	(1.6)	(0.3)	(1.3)	(0.2)	(1.3)	(0.5)	(2.1)	(0.1)	(0.68)
Patients with infections ($n=21$)	1.89	0.56	1.20	0.95	1.21	1.34	1.90	0.70	6.54
	(1.2)	(0.2)	(1.1)	(0.2)	(1.1)	(0.4)	(1.7)	(0.1)	(0.47)
Patients with depression ($n=21$)	2.47	0.64	2.45	1.07	1.35	1.46	3.52	0.73	6.97
	(1.9)	(0.2)	(1.4)	(0.2)	(0.9)	(0.3)	(1.7)	(0.1)	(0.61)
Healthy subjects ($n=21$)	1.83	0.51	1.60	0.84	0.79	1.23	1.15	0.67	6.31
	(1.2)	(0.5)	(1.4)	(0.1)	(0.6)	(0.3)	(1.1)	(0.1)	(0.4)

Mean log scores (s.d.) for tracking ability (as mean delay in screen movements, ms); and for error rates (Errors) and reaction times (RT) on tasks involving auditory discrimination (Beeps), short-term memory (STM), left–right discrimination ('Little Man'), and vigilance. Statistical tests were performed on summed data, or between different task components (e.g. easy v. difficult, see text).

analysis of the performance decrement associated with the change in task difficulty. All subjects displayed considerably more difficulty in performing auditory discriminations as well as pursuit-tracking under divided attention (i.e. difficult) conditions than when each of these tasks were performed separately (increase in error rate: $F=25.48$; decline in tracking ability: $F=1323.09$). The magnitude of these performance decrements did not differ between the four groups ($Fs < 1$). Similarly, left–right discriminations were performed less accurately ($F=6.59$) and more slowly ($F=24.24$) by all subjects under difficult (figure oriented upside-down) than under easy (figure oriented head-up) conditions. The four groups were not differentially affected by the increase in task difficulty (errors: $Fs < 3.44$, reaction times: $Fs < 1.70$). Set membership decisions required more time when this task was interspersed with arithmetical exercises ($F=228.78$). This increase in reaction times was greater in patients with CFS and those with depression than in patients suffering from an acute infective illness ($F=7.73$).

Effects of task duration

Trend analyses revealed a significant, linear increase in errors ($F=38.88$) and response latencies ($F=28.66$) over time. The four groups did not differ with regard to the rate of increase in error scores ($Fs < 2.53$) or reaction times ($Fs < 2.31$).

Stability of performance

Tracking performance typically shows a negatively accelerated curve to the subject's maximal performance. This occurs because the test begins with a relatively large delay in screen movements (i.e. 80 ms). This delay is progressively reduced until the subject is making approximately one tracking error every five seconds. Healthy subjects tend to maintain maximal performance for the remainder of the 120 seconds. The performance of patients with CFS and depressive patients tended to vary cyclically throughout the session. Fourier analysis quantifies cyclic variation as the relative power (amplitude) of the sine wave components of that variation in successive frequency bands. The cut-off of 0.016 Hz was chosen to remove the component of variation which resulted from the normal decrease in delay to maximal performance. Table 3 shows the mean total power scores, summed across all frequency intervals, for each group of

Table 3 Performance stability

	Task conditions	
	Easy	Difficult
Patients with CFS ($n=21$)	2.22	2.33
	(0.69)	(0.83)
Patients with infections ($n=21$)	1.65	1.69
	(0.66)	(0.54)
Patients with depression ($n=21$)	2.01	2.19
	(0.61)	(0.87)
Healthy subjects ($n=21$)	1.45	1.47
	(0.47)	(0.48)

Mean total log scores (s.d.) of subjects under easy and difficult (divided attention) tracking conditions.

subjects under both task conditions. Higher scores signify greater instability in tracking performance.

The performance of the three patient groups was considerably more unstable than that of healthy subjects, whether tracking was performed by itself ($F=8.42$) or as part of a divided attention task ($F=7.19$). Patients with CFS and those with depression showed significantly more fluctuation in the tracking performance under difficult ($F=8.87$), but not easy ($F=5.32$) task conditions than patients with acute infective illnesses. Patients with CFS did not differ from depressive patients under either task condition ($F < 1.63$). There was no significant change in subjects' performance stability as a function of task difficulty (main effect: $F=5.22$, between-group differences: $Fs < 1$).

Subjective workload

Subjects in all three patient groups generally reported higher levels of workload for the different tasks than did healthy subjects ($F=10.52$). No other between-group differences were evident ($Fs < 3.34$). There was a linear increase in reported workload as a function of the number of completed tasks ($F=15.84$), but the rate of increase in perceived workload did not differ reliably between the four groups of subjects ($Fs < 4.26$). Correlational analyses were performed to examine the relationship between perceived workload and objective performance (total reaction time, total error rate, and average tracking ability). No reliable relationship between reported workload and any of the performance indices was demonstrated in any of the three patient groups. In contrast, the workload rating of healthy

subjects correlated well with their total error rate ($r=0.59$, $P < 0.01$) and average tracking performance ($r=0.52$, $P < 0.05$) but not with reaction times. Possible associations between workload experience and negative mood were also examined. We found no significant correlations between perceived workload and any of the POMS subscales in patients with CFS, depression, or healthy subjects. In patients with acute infective illness, however, reported workload was related to scores on the subscales of depression ($r=0.72$, $P < 0.01$), tension ($r=0.66$, $P < 0.01$), and confusion ($r=0.44$, $P < 0.05$; results not corrected for multiple comparisons).

Measures of mood state

All three patient groups scored significantly higher than healthy subjects on each of the POMS factors (tension: $F=32.47$, depression: $F=28.32$, confusion: $F=42.23$, and fatigue: $F=111.13$; see Fig. 1). There were no significant differences between the three patient groups in the reported level of fatigue ($F=2.72$). However, the ratings of patients with depression were significantly higher than those of patients with CFS and acute infective illness on the tension ($F=13.65$), depression ($F=39.41$) and confusion ($F=5.58$) subscales. The scores of patients with CFS and those with acute infective illness did not differ on any of the subscales ($Fs < 4.0$).

Analysis of the multiple possible associations between subjects' scores on the four POMS subscales and three performance indices, in patients with CFS or depression, and healthy controls, revealed no significant relationships. Without correcting for multiple comparisons, in patients with acute infections only, POMS depression scores were correlated with their total error rate ($r=0.47$, $P < 0.05$), and tension scores related

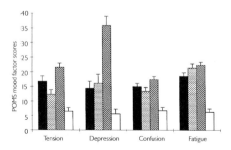

Fig. 1 Measures of mood state. Mean scores obtained from four POMS subscales for patients with CFS (■), acute infective illness (▨) or depression (▨), and healthy subjects (□). Error bars represent s.e.m.

to both their error rate ($r=0.69$, $P<0.01$) and reaction times ($r=0.47$, $P<0.05$).

DISCUSSION

Our results demonstrate differences between a sample of healthy subjects and patients suffering from either CFS, major (non-melancholic) depression or acute infective illnesses in cognitive performance, workload experience and mood. Subjects in all three patient groups were impaired on tasks assessing a range of cognitive capacities, including selective and divided attention, visuo-motor coordination, spatial discrimination, vigilance and short-term memory. The performance level of patients suffering from an acute infective illness was higher than that of patients with CFS or major depression. The latter two groups did not differ. The impairments in all three of the patient groups were more evident in the overall level, rather than the pattern of performance. Performance decrements were observed in all four groups of subjects as a function of task complexity and task duration, however, there was little evidence that the performance of specific patient groups was more affected than that of healthy subjects.

Subjects in all three patient groups demonstrated considerable instability throughout their tracking performance, relative to healthy subjects. The performance of patients with acute infections was significantly more stable than that of patients with CFS or depression. The latter two groups did not differ. Thus, all three patient groups, but especially those with CFS and depression, showed a fluctuating, on–off, performance pattern, the level of which was not disproportionately affected by an increase in task difficulty.

Reported workload was higher in the three patient groups compared with healthy controls. However, there were no notable differences among the patient groups with regard to workload experience, nor was there any relationship between their workload ratings and the difficulties encountered while performing the tasks. Thus, we were unable to document the 'process of fatigue' whether as a decline in objective performance or as a substantial increase in patients' experience of workload over time.

Discrepancies between subjective reports of difficulty and measures of objective performance are commonly reported in patients with CFS (Moss-Morris et al, 1996; Wearden & Appleby, 1997).

CLINICAL IMPLICATIONS

■ Patients with CFS, depression or acute infective illness demonstrate a non-specific impairment of attention.

■ Cognitive impairment in patients with CFS appears to be independent of severity of depressed mood.

■ All patient groups reported increased mental effort to complete attention tasks.

LIMITATIONS

■ The effects of other relevant factors, such as the prevalence of sleep disturbance, were not studied directly.

■ The non-specific nature of available diagnostic criteria for CFS introduces a degree of heterogeneity even in carefully selected patient samples.

■ Our best results are reliant on subjects' cooperation and motivation.

UTE VOLLMER-CONNA, PhD, DENIS WAKEFIELD, MD, ANDREW LLOYD, MD, Inflammation Research Unit, School of Pathology, University of New South Wales; IAN HICKIE, MD, School of Psychiatry, University of New South Wales; KEVIN BIRD, PhD, REGINALD WESTBROOK, DPhil, JIM LEMON, PhD, School of Psychology, University of New South Wales, Sydney

Correspondence: Dr Ute Vollmer-Conna, Inflammation Research Unit, School of Pathology, University of New South Wales, Sydney 2052 NSW, Australia. Fax: (61-2) 9385 1389; e-mail: u.vollmer-conna@unsw.edu.au

(First received 30 September 1996, final revision 7 April 1997, accepted 14 April 1997)

Although subjective complaint of difficulty has previously been linked to mood disturbance (Grafman et al, 1993), we did not detect such a relationship.

Generalised rather than specific impairment

The performance deficits shown by the three patient groups suggest a general cognitive impairment rather than specific deficits related to a sensory modality and/or mental activity. The fluctuating, on–off, performance pattern, evident from the analysis of patient's tracking ability, points to a continuous struggle to keep attention focused on the task in hand. This performance pattern also reflects the patients' repeated efforts to focus their attention after each lapse. A primary impairment in maintaining selective attention, albeit more pronounced in patients with CFS and depression than in those with acute infections, would affect performance across cognitive domains and may offer a plausi-

ble explanation for our results. Difficulty in maintaining attention also may be responsible for the overall slowing in response speed found by us and other researchers (Prasher et al, 1990; Scheffers et al, 1992; Smith et al, 1993).

Recent proposals that a single and/or non-specific deficit, such as impaired attention or information processing speed, may be responsible for most of the performance deficits reported in patients with CFS (DeLuca et al, 1995; Moss-Morris et al, 1996), and for patients with depression (Mialet et al, 1996) are consistent with our own interpretation of the data.

The role of depression

As depression is common in patients with CFS, it has been suggested that the reported fatigue and cognitive impairment may result simply from associated mood disturbance (see Wessely, 1993, for review). Our results do indeed document similarities in the cognitive profiles of patients with CFS and non-melancholic depression, but the two groups differ markedly in terms of severity of depressed mood. Further, correlational data within each of these groups do not support the general proposition that the severity of depressed mood accounts for the degree of observed cognitive impairment. These results are consistent with most (see Moss-Morris *et al*, 1996, for review), but not all (Wearden & Appleby, 1997) studies which have assessed the relationship between cognitive dysfunction and depressed mood in patients with CFS.

CONCLUSIONS

The neurocognitive deficits shown by the patient groups in this study are similar in form, with deficits in attention, response speed, and performance accuracy being notable. Patients with CFS and patients with depression showed greater impairment than patients with acute infection. The similar impairments of concentration and attention may reflect a common pathophysiological process in the various illness groups, although in patients with CFS this process appears to be independent of depressed mood.

ACKNOWLEDGEMENT

This research was supported by funding from the CFS/ME Society of New South Wales.

REFERENCES

American Psychiatric Association (1987) *Diagnostic and Statistical Manual of Mental Disorders* (3rd edn, revised) (DSM–III–R). Washington, DC: APA.

DeLuca, J., Johnson, S. K. & Natelson, B. H. (1993) Information processing efficiency in chronic fatigue syndrome and multiple sclerosis. *Archives of Neurology*, **50**, 301–304.

—, —, Beldowicz, D., et al (1995) Neuropsychological impairments in chronic fatigue syndrome, multiple sclerosis, and depression. *Journal of Neurology, Neurosurgery, and Psychiatry*, **58**, 38–43.

Grafman, J., Schwartz, V., Dale, J. K., et al (1993) Analysis of neuropsychological functioning in patients with chronic fatigue syndrome. *Journal of Neurology, Neurosurgery, and Psychiatry*, **56**, 684–689.

Hart, S. G. & Staveland, L. E. (1988) Development of NASA-TLX (task load index): Results from empirical and theoretical research. In *Human Mental Workload* (eds P. A. Hancock & N. Meshkati), pp. 139–183. Amsterdam: Elsevier.

Lemon, J. (1990) *The Rozelle Test Battery: A Computerized Testing Instrument for Visuomotor and Cognitive Testing.* (Technical report No. 9). Sydney: National Drug and Alcohol Research Centre.

Lloyd, A., Hickie, I., Boughton, C. R., et al (1990) The prevalence of chronic fatigue syndrome in an Australian population. *Medical Journal of Australia*, **153**, 522–528.

Mackworth, N. H. (1948) The breakdown of vigilance during prolonged visual search. *Quarterly Journal of Experimental Psychology*, **1**, 7–11.

McNair, D. M., Lorr, M. & Droppleman, L. F. (1981) Impaired attention in depressive states: a non-specific deficit? *Psychological Medicine*, **26**, 1009–1020.

Moss-Morris, R., Petrie, K. J., Large, R. G., et al (1996) Neuropsychological deficits in chronic fatigue syndrome:

artifact or reality? *Journal of Neurology, Neurosurgery, and Psychiatry*, **60**, 474–477.

Nelson, H. E. (1982) *National Adult Reading Test (NART).* Windsor, Berks: NFER–Nelson.

Prasher, D., Smith, A. & Findley, L. (1990) Sensory and cognitive event-related potentials in myalgic encephalomyelitis. *Journal of Neurology, Neurosurgery, and Psychiatry*, **53**, 247–253.

Quinn-Curtis (1990) *Sciences/Engineering/Graphics Tools for Turbo C, Revision 7.* Needham, MA: Quinn-Curtis.

Raven, J. C. (1962) *Advanced Progressive Matrices.* London: H. K. Lewis & Co.

Rodger, R. S. (1967) Type II errors and their decision basis. *British Journal of Mathematical and Statistical Psychology*, **20**, 187–204.

Sandman, C. A., Barron, J. L., Nackoul, K., et al (1993) Memory deficits associated with chronic fatigue immune dysfunction syndrome. *Biological Psychiatry*, **33**, 618–623.

Scheffers, M. K., Johnson, R., Grafman, J., et al (1992) Attention and short-term memory in chronic fatigue syndrome patients: An event-related potential analysis. *Neurology*, **42**, 1667–1675.

Smith, A. P., Behan, P. O., Bell, W., et al (1993) Behavioural problems associated with the chronic fatigue syndrome. *British Journal of Psychology*, **84**, 411–423.

Sternberg, S. (1966) High speed scanning in human memory. *Science*, **153**, 652–654.

Wearden, A. & Appleby, L. (1997) Cognitive performance and complaints of cognitive impairment in chronic fatigue syndrome (CFS). *Psychological Medicine*, **27**, 81–90.

Wessely, S. (1993) The neuropsychiatry of chronic fatigue syndrome. In *Chronic Fatigue Syndrome* (eds G. R. Bock & J. Whelan). Ciba Foundation Symposium No. 173, pp. 212–237. Chichester: Wiley.

Wilkinson, L. (1990) *Systat: The System for Statistics.* Evanston, IL: Systat Inc.

London–East Anglia randomised controlled trial of cognitive–behavioural therapy for psychosis

I: Effects of the treatment phase

ELIZABETH KUIPERS, PHILIPPA GARETY, DAVID FOWLER, GRAHAM DUNN, PAUL BEBBINGTON, DANIEL FREEMAN and CLARE HADLEY

Background A series of small, mainly uncontrolled, studies have suggested that techniques adapted from cognitive–behavioural therapy (CBT) for depression can improve outcome in psychosis, but no large randomised controlled trial of intensive treatment for medication-resistant symptoms of psychosis has previously been published.

Method Sixty participants who each had at least one positive and distressing symptom of psychosis that was medication-resistant were randomly allocated between a CBT and standard care condition ($n=28$) and a standard care only control condition ($n=32$). Therapy was individualised, and lasted for nine months. Multiple assessments of outcome were used.

Results Over nine months, improvement was significant only in the treatment group, who showed a 25% reduction on the BPRS. No other clinical, symptomatic or functioning measure changed significantly. Participants had a low drop-out rate from therapy (11%), and expressed high levels of satisfaction with treatment (80%). Fifty per cent of the CBT group were treatment responders (one person became worse), compared with 31% of the control group (three people became worse and another committed suicide).

Conclusions CBT for psychosis can improve overall symptomatology. The findings provide evidence that even a refractory group of clients with a long history of psychosis can engage in talking about psychotic symptoms and their meaning, and this can improve outcome.

Traditionally, it has been thought that the experiences of psychosis were categorically different from normal experiences. Symptoms such as delusions have been defined in terms of being unresponsive to rational argument (Jaspers, 1963) and thus unamenable to 'talking' therapies. However, since the 1950s a small number of single case studies have indicated that if specific techniques are used, talking to people about their psychotic experiences can be productive and improve symptomatology (Beck, 1952; Watts *et al*, 1973). More recently, other studies have shown that gentle challenge of evidence, presenting alternative possible viewpoints, reality-testing and enhancing coping strategies may be helpful, particularly for those with distressing positive symptoms (Fowler & Morley, 1989; Chadwick & Lowe, 1990; Kingdon & Turkington, 1991; Fowler, 1992; Tarrier *et al*, 1993; Garety *et al*, 1994; Haddock *et al*, 1996), even for those with acute episodes (Drury *et al*, 1996).

Despite the promise of the studies so far published (Bouchard *et al*, 1996), there have been only two randomised controlled trials (RCTs) (Tarrier *et al*, 1993; Drury *et al*, 1996) neither of which offered long-term treatment. Therefore, we aimed to offer cognitive–behavioural therapy (CBT) for a period of nine months to those with persistent, distressing, medication-resistant symptoms of psychosis, and to evaluate any changes in outcome using multiple criteria, and an RCT design. A further aim was to engage as many clients in therapy as possible, as we did in our earlier study (Garety *et al*, 1994). This is because failure to engage clients in therapy, while a well documented problem for this client group, would obviously limit the usefulness of any psychological treatment for psychosis. In this paper we present the results of the treatment phase of a three-centre study, based in London and East Anglia.

METHOD

Participants

The study was conducted at three major sites; at the Maudsley Trust, London; at Addenbrooke's Hospital Trust, Cambridge; and at Norfolk Mental Health Trust, Norwich. Participants were catchment area clients who were recruited by asking for referrals from community teams and in-patient units.

Criteria for referral were: at least one current positive psychotic symptom (such as delusions or hallucinations) that was distressing, unremitting (at least the past six months) and medication resistant, that is had not responded to a previous trial of at least six months of appropriate neuroleptic medication. Clients prescribed clozapine needed to have been stable on this for at least one year (to allow time for all benefit to occur). People who had drug, alcohol or organic problems as primary features were excluded.

Procedures and randomisation

Once referred, all possible participants were seen for a screening interview by an independent evaluator to establish whether they met our criteria. Once this was confirmed and informed consent had been obtained, randomisation was carried out separately within each treatment centre by the trial statistician (G.D.), using randomised permuted blocking (Pocock, 1983) and a block size of six. Participants then entered either the control condition or the treatment group, and baseline assessments were carried out. Considerable efforts were made to collect data from all participants in the trial from the time of randomisation onwards.

Prior power calculations, based on the results of the pilot study (Garety *et al*, 1994), had indicated that a trial with a total of 60 people would have a power of at least 0.80 to detect an effect size of 0.516 using a two-group *t*-test with a 0.05 two-tailed significance level.

Assessments

A wide range of assessments was administered to participants at baseline, three months, six months, and nine months (which was the end of the treatment condition). A follow-up at 18 months after entry into the trial is still continuing. This paper will present only the results of the treatment phase of the trial. In a trial of psychological treatment it is extremely difficult to make assessments that are totally blind to the treatment condition and this was not attempted. However, all assessments were carried out by independent research workers (D. Freeman and C. Hadley) who were not involved in the treatments.

Measures

Our previous study had established that participants were able to cope with our assessments. These were administered over several sessions. We wished to look in detail at symptoms, functioning, and cognitive and emotional variables because we wanted not only to monitor outcome, but also to find out whether there were predictors of good or poor treatment response and correlations between outcome measures. These will be reported separately (Garety *et al*, 1997).

Symptom and functioning measures

We used the Present State Examination (PSE–10; World Health Organization, 1992) to establish psychotic symptomatology, using the associated CATEGO–V programme to derive diagnostic categories according to DSM– III–R (American Psychiatric Association, 1987) at baseline. The Brief Psychiatric Rating Scale (19-item, 0–6 scale) (BPRS; Overall & Gorham, 1962) was administered to assess overall mental state (baseline and three-monthly). The research workers in the separate centres achieved a high level of interrater reliability on the BPRS (intra-class correlation coefficient= 0.92). We used Personal Questionnaires every three months to monitor changes in key symptoms identified by the PSE, as this methodology has proved to be both reliable and sensitive (Brett-Jones *et al*, 1987). For delusions we measured conviction, preoccupation and distress; for hallucinations we measured frequency, intensity and distress. We also assessed hallucinations (Hustig & Hafner, 1990) three-monthly, and used the Maudsley Assessment of Delusions Schedule (MADS; Buchanan *et al*, 1993) (baseline and nine months).

Insight (Amador *et al*, 1993) was measured at baseline and at nine months. The Beck Depression Inventory (BDI; Beck *et al*, 1961) (three-monthly) the Beck Anxiety Inventory (BAI; Beck *et al*, 1988) (baseline and nine months), Beck Hopelessness Scale (BHS; Beck *et al*, 1974) (baseline and nine months), and the Social Functioning Scale (Birchwood *et al*, 1990) (baseline and nine months) were also completed.

Cognitive measures

The National Adult Reading Test (NART; Nelson, 1982) and the Quick Test (Ammons & Ammons, 1962) are estimates of premorbid and current IQ, respectively. Cognitive deficits and biases were investigated using tasks involving cognitive estimations (Shallice & Evans, 1978), verbal fluency (Miller, 1984) and probabilistic reasoning (Garety *et al*, 1991). All of these were measured at baseline only.

Other measures

The Self Concept Questionnaire (Robson, 1989) is a measure of self-esteem (baseline and nine months). The Dysfunctional Attitudes Scale investigates underlying beliefs about the self (described in Williams, 1992) (baseline and nine months). The Autobiographical Memory Task (Williams & Dritschel, 1988) (baseline), the Recall of Adjectives Task (Bellew, 1990) (baseline), and a Satisfaction with Therapy Questionnaire (nine months) were also completed.

Treatment condition

Participants randomised into the treatment group received up to nine months of individual CBT for psychosis. Sessions were conducted weekly initially, and then fortnightly, for up to an hour. Therapy was designed to achieve the following aims:

(a) to reduce the distress and interference that can arise from the experience of psychotic symptomatology;

(b) to reduce emotional disturbance such as depression, anxiety and hopelessness, and to modify dysfunctional schemas if they existed; and

(c) to promote the active participation of the individual in the regulation of their risk of relapse and social disability.

The methods used to achieve these aims have been discussed in detail in our manual (Fowler *et al*, 1995). Specific interventions were individualised from the assessment phase of the treatment. Initial sessions were focused on facilitating engagement in treatment. Considerable effort was spent on building and maintaining a good basic therapeutic relationship, and this relationship was characterised by considerable flexibility on the part of the therapist. When necessary, treatment was arranged in locations convenient to the client, including home visits and proactive outreach following

non-attendance. Within sessions the therapist was highly sensitive to changes in mental state and in particular the occurrence of paranoia. Active attempts were made to manage such problems so as to ensure that clients did not feel unduly pressured and to prevent treatment from becoming aversive. If necessary, sessions were cut short or rearranged. Difficult topics were discussed only when clients felt able to do so. During the early sessions the therapist conducted a detailed analysis of the client's problems. This involved eliciting in detail the client's interpretation of the development of their problems over time, in particular the development of delusional ideas and voices from their first emergence, and the client's appraisals of psychotic experiences occurring in different episodes. The therapist also attempted a detailed analysis of the current problems that the client had prioritised. Such analysis aimed to elucidate triggering factors, current coping responses and the context in which psychotic experiences were embedded. Following this, treatment involved the use of several of the following strategies according to an individualised case formulation.

Improving coping strategies and developing and practising new ones

This involved using a variety of widely known behavioural therapy techniques, including activity scheduling, relaxation and skills training. The aim was to build on the client's own coping repertoire to manage current problems. Such techniques were used primarily to assist clients to engage in functional activities such as going shopping or socialising, or to manage the behavioural consequences of psychotic symptoms such as impulses deriving from voice commands, or self-harm.

Clients' own coping repertoires were delineated, and they were encouraged to use strategies such as distraction or avoidance more specifically and consistently. Other strategies such as alcohol use and high levels of social withdrawal were discussed in terms of their long-term costs, and discouraged. New strategies such as reading aloud to combat auditory hallucinations were suggested for the client to try out and report back on.

Developing a shared model in collaboration with the client

Therapists engaged in collaborative discussion with clients about the nature of psychotic symptoms and the effects on their lives. Information was offered to enable clients to understand what had happened to them in the context of current ideas about the basis of psychotic experiences. The aim was to assist clients to a new interpretation of their problems which had a less distressing meaning for them, and which was more likely to lead to engaging in health-promoting behaviour such as taking medication. Some clients wished for complex discussion of the interaction between biological, social and cognitive factors, others preferred using more basic concepts. The therapists were open-minded about the degree to which clients preferred or accepted a medical model of events, and tolerant of their rejection of diagnoses. In cases where clients were particularly resistant to changing delusional beliefs, therapists worked 'within' the delusional system by fostering less distressing and more functional specific meanings while not directly tackling the delusional belief itself.

Modifying delusional beliefs and beliefs about hallucinations

Therapists helped clients to review the evidence for their beliefs. Gentle challenge and the presentation of possible alternative explanations were used, together with reality-testing where appropriate. Beliefs held with less conviction were discussed first. Beliefs about hallucinations were looked at in detail in the same way, but more particularly, the meaning attributed to voices was examined. While links between current voices, especially distressing ones, and earlier incidents in clients' lives were not always evident, they could sometimes be uncovered and this was often helpful. If possible, voices and other hallucinations were discussed as internal events, which were experienced as real by clients, but were not part of the experience of others. If feasible, reality-testing was undertaken, such as testing out the actual rather than the feared consequences of not always obeying a command hallucination.

Modifying dysfunctional schemas
(Beck et al, 1979)

In the context of a life review (Young, 1990) clients' negative views or dysfunctional assumptions about themselves were identified, and the evidence for their veracity was re-examined in light of a current review of their circumstances; for example, was it always true that the individual was a 'bad person' or 'worthless'?

Management of social disability and relapse

This included discussion of relapse signatures (Birchwood, 1996), issues of stigma and the need to make changes as small as possible, given the clients' history of vulnerability. The clients' ability to identify triggers that might exacerbate psychotic phenomena was discussed and they were encouraged to take appropriate avoidant or coping measures such as increased medication, seeking help, supportive discussion or distraction techniques. These issues were often discussed later on in treatment, after work on specific symptoms had either been completed or had proceeded as far as possible.

Therapists

Therapists in the trial were experienced clinical psychologists. They met regularly during the treatment phase (at least monthly), either for peer supervision (E. Kuipers, P. Garety, D. Fowler and Steve Jones) or for therapy supervision with D. Fowler (Nina Dick, Erik Kuiper, Michelle Painter and Mark Westacott). Strenuous attempts were made at all times to follow procedures as laid down in the treatment manual (Fowler et al, 1995).

All clients in the treatment condition also received routine care from their clinical teams. In most instances, this included case management and medication. Where the former was not routinely available, the therapist negotiated with the clinical team to provide the monitoring and review appropriate to case management. Thus, participants in the trial had a designated keyworker who saw them regularly and was responsible for coordinating their care. Clinical teams were asked, if at all possible, not to change clients' medication during the trial, and to inform us of changes that were unavoidable. This was monitored as closely as possible.

Control condition

Participants randomised into this condition received routine care from their clinical team, which as part of our entry criteria consisted of case management and medication. As above, the research team negotiated with the clinical team to ensure that clients had an allocated keyworker responsible for coordinating their care and setting goals for them. All control group keyworkers were also given feedback from the initial assessments, and were encouraged to review the client's progress every three months.

Measures of contact with the clinical team, days spent in hospital and other aspects of the costs of each group were collected and will be presented separately.

Statistical analysis

All statistical analyses were carried out using SPSS for Windows (Version 6.0) or BMDP PC–90. Changes over time (baseline, three, six and nine months) were assessed by the separate estimation of a linear trend for each person in the trial (using the data available for that person, even though they may not have provided data for all four assessments). These estimates were then used as the response variable in further analyses, as recommended by Matthews et al (1990). The linear trend was constructed (e.g. BPRS units/3 months) so that a negative value indicated an improvement (that is, there was an overall decrease in the measured score, BPRS total, say, over time) with a larger absolute value indicating a greater improvement (-5, for example, being a better outcome than -3). Typically we used a two-way analysis of variance (ANOVA) with the 'experimental' sums of squares option in SPSS; the two explanatory factors being treatment centre (London, Cambridge or Norwich) and treatment group (CBT or control).

RESULTS

Participants

One hundred and fifty-two people were referred for possible inclusion in the trial. Of these, 47 had no distressing positive symptom present at the screening interview. Ten had not been stabilised on medication, and 26 were not suitable for practical reasons such as living out of the catchment area. Nine people met the criteria but did not agree to participate (9 of 69; 8%). Thus a total of 60 people met the criteria, consented, and were entered into the trial. Of these, all were on medication apart from three whose symptoms had been medication-resistant in the past, but who consistently refused to take any at the beginning of the trial. After randomisation, 28 people entered the treatment group and 32 the control group. Demographic and clinical information on participants in the two groups are presented in Tables 1 and 2.

From Table 1 it can be seen that the total sample was middle-aged, had a preponderance of men, a long history of illness, and average scores on an estimate of current IQ. The only difference between the

Table 1 Demographic data on participants who entered the therapy trial

Variable	CBT group			Control group		
	n	Mean	Range	n	Mean	Range
Age (years)	28	38.5	19–65	32	41.8	18–63
Duration of illness (years)	25	12.1	1–26	30	14.0	1–33
Number of admissions	24	5.2	0–30	29	4.3	0–12
Predicted IQ (NART)	25	102.9	69–129	25	98.7	71–131
Current IQ (Quick Test)	25	99.8	72–130	29	91.5	70–116
Gender						
Male	15			23		
Female	13			9		

NART, National Adult Reading Test.

treatment and control groups was that the latter had a somewhat lower current IQ.

The clinical data presented in Table 2 show the scores on the symptoms and functioning measures that we used. As expected, the group as a whole was symptomatic, with moderate levels of depression, anxiety and hopelessness. By chance, the CBT group had lower levels of self-esteem than the control group at baseline, but both groups scored within the range for those with clinical problems. Social functioning was comparable to norms found in an unemployed group of people with schizophrenia (Birchwood et al, 1990).

Table 3 itemises the range of psychotic symptoms found in both groups, which did not differ appreciably. Most participants had delusions, and a majority also had hallucinations, particularly in the treatment group. Diagnostic classification showed a preponderance of paranoid schizophrenia.

Withdrawals

Out of the 60 people who gave their consent for the trial, a total of 11 people (18%) withdrew from assessments over nine months, four (14%) from the CBT condition and seven (22%) from the control group (five of whom withdrew immediately after randomisation). Of the four people who dropped out of the treatment condition by nine months, only three (11%) attended for fewer than 10 sessions.

Number of therapy sessions received

The median number of therapy sessions given to the treatment group was 15, and the mean was 18.6 (range 0–50). One person did not attend any therapy appointments, one had fewer than five sessions, six had 'brief therapy' (12 sessions or fewer). The rest of the treatment group ($n=20$) had what we defined as 'full therapy' (more than 12 sessions). Treatment sessions usually lasted for an hour, but were kept flexible (could be shortened) depending on a client's current mental state. Most sessions were conducted in out-patient clinic settings, but some were home visits or ward visits to maximise the likelihood of engagement in

treatment, by offering sessions that were in a convenient location for clients (e.g. one client was physically disabled and was always seen at home).

Outcome measures

Symptoms and functioning

All available data were analysed. The only participants who did not contribute either refused assessments after randomisation (withdrawals) or provided only one assessment and thus could not contribute to a trend estimate. Of the 53 people who did provide sufficient outcome data on the BPRS to estimate trends, two provided information on two time points, five provided three of the four BPRS total scores, and the remainder (46) provided complete data (that is, BPRS scores at all four times). The means for the BPRS linear trends and raw scores can be seen in Tables 4 and 5.

The CBT group did significantly better than the controls ($F_{1,47}=7.41$; $P=0.009$). There was little evidence that the difference between the CBT and control groups depended on centre (the test for the group by centre interaction: $F_{2,47}=0.59$; $P=0.561$). Although there seemed to be an improvement in the control clients, particularly in Norwich, neither the centre effect nor the overall change in the control group was statistically significant. It should, however, be noted that there appears to be a lack of homogeneity of the standard deviations (Cochrane's $C_{8,6}=0.46$; $P=0.06$), with both Cambridge groups being considerably more variable than the others. As there appears to be no simple relationship between the mean trend and its standard deviation, a simple transformation of the data would not remove this heterogeneity. The results appear to be robust, however, since dropping both the Cambridge groups from the analysis yields homogeneous standard deviations in the remaining four groups, and a statistically significant group effect remains ($P=0.01$).

The analysis was repeated after setting the BPRS trend at zero (i.e. no change) for those seven patients (two from the CBT group and five controls) for which a trend estimate was not available (i.e. they provided fewer than two of the repeated assessments) to provide a full 'decision to treat' analysis using the standard 'carry forward' method to impute missing values. A two-group t-test for the last row of Table 5 gave $t=-2.55$ with 51 d.f. ($P=0.014$). Inserting zeros for missing participants and repeating the t-test gave $t=-2.70$ with 58 d.f. ($P=0.009$). The mean

Table 2 Clinical data on participants who entered the therapy trial

Variable	CBT group			Control group		
	n	Mean	s.d.	n	Mean	s.d.
BPRS	27	26.4	6.5	26	24.5	7.1
BDI	27	23.6	10.1	26	20.0	10.1
BHS	27	11.6	4.8	27	9.8	5.2
BAI	27	17.5	11.0	26	17.3	14.8
Self-esteem	25	90.1	29.6	28	107.3	23.3
Social Functioning Scale	27	103.3	7.2	30	101.6	9.0

BPRS, Brief Psychiatric Rating Scale; BDI, Beck Depression Inventory; BHS, Beck Hopelessness Scale; BAI, Beck Anxiety Inventory.

Table 3 DSM–III–R diagnoses and positive symptoms present in participants

Variable	CBT group (n=27)	Control group (n=27)
DSM–III–R diagnosis		
Schizophrenia (paranoid type)	19	20
Delusional disorder	6	7[1]
Schizoaffective disorder	2	0
	(n=27)	(n=29)[2]
Positive symptoms		
PSE: One or more delusions	20	28
PSE: One or more hallucinations	22	18
PSE: Perceptual disorders other than hallucinations	1	4
PSE: Subjective thought disorder and/or replacement of will	5	7

1. The diagnosis for one person was confirmed at the three-month assessment because of a lack of information from the initial assessment.
2. Information is included concerning positive symptoms present in two participants who withdrew from the research partway through collection of PSE–10 data.

Table 4 Brief Psychiatric Rating Scale linear trends in each centre

Centre	CBT group			Control group		
	n	Mean	s.d.	n	Mean	s.d.
London	14	−1.49	1.57	12	0.18	1.66
Cambridge	6	−2.90	3.99	8	−0.35	3.08
Norwich	6	−2.37	1.60	7	−1.67	1.21
Combined	26	−2.02	2.31	27	−0.46	2.15

Significant difference between CBT and control groups ($P=0.009$).

Table 5 Mean Brief Psychiatric Rating Scale scores

Assessment	CBT group			Control group		
	n	Mean	s.d.	n	Mean	s.d.
Initial	27	26.4	6.5	26	24.5	7.1
Three-month	25	22.2	8.2	27	22.3	7.2
Six-month	25	21.2	7.3	27	22.9	6.2
Nine-month	23	19.9	8.5	24	22.7	7.6

trend for the CBT group ($n=28$) was then −1.87 (s.d. 2.89) and for the controls $n=32$ −0.38 (s.d. 1.98).

Visual inspection showed that items on the BPRS which changed most in comparison with the control group were suspiciousness (ideas of reference and persecution), unusual thought content (delusional ideas) and hallucinations. The self-reported reduction in delusional conviction, measured by linear trend, was −0.65 for the CBT group and −0.30 for the controls. Delusional distress was −0.61 for CBT and −0.39 for controls. The linear trend for the frequency of hallucinations was −0.24 for the CBT group and −0.01 for the control group. None of these reached significance at conventional levels, although all favoured the CBT condition. Change on all other symptom and functioning measures was not significantly different between conditions at this stage of the trial.

Clinical outcome

In comparison with others who have tended to determine indices of clinical response on arbitrary grounds, we decided to adopt an approach which aimed to take account of the degree of natural variability in BPRS scores over time. An estimate of the average variability in BPRS scores in the control group was therefore calculated (taken as the root mean sum of the squared standard deviation of individual BPRS scores for each case in the control group). This equated to five points. An improvement or worsening of greater than or equal to five points on the BPRS was then taken as indicating a reliable clinical change, and an improvement or worsening of greater than or equal to 10 points on the BPRS as indicating a large clinical change. (A five-point change on the BPRS is similar to the criterion of a 20% improvement taken to be an index of clinical response on the BPRS by Breier *et al* (1994)). In these terms, 6/28 (21%) achieved a large clinical improvement, and a further 8/28 (29%) of the treatment group achieved a reliable clinical improvement. One person of the 28 (3%) in the treatment group showed a reliable worsening of symptoms on the BPRS. In the control group, 1/32 (3%) showed a large clinical improvement and 9/32 (28%) of cases achieved reliable clinical improvements. Three of the 32 (9%) of the control group showed a clinically significant worsening of symptoms over the nine months.

If we widen the criteria to include clinically significant response in the client's primary presenting problem as measured by the Personal Questionnaires, then 18/28 (64%) of treatment and 15/32 (47%) of controls achieved clinically significant improvements. If cases with no clear linear trend in the scores are excluded (i.e. where there is little obvious evidence of trend), then the number in the control group who changed drops to 12/32 (37%).

One person in the control condition had committed suicide by the end of nine months. No one in the treatment condition had done this.

Medication

Medication regimes were complex and information was sometimes incomplete. We calculated chlorpromazine equivalents (CPZ) following the guidelines in the *British National Formulary*. Full data were available for the London participants, but data were more limited for East Anglia. We classified these into no medication, low (less than 300 mg CPZ/day), medium (300–600 mg CPZ/day) and high (more than 600 mg CPZ/day). We also divided participants into those receiving constant, fluctuating, decreasing or increasing doses. Four clients were switched to clozapine before the final assessment. Three of these were in the control group, and the change occurred between the three and six month assessments. One person was in the CBT group and the change only occurred after the six month assessment.

Inspection of the data at baseline in Table 6, suggests that there were no particular differences in medication between the treatment and control conditions. However, over the nine months of the trial more control participants had their medication increased, whereas two of the CBT group and none of the controls had it decreased. This meant that as the trial progressed more of the control group moved into the high-dose category and fewer of them received low doses or no medication compared with the CBT group.

Table 6 Medication levels based on chlorpromazine equivalents

	CBT group	Control group
Level of neuroleptic dose at start of trial		
None	2	1
Low	5	4
Medium	3	10
High	8	5
Changes in medication during trial		
No change	11	10
Fluctuating	1	2
Increasing	2	7
Decreasing	2	0
Level of neuroleptic medication throughout the trial		
None	4	0
Low	2	2
Medium	4	8
High	6	9

Levels of neuroleptic medication: Low: less than 300 mg chlorpromazine; medium: 300 to 600 mg of chlorpromazine; high: greater than 600 mg chlorpromazine.
All available data on medication are included. These were predominantly from the London sample, which when considered on its own did not have a discernibly different pattern.

Table 7 Satisfaction with cognitive–behavioural therapy

	CBT group (n=20)
How satisfied are you with the therapy?	
Very satisfied	5
Satisfied	11
Indifferent	3
Dissatisfied	1
During therapy how much progress do you feel you actually made?	
Much progress	4
Some progress	13
No progress	2
Things got worse	1
In future, how much progress do you think you will be able to make in dealing with your problem?[1]	
Much progress	9
Some progress	8
No progress	1
Things will get worse	1

1. One participant did not answer this question.

Satisfaction

Twenty of the 28 in the treatment group completed a satisfaction with therapy questionnaire at nine months. As can be seen in Table 7, 16 (80%) were satisfied or very satisfied with the therapy, 17 felt they had made some or much progress, and 17 felt they would be able to make some or much progress in the future. One client reported that 'things got worse', and this person was also dissatisfied with treatment.

DISCUSSION

The results of this trial show that at the end of nine months of CBT it is possible to improve the overall symptomatology of people with medication-resistant, distressing symptoms of psychosis. This group still exists even after the introduction of the new neuroleptics (Kane, 1996). We showed a decrease in BPRS scores of 25% and this was produced mainly by changes in our targeted symptoms of delusions and hallucinations. There were no appreciable improvements in the level of depression. At this stage, the specific improvements observed in conviction for delusional ideas, were not statistically significant, in contrast to the results from our previous waiting list control trial. This is at least partly because of the more stringent methodology of an RCT design compared to uncontrolled or less well controlled trials. Further support for the specific effects of CBT is provided by a finding that only in the CBT group was outcome predicted by a cognitive measure linked to delusional thinking (Garety et al, 1997).

Engagement

The therapy was acceptable to clients, who expressed high levels of satisfaction and did not show demonstrable negative consequences. Our results illustrate that psychological treatments can be offered to clients even when they have long histories of illness, and continuing distressing symptoms of psychosis. Our drop-out rates, which remained low, are particularly encouraging, and suggest that if engagement issues are dealt with, then even this client group can accept demanding interventions. This has also been demonstrated in a recent study of compliance therapy (Kemp *et al*, 1996), which addressed client-centred concerns in a similar way, but has often previously been problematic (e.g. Tarrier *et al*, 1993).

Rate of improvement

The rate of improvement in overall symptomatology (BPRS scores) that we have demonstrated, is around the same level as that found in studies on the effects on clozapine on clinically similar samples of people who have failed to respond to standard medication. While relatively few RCTs of clozapine have been completed, those in the literature are usually six-week trials, on large numbers of clients, comparing clozapine to chlorpromazine (Kane *et al*, 1988) or to haloperidol (Breier *et al*, 1994). These showed changes on the BPRS of between 11 and 26% in the clozapine group. Interestingly, the Kane *et al* study (n=268) showed a 26% change in the clozapine group, compared with an 8% change in the chlorpromazine group, that is both groups improved with intensive monitoring and optimal medication.

The advantage of a talking therapy is that it does not have physical side-effects, and can produce change that is both clinically noticeable and significant. The disadvantages of such treatments include intensive input by experienced clinicians (around 19 hours over nine months) and the extra training and supervision that is required to support therapists. A further disadvantage of this intervention so far, is that at this stage we have shown change only in BPRS scores, not in social functioning or any of our other measures.

Methodological problems

Our study suffered from methodological problems that are common to virtually all trials of psychological treatments. Most problematic was the view that we could not ensure our evaluators would remain blind to the treatment condition. Contacting and assessing 60 individuals over nine months requires considerable persistence and

sensitivity, and from the experience of our pilot study we did not feel it was realistic or reasonable to assume that we could prevent details of therapy or control conditions emerging during assessment meetings with evaluators. We may have been mistaken about this, and it does weaken the methodology. However, we decided before the trial started that while we could maintain the independence of our evaluators by not involving them in treatment, we would not attempt to keep them blind to treatment type. This decision is endorsed by Shapiro (1996), who comments that blind evaluation is virtually impossible with psychological treatment trials: "Personnel employed to interview patients to assess their progress are seldom able to avoid exposure to information (especially within patients' accounts of their experiences) that gives away the nature of the treatment they have undergone" (p. 204).

Second, although we monitored medication and medication changes in both groups, it was not possible to keep all individuals stable or on the same medication regime. It remains a possibility that some improvements were due to medication effects, particularly in the control group. Clinicians increased standard medication or changed to clozapine more often for control patients.

Third, the selection of a viable control condition can be seen as problematic. In this study, we decided to compare CBT with the best current routine treatment, case management and medication. These cannot ethically be withdrawn from the treatment group (nor would we wish it), so in effect we evaluated CBT as added to the best standard treatment compared with this standard treatment alone. It is obviously a possibility that the extra 19 hours (mean) of treatment effected improvement because of non-specific attention. The fact that our results showed specific symptomatic change predicted by related cognitive measures (Garety *et al*, 1997) mitigates against this, but lack of change in delusional conviction or depression at this stage suggests that we cannot assume our CBT interventions were the effective ingredients in improvement. On the other hand, there is a case for arguing that the detailed assessments the control group received in itself comprised elements of an attentional control condition. The control group had equally sustained contact with the assessors over time; the assessors had to engage the patients, and at the beginning patients

received a detailed assessment phase involving around six sessions. Patients then had regular assessment contacts at three-month intervals. Some patients reported that they believed the assessors were part of their treatment team. The process of conducting assessments involved specific discussion of symptoms in a supportive atmosphere, and it is possible that such assessments were themselves a minimal focusing intervention. However, this still does not control for the therapy time in the CBT condition, and further controlled studies are required to clarify the issue of specific versus non-specific effects of therapy.

Fourth, we did not aim in this study to examine which aspects of CBT were effective, or to look at an optimal number of sessions for this kind of treatment. Some patients would attend only for 'brief therapy', despite efforts to visit them at home or reorganise appointments. Others attended for maximum or even excessive numbers of sessions, without much apparent benefit. Thus, individuals varied considerably in how long they took to show change, and this issue remains to be clarified.

Clinical implications

Finally, it is clear that even though we demonstrated changes in our treatment group, only 50% of them were treatment responders. Assessing change in patients with very long-standing and treatment-resistant psychotic symptoms poses the problem that even clinically noticeable change does not place people back in the 'normal' range. On the other hand, even small changes in symptom levels might signify important differences in an individual's ability to cope with problems, or cope in the future. We will be able to discuss any maintenance or prevention effects when we have completed the follow-up phase of the study. Predictors of outcome are discussed in a subsequent paper (Garety *et al*, 1997). However, our research seems to indicate that talking to patients about psychotic symptoms and their meaning to the individual is a skill that clinicians working in this area should develop.

ACKNOWLEDGEMENTS

We thank all the patients who participated in this study and the clinicians and clinical teams in London and East Anglia who cooperated in referring and

Shapiro, D. A. (1996) Outcome research. In *Behavioural and Mental Health Research* (2nd edn) (eds G. Parry & F. Watts). Hove: Lawrence Erlbaum.

Tarrier, N., Beckett, R., Harwood, S., *et al* (1993) A trial of two cognitive–behavioural methods of treating drug-resistant psychotic symptoms in schizophrenic patients. I: Outcome. *British Journal of Psychiatry*, **162**, 524–532.

Watts, F. N., Powell, G. E. & Austin, S. V. (1973) The modification of abnormal beliefs. *British Journal of Medical Psychology*, **46**, 359–363.

Williams, J. M. G. (1992) *The Psychological Treatment of Depression. A Guide to Theory and Practice of Cognitive Behaviour Therapy*. London: Routledge.

___ & Dritschel B. H. (1988) Emotional disturbance and the specificity of autobiographical memory. *Cognition and Emotion*, **2**, 221–234.

World Health Organization (1992) *SCAN Schedules for Clinical Assessment in Neuropsychiatry*. Geneva: WHO.

Young, J. (1990) *Cognitive Therapy for Personality Disorder*. Sarasota, FL: Professional Resource Exchange Inc.

The predictive validity of a diagnosis of schizophrenia

A report from the International Study of Schizophrenia (ISoS)
coordinated by the World Health Organization and the
Department of Psychiatry, University of Nottingham

PETER MASON, GLYNN HARRISON, TIM CROUDACE,
CRISTINE GLAZEBROOK and IAN MEDLEY

Background Outcome is important in the validation of psychiatric diagnosis, as most disorders lack clinicopathological correlates. We describe the predictive validity of four definitions of schizophrenia (DSM–III–R, ICD–10, ICD–9 and CATEGO S+), in a representative cohort of patients selected during their first episode of psychosis.

Method Each definition of schizophrenia was applied to 99 patients. Their respective ability to predict 13-year outcome (Global Assessment of Functioning scales) was assessed.

Results DSM–III–R and ICD–10 diagnoses of schizophrenia have high predictive validity for long-term outcome, and both provide relatively stable diagnoses. ICD–9 is reasonably good at predicting disability, but not symptoms, and CATEGO S+ showed no predictive validity. Adding six-month duration criteria to ICD–10, ICD–9 and CATEGO S+ improved their predictive validity, and removing the six-month duration criterion from DSM–III–R commensurately reduced predictive validity.

Conclusions Modern diagnostic systems (DSM–III–R and ICD–10) have high predictive validity, and are superior to ICD–9. The six-month duration criterion of DSM–III–R schizophrenia accounts for its predictive validity and stability over 13 years, but restricts its use in first-episode studies. The one-month duration criterion of ICD–10 is less restrictive, without major compromises in predictive validity or stability.

In the absence of clinicopathological correlates, it is difficult to validate diagnoses in psychiatry. Robins & Guze (1970) proposed a systematic approach for the validation of psychiatric diagnoses and included outcome as one of five suggested validating criteria. Outcome is of particular relevance in schizophrenia, since early concepts of the disorder (dementia praecox) were characterised by a chronic course and poor outcome (Kraepelin, 1919). Bleuler (1950) also observed poor outcome in "the group of schizophrenias", despite focusing primarily on signs and symptoms rather than on course and outcome. Some authors (Kleist, 1960; Leonhard, 1961) believed that recovery precluded a diagnosis of schizophrenia, and redefined patients with better outcome as suffering from the cycloid psychoses. Langfeldt (1969), continuing the conceptualisation of poor outcome as a validating factor for a diagnosis of schizophrenia, coined the term schizophreniform psychosis for those patients symptomatically resembling schizophrenia but having better outcome. Attempts have been made to define certain symptoms that are typical of schizophrenia, for example Schneider's First Rank Symptoms (Schneider, 1959), but their ability to define poor prognosis schizophrenia has not been proven (Hawk et al, 1975; Kendell et al, 1979; Bland & Orn, 1979; World Health Organization, 1979). However, the addition of duration criteria, as in Feighner et al (1972) and DSM–III (American Psychiatric Association, 1980), has significantly increased the predictive validity of the diagnosis of schizophrenia (Stephens et al, 1980, 1982; Helzer et al, 1981, 1983; Endicott et al, 1986).

The stability of diagnosis over time may also be considered to add to the validity of a diagnosis (Robins & Guze, 1970). The more stable a diagnosis, the more likely it is to reflect a basic and consistent psychopathological or patho-

physiological process (Fennig et al, 1994). McGlashan (1984) found that the New Haven Schizophrenia Index (Astrachan et al, 1972) produced a less stable diagnosis of schizophrenia over 15 years than Feighner criteria, and suggested that the incorporation of duration criteria into the latter are partly responsible for this difference. Tsuang et al (1981) reported that a diagnosis of schizophrenia, according to Feighner criteria, remains stable over 30–40 years in 92.5% of cases.

In the present study we aimed to test the predictive validity of three major diagnostic classifications of schizophrenia: DSM–III–R (American Psychiatric Association, 1987), ICD–10 (World Health Organization, 1992a) and ICD–9 (World Health Organization, 1978a), and a 'restrictive' CATEGO S+ definition of schizophrenia (which relies heavily upon Schneider's first rank symptoms). A 13-year follow-up was conducted with a complete and representative sample of first-onset psychoses. The contribution of a six-month duration criterion is specifically tested, and the stability of ICD–10 and DSM–III–R schizophrenia is also studied. The cohort under investigation was part of the International Study of Schizophrenia (ISoS), which is a transcultural investigation in 20 centres in 15 countries coordinated by the World Health Organization (WHO). It was designed to explain findings of previous WHO studies in this area; to identify patterns of long-term course and outcome of severe mental disorders in different cultures; to further develop methods for the study of characteristics of mental disorders and their course in different settings; and to strengthen the scientific basis for future international multidisciplinary research on schizophrenia and other psychiatric disorders seen in a public health perspective. The cohort described in this paper was identified in the WHO's Determinants of Outcome of Severe Mental Disorder Study (1978–80) for which Nottingham was the UK field centre (Jablensky et al, 1992).

METHOD

The methods of case ascertainment, assessments and follow-up have been described previously (Harrison et al, 1994; Mason et al, 1995; Sartorius et al, 1996).

The sample

The sample comprised all patients (aged 15–54) making their first contact (out- and in-patients) from a defined catchment area (population 390 000) between 1 August 1978 and 31 July 1980. An over-inclusive screening schedule for psychosis identified the subjects, who were then assessed using several semi-structured interviews by the project team. Ninety-nine subjects were identified, comprising 65 men and 34 women, with a mean age of 29.60 (s.d. 10.12).

Follow-up information was available on 96% of the original sample. Four patients could not be traced and nine were dead. Sixty-nine subjects had full assessments, and for the remaining 17 subjects, high-quality information was available from records and informants. The 86 subjects available for follow-up did not differ significantly from those dead or lost to follow-up, with respect to their gender, age, type of onset, duration of symptoms and diagnosis (schizophrenia or not) for DSM–III–R, ICD–10, ICD–9 and CATEGO S+.

Initial assessments

All subjects were interviewed by a project psychiatrist using the Present State Examination (PSE; Wing et al, 1974) and the Psychological Impairments Rating Scale (PIRS; Jablensky et al, 1980). Other schedules covering the psychiatric, personal, family and social background (Psychiatric and Personal History Schedule (PPHS; World Health Organization, 1978b)) and social disability (Disability Assessment Schedule (DAS; Jablensky et al, 1980)) were completed by a different interviewer with a close relative of the patient, or other informant.

Follow-up assessment

Assessments were carried out with both patients and a key informant, and further information was elicited from general practice and hospital records. For comparability with earlier measures, assessments including the PSE, the PIRS and the DAS, and other instruments were developed by the WHO to measure long-term outcome (Life Chart Schedule; WHO, 1992c; Broad Rating Schedule; WHO, 1992b).

For the purposes of this paper, data from the Global Assessment of Functioning scales (GAF) for symptoms and disability, derived from the Global Assessment Scale (Endicott et al, 1976), were selected from the range of follow-up assessments. These scales rate the severity of symptoms and the severity of disability in the past month on an ordinal scale from 1 (most severe) to 90 (no symptoms/disability). Pre-study and maintenance reliability exercises were conducted (Mason et al, 1995). Pre-study intraclass correlation coefficients (ICC) for GAF symptoms and disability were 0.85 and 0.94, respectively. Maintenance ICC for GAF symptoms and disability were 0.96 and 0.89, respectively.

Diagnoses

ICD–9

On completion of the initial assessments (between 1978 and 1980), at least two project psychiatrists reviewed the available data and assigned a project ICD–9 diagnosis to each subject.

CATEGO S+

The CATEGO Diagnostic Program (Wing et al, 1974) was used to determine the subjects meeting the restrictive definition of S+ schizophrenia based upon the original PSE ratings.

DSM–III–R and ICD–10

A re-diagnosis exercise was conducted at the point of 13-year follow-up. The original schedules and narratives were reviewed by G. H., blind to outcome, who assigned a diagnosis according to DSM–III–R Research Diagnostic Criteria, using a diagnostic decision instrument which systematically checked criteria for every possible psychotic disorder in DSM–III–R and ICD–10 (available from the authors). The re-diagnosis exercise was possible given the extensive baseline clinical data collected at entry to the study. A reliability exercise was carried out with I. M., who independently diagnosed 20 cases, also blind to outcome. Pairwise agreement between G. H. and I. M. for a classification of schizophrenia versus other psychotic disorder was 100% for both ICD–10 and DSM–III–R.

Duration criteria

To study the effects of six-month duration criteria, 'duration adjusted' definitions of schizophrenia were created for ICD–10, ICD–9, DSM–III–R and CATEGO S+. Information about duration, recorded in the PPHS, was used to add six-month duration criteria to the ICD–10, ICD–9 and S+ definitions. For DSM–III–R, the six-month duration criterion was removed by adding those subjects classified as having a schizophreniform disorder (meets criteria for schizophrenia, but episode lasts less than six months) to those meeting full DSM–III–R criteria for schizophrenia at intake into the study.

Diagnosis stability

For the purposes of assessing the stability of diagnosis over 13 years, a 'main overall diagnosis' for both DSM–III–R and ICD–10 was assigned to each subject. This diagnostic exercise was conducted by G. H. using the same diagnostic decision instrument as in the re-diagnosis exercise. The main overall diagnosis was made immediately after the re-diagnosis exercise and was based on all data collected at onset and at follow-up. This exercise attempted to assign an overall diagnosis taking into account the 13-year course of the disorder and the 'final' outcome in terms of symptoms and social disability. A reliability exercise was carried out with I. M. who independently diagnosed 20 cases. Pairwise agreement between G. H. and I. M. for a diagnosis of schizophrenia was 100% for both ICD–10 and DSM–III–R.

ANALYSES

The data were analysed using SPSS for UNIX. The degree of concordance between the eight definitions of schizophrenia was examined using Cohen's kappa, with 95% confidence intervals. To examine the predictive validity of a diagnosis of schizophrenia at 13 years, median scores and interquartile ranges were calculated for the two outcome measures (GAF symptoms and GAF disability) for each definition of schizophrenia. The median scores and interquartile ranges for those subjects not meeting criteria for schizophrenia were also calculated. Mann–Whitney U tests were used to test the null hypothesis that a diagnosis of schizophrenia is no better at predicting poor outcome than a non-schizophrenia psychotic disorder, for the eight definitions of schizophrenia.

The matrix of kappa values for diagnostic agreement between the diagnoses was subjected to exploratory, non-metric multidimensional scaling (using the ALSCAL procedure in SPSS). Since there were in total only eight diagnoses, a two-dimensional configuration was chosen.

Finally, kappa values were also calculated to demonstrate the degree of concordance between an onset diagnosis of schizophrenia and the final 'main overall diagnosis' of schizophrenia, for DSM–III–R and ICD–10. Sensitivities and specificities were calculated to determine their predictive relationships.

RESULTS

Diagnostic concordance

Table 1 shows the concordance between standard and 'duration adjusted' definitions of schizophrenia applied at first episode. There is high concordance between definitions sharing six-month duration criteria, and between ICD–9, ICD–10 and 'duration adjusted' DSM–III–R. Table 1 also shows that inclusion of six-month duration criteria restricts the diagnosis to between 23 and 31 cases. Of the standard diagnoses, DSM–III–R provides the most restrictive definition of schizophrenia, with only 31 subjects fulfilling DSM–III–R criteria compared with 56 and 67 subjects fulfilling ICD–10 and ICD–9 criteria for schizophrenia, respectively.

Predictive validity of diagnosis

Tables 2 and 3 show that a diagnosis of schizophrenia has significantly greater predictive validity at 13 years, in terms of symptoms and disability, than a non-schizophrenia psychotic disorder, for the DSM–III–R and ICD–10 systems of classification. An ICD–9 diagnosis of schizophrenia is less discriminating (especially for symptoms), and a CATEGO S+ definition of schizophrenia has no predictive validity. Tables 2 and 3 also show that the addition of six-month duration criteria improves the predictive validity of ICD–10 and ICD–9, but this improvement is much less for CATEGO S+. Removing the duration criterion from DSM–III–R makes it a much broader diagnosis, but reduces its predictive validity, particularly for symptomatic outcome.

The two-dimensional scaling solution (Fig. 1) fitted the data well (r-squared=0.99, s-stress=0.01), but this is not surprising given that there are only eight data points. The plot displays the relationships between diagnoses through the spatial proximity of their points. Two clusters are observed; the first (top left) includes the two ICD classifications and DSM–III–R with the duration criteria removed, and the second (top right) includes DSM–III–R and the two ICD classifications supplemented by six-month duration criteria. The final points for CATEGO S+ and 'duration adjusted' CATEGO S+ are distant from both of these.

Stability of diagnosis

For DSM–III–R an onset diagnosis of schizophrenia proved to be very stable over 13 years, with all 31 subjects retaining schizophrenia as a main overall diagnosis (specificity 100%).

ICD–10 proved to be less specific (specificity 88.64%), with five subjects who were given an onset diagnosis of schizophrenia changing to a non-schizophrenia main overall diagnosis. These included four subjects with a main overall diagnosis of bipolar affective disorder, and one subject with a psychotic disorder due to use of alcohol (schizophrenia-like). In terms of the ability to predict a main overall diagnosis of schizophrenia, DSM–III–R proved to be considerably less sensitive than ICD–10 (60.78 and 92.73%, respectively). In addition to the 31 subjects meeting DSM–III–R criteria at onset, an additional 20 subjects received a main overall diagnosis of schizophrenia. Of these, 17 were initially assigned a diagnosis of schizophreniform psychosis, one a bipolar disorder (manic with psychotic features), one had a psychotic disorder 'not otherwise specified', and the last had major depression (single episode with psychotic features). For ICD–10, an additional four subjects given a non-schizophrenia diagnosis at onset received a main overall diagnosis of schizophrenia. Of these, one was initially assigned a diagnosis of acute polymorphic disorder with symptoms of schizophrenia, one had a schizoaffective disorder (manic type), one had an unspecified non-organic psychosis, and one had a severe depressive episode (with psychotic symptoms). For DSM–III–R there were 48 subjects who received a non-schizophrenia diagnosis at onset who retained this as a main overall diagnosis, and for ICD–10 there were 39. The

Table I Concordance (Cohen's kappa) between standard and 'duration adjusted' definitions of schizophrenia, with 95% confidence intervals

Diagnosis	n	Male/female ratio	DSM–III–R	ICD–10	ICD–9	CATEGO S+	'Duration adjusted' DSM–III–R	'Duration adjusted' ICD–10	'Duration adjusted' ICD–9
DSM–III–R	31	20/11 (1.82)	–	–	–	–	–	–	–
ICD–10	56	37/19 (1.95)	0.52 (0.36–0.68)*	–	–	–	–	–	–
ICD–9	67	45/22 (2.05)	0.36 (0.18–0.54)*	0.77 (0.63–0.91)*	–	–	–	–	–
CATEGO S+	59	35/24 (1.46)	0.13 (−0.05–0.31)	0.32 (0.12–0.52)*	0.31 (0.11–0.51)*	–	–	–	–
'Duration adjusted' DSM–III–R	59	38/21 (1.81)	0.47 (0.31–0.63)*	0.90 (0.80–1.00)*	0.83 (0.71–0.95)*	0.37 (0.17–0.57)*	–	–	–
'Duration adjusted' ICD–10	27	16/11 (1.45)	0.85 (0.73–0.97)*	0.45 (0.27–0.63)*	0.30 (0.14–0.46)*	0.15 (−0.03–0.33)	0.37 (0.19–0.55)*	–	–
'Duration adjusted' ICD–9	31	20/11 (1.82)	0.77 (0.63–0.91)*	0.36 (0.18–0.54)*	0.36 (0.18–0.54)*	0.06 (−0.12–0.24)	0.28 (0.10–0.46)*	0.90 (0.80–1.00)*	–
'Duration adjusted' CATEGO S+	23	12/11 (1.09)	0.65 (0.47–0.83)*	0.26 (0.08–0.44)*	0.15 (−0.01–0.31)	0.34 (0.16–0.52)*	0.23 (0.05–0.41)*	0.73 (0.57–0.89)*	0.65 (0.47–0.83)*

*Confidence intervals that do not include zero are significant at $P < 0.05$.

concordance (Cohen's kappa) between onset diagnoses and main overall diagnoses (schizophrenia and non-schizophrenia) was 0.60 (95% CI 0.44–0.76) for DSM–III–R and 0.82 (95% CI 0.70–0.94) for ICD–10.

DISCUSSION

Methodology

This study was based on an epidemiologically defined cohort of patients homogeneous for the stage of their illness. Diagnoses were applied blind to outcome status, and satisfactory reliability was established for diagnosis and follow-up assessments. The high follow-up rate suggests that selection

Table 2 Prediction of symptoms (GAF) at 13 years by diagnosis

Diagnosis		n^1	Median (IQ range)	Mann–Whitney U test (corrected for ties)				2-tailed P
				Mean rank	U	W	Z	
DSM–III–R	Schizophrenia	26	40 (34.25–70.25)	30.60	444.5	795.5	−3.0933	0.0020
	Other psychosis	59	75 (50–85)	48.47				
ICD–10	Schizophrenia	47	55 (35–80)	37.59	638.5	1888.5	−2.2623	0.0237
	Other psychosis	38	75 (50–85)	49.70				
ICD–9	Schizophrenia	57	60 (37.5–81)	40.48	654.5	1347.5	−1.3494	0.1772
	Other psychosis	28	72.5 (50–85)	48.13				
CATEGO S+	Schizophrenia	50	70 (40–82)	44.61	794.5	1424.5	−0.7229	0.4697
	Other psychosis	35	55 (35–81)	40.70				
'Duration adjusted' DSM–III–R	Schizophrenia	50	60 (38.75–80.25)	39.88	719.0	1661.0	−1.4009	0.1612
	Other psychosis	35	75 (50–85)	47.46				
'Duration adjusted' ICD–10	Schizophrenia	22	47.5 (31.5–72.5)	31.14	432.0	685.0	−2.6337	0.0084
	Other psychosis	63	70 (40–85)	47.14				
'Duration adjusted' ICD–9	Schizophrenia	25	50 (33.5–73)	32.18	479.5	804.5	−2.6238	0.0087
	Other psychosis	60	72.5 (41.25–85)	47.51				
'Duration adjusted' CATEGO S+	Schizophrenia	19	60 (35–80)	36.53	504.0	694.0	−1.3049	0.1919
	Other psychosis	66	70 (40–85)	44.86				

1. 14 cases missing (nine dead, four lost and one cerebrovascular accident).

Table 3 Prediction of disability (GAF) at 13 years by diagnosis

Diagnosis		n^1	Median (IQ range)	Mann–Whitney U test (corrected for ties)				2-tailed P
				Mean rank	U	W	Z	
DSM–III–R	Schizophrenia	27	45 (40–75)	32.41	497.0	875.0	−2.8026	0.0051
	Other psychosis	59	75 (45–85)	48.58				
ICD–10	Schizophrenia	48	55 (40.25–80.75)	37.55	626.5	1938.5	−2.4967	0.0125
	Other psychosis	38	80 (50–85)	51.01				
ICD–9	Schizophrenia	58	58 (44–81)	39.94	605.5	1424.5	−1.9138	0.0556
	Other psychosis	28	77.5 (51.25–85)	50.88				
CATEGO S+	Schizophrenia	51	75 (45–81)	43.95	869.5	1499.5	−0.2033	0.8389
	Other psychosis	35	61 (45–81)	42.84				
'Duration adjusted' DSM–III–R	Schizophrenia	51	55 (45–81)	39.55	691.0	1724.0	−1.7813	0.0749
	Other psychosis	35	80 (50–85)	49.26				
'Duration adjusted' ICD–10	Schizophrenia	23	45 (40–75)	32.61	474.0	750.0	−2.4578	0.014
	Other psychosis	63	75 (45–85)	47.48				
'Duration adjusted' ICD–9	Schizophrenia	26	45 (38.75–75)	32.15	485.0	836.0	−2.7895	0.0053
	Other psychosis	60	75 (46.25–85)	48.42				
'Duration adjusted' CATEGO S+	Schizophrenia	20	72.5 (40.25–78.75)	38.28	555.5	765.5	−1.0742	0.2827
	Other psychosis	66	67.5 (45–85)	45.08				

1. 13 cases missing (nine dead and four lost).

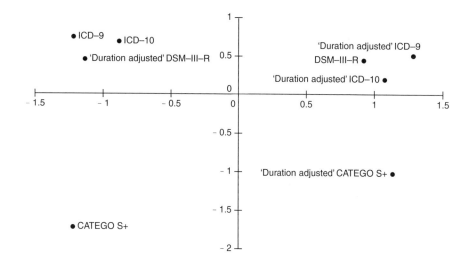

Fig. I Multidimensional scaling of eight definitions of schizophrenia

phrenia. They similarly concluded that while the six-month component is important, it is not the sole reason for the predictive ability of these criteria, since many patients who had psychotic symptoms for more than six months but who did not fulfil other DSM–III criteria went on to have relatively good outcomes. These authors went on to suggest that the inclusion of prodromal symptoms, which may be viewed more appropriately as insidious onset rather than established chronicity, in addition to the six-month duration criterion, is responsible for the high predictive validity of DSM–III.

Stability of diagnosis

The stability of a DSM–III–R diagnosis of schizophrenia over 13 years is in keeping with other diagnostic criteria using six-month inclusion criteria, such as Feighner criteria and DSM–III (Tsuang *et al*, 1981; McGlashan, 1984). However, DSM–III–R is stringent in its selection of subjects, given the large proportion of cases later reclassified as schizophrenia. Seventeen of these subjects did not receive an onset diagnosis of schizophrenia because they failed to meet the duration criteria. ICD–10 proves less restrictive, and remains reasonably stable over 13 years with only five out of 56 subjects (9%) losing schizophrenia as a final overall diagnosis. It demonstrates better stability than diagnostic criteria that rely on less-specific signs and symptoms. For example, a diagnosis of schizophrenia using the New Haven Schizophrenia Index has a stability of only 64% over 15 years (McGlashan, 1984). Fennig *et al* (1994) reported the six-month stability of psychiatric diagnoses in 278 first-admission patients with psychosis, and found that only 75.4% of patients initially given a DMS–III–R diagnosis of schizophrenia retained that diagnosis at six-month follow-up. Of those patients given a schizophreniform diagnosis at entry, only 27.3% were re-diagnosed as schizophrenic. These findings are inconsistent with those of the present study, and probably reflect differences in the duration of follow-up.

CONCLUSIONS

Diagnoses that rely upon certain 'characteristic' cross-sectional symptoms of schizophrenia (CATEGO S+) are unable to define an illness with a poor prognosis. Modern diagnostic systems (DSM–III–R and ICD–10)

biases have not seriously compromised the findings.

Predictive validity of diagnosis

These data show that DSM–III–R and ICD–10 definitions of schizophrenia are good predictors of outcome at 13 years for both symptoms and disability. DSM–III–R is a better predictor of 13-year outcome than ICD–10, but ICD–10 performs well and is less restrictive when applied at first episode. In addition, an ICD–10 diagnosis is based upon information which may be more reliably attained, since it uses symptoms and signs present over one month and does not include a retrospective assessment of prodromal symptoms, which may be included in DSM–III–R schizophrenia. The ICD–9 classification performs well as a predictor of disability at 13 years, but is a poor predictor of symptoms.

Pope & Lipinski (1978) concluded in their review that schizophrenic symptoms, taken alone and in cross-section, have little validity in determining prognosis. This conclusion is supported by our data for the S+ classification, although it should be emphasised that the class S+ is only one of the range of schizophrenic classes generated by the CATEGO programme. Hawk *et al* (1975), Bland & Orn (1979) and the World Health Organization (1979) have all noted the poor predictive validity of first rank symptoms, and Kendell *et al* (1979) reported similar findings using the CATEGO programme.

Contribution of duration criteria

The removal of the duration criterion from DSM–III–R and the addition of six-month criteria to ICD–10 and ICD–9 serves to confirm the conclusions of previous studies that a six-month duration criterion improves the predictive validity of a diagnosis of schizophrenia (Stephens *et al*, 1980, 1982; Helzer *et al*, 1981, 1983; Endicott *et al*, 1986). It is probable, however, that adding duration criteria merely creates a tautology that the longer one has an illness, the more likely ones is to have it for a long time. In a separate analysis of the subjects with an ICD–10 diagnosis of schizophrenia, Harrison *et al* (1996) found that the addition of two-year course type to other predictor variables (gender, mode of onset, marital status, age and duration of illness at entry to the study) could add as much as 21% to the outcome variance, providing further evidence to support this tautology.

The pattern of diagnostic concordance observed and its visual representation in multidimensional scaling suggest that different definitions of schizophrenia fall into three main groups: diagnoses based on cross-sectional symptoms only; broader definitions independent of long duration criteria; and diagnoses emphasising duration criteria. Our data validate these apparent differences and suggest that duration criteria are not the only components of a definition of schizophrenia that can confer predictive validity for outcome at 13 years. Helzer *et al* (1983) specifically studied the contribution of the six-month duration criterion to the predictive validity of DSM–III schizohave relatively high predictive validity, and are superior to ICD–9 in this respect. The six-month duration criterion of DSM–III–R schizophrenia accounts for most of its predictive validity and its stability over 13 years, but render it highly restrictive for first-episode studies. ICD–10 schizophrenia is much less restrictive for use in first-episode studies compared with DSM–III–R, without major compromises in predictive validity or stability over time.

ACKNOWLEDGEMENTS

This paper is based on the data and experience obtained during the participation of the authors in the project on Long-Term Course and Outcome of Schizophrenia, a project sponsored by the World Health Organization, and funded by the World Health Organization, the Laureate Foundation (US) and the participating field research centres.

The chief collaborating investigators in the 20 field research centres of this study are as follows. Aarhus: A. Bertelsen; Agra: K. C. Dube; Beijing: Shen Yucun; Cali: C. Leon; Chandigarh: V. Varma; Dublin: D Walsh; Groningen: R. Giel; Hong Kong: P. Lee; Honolulu: A. J. Marsella; Ibadan: M. Olatawura; Khartoum: T. Baasher; Madras: D. Thara; Mannheim: H. Hafner; Moscow: S. J. Tsirkin; Nagasaki: Y. Nakane; Nottingham: G. Harrison; Orangeburg: E. Laska; Prague: S. Skoda; Rochester: L. Wynne; Sofia: K. Ganev. At WHO Headquarters, Geneva, the study is coordinated by N. Sartorius (until August 1993), W. Gulbinat (1993–1995) and A. Janca (1996–).

We thank Professor J. E. Cooper for allowing access to these data and for help with this project. The authors are grateful to the Mental Health Foundation who supported this study.

CLINICAL IMPLICATIONS

■ Diagnoses of schizophrenia based upon Schneider's first rank symptoms alone are unable to define an illness with a poor prognosis.

■ Definitions of schizophrenia that include six-month duration criteria, such as DSM–III–R, have high predictive validity and stability over 13 years, but are compromised by relatively low sensitivity.

■ An ICD–10 definition of schizophrenia has high predictive validity and good stability over 13 years. It also has high specificity and sensitivity, and probably represents the most clinically useful definition for first-episode studies.

LIMITATIONS

■ The sample size is modest and the number of patients meeting DSM–III–R criteria for schizophrenia is particularly small.

■ There is no information on outcome for four subjects who were lost to follow-up.

■ The findings may have limited generalisability, since the community-oriented nature of the Nottingham Psychiatric Services may influence outcomes.

P. MASON, MRCPsych, G. HARRISON, FRCPsych, T. CROUDACE, PhD, C. GLAZEBROOK, PhD, Academic Department of Psychiatry, University of Nottingham; I. MEDLEY, MRCPsych, Mandala Centre, Nottingham, UK

Correspondence: Dr P. Mason, Department of Psychiatry, Royal Liverpool University Hospital, Liverpool L69 3BX

(First received 30 May 1996, final revision 19 September 1996, accepted 24 October 1996)

REFERENCES

American Psychiatric Association (1980) *Diagnostic and Statistical Manual of Mental Disorders* (3rd edn) (DSM–III). Washington, DC: APA.

__ **(1987)** *Diagnostic and Statistical Manual of Mental Disorders* (3rd edn, revised) (DSM–III–R). Washington, DC: APA.

Astrachan, B. M., Harrow, M., Adler, D., et al (1972) A checklist for the diagnosis of schizophrenia. *British Journal of Psychiatry,* **121,** 529–539.

Bland, R. C. & Orn, H. (1979) Schizophrenia: diagnostic criteria and outcome. *British Journal of Psychiatry,* **134,** 34–38.

Bleuler, E. (1950) *Dementia Praecox or the Group of Schizophrenias* (trans. J. Zint). New York: International University Press.

Endicott, J., Spitzer, R. L., Fleiss, J. L., et al (1976) The Global Assessment Scale. A procedure of measuring overall severity of psychiatric disturbance. *Archives of General Psychiatry,* **33,** 766–771.

__ **, Nee, J., Cohen, J., et al (1986)** Diagnosis of schizophrenia: prediction of short-term outcome. *Archives of General Psychiatry,* **43,** 13–19.

Feighner, J. P., Robins, E., Guze, S. B., et al (1972) Diagnostic criteria for use in psychiatric research. *Archives of General Psychiatry,* **26,** 57–63.

Fennig, S., Kovasznay, B., Rich, C., et al (1994) Six-month stability of psychiatric diagnoses in first-admission patients with psychosis. *American Journal of Psychiatry,* **151,** 1200–1208.

Harrison, G., Mason, P., Glazebrook, C., et al (1994) Residence of incident cohort of psychotic patients after 13 years of follow-up. *British Medical Journal,* **308,** 813–816.

__ **, Croudace, T., Mason, P., et al (1996)** Predicting the long-term outcome of schizophrenia. *Psychological Medicine,* **26,** 697–705.

Hawk, A. B., Carpenter, W. T. & Strauss, J. S. (1975) Diagnostic criteria and five-year outcome in schizophrenia. *Archives of General Psychiatry,* **32,** 343–347.

Helzer, J. E., Brockington, I. F. & Kendell, R. E. (1981) Predictive validity of DSM–III and Feighner definitions of schizophrenia. A comparison with research diagnostic criteria and CATEGO. *Archives of General Psychiatry,* **38,** 791–797.

__ **, Kendell, R. E. & Brockington, I. F. (1983)** Contributions of the six-month criterion to the predictive validity of the DSM–III definition of schizophrenia. *Archives of General Psychiatry,* **40,** 1277–1280.

Jablensky, A., Schwarz, R. & Tomov, T. (1980) WHO collaborative study on impairments and disabilities associated with schizophrenic disorders. *Acta Psychiatrica Scandinavica* **62,** (suppl. 285), 152–163.

__ **, Sartorius, N., Ernberg, E., et al (1992)** Schizophrenia: manifestations, incidence and course in different cultures. A World Health Organisation Ten Country Study. *Psychological Medicine,* Monograph Supplement 20. Cambridge: Cambridge University Press.

Kendell, R. E., Brockington, I. F. & Leff, J. P. (1979) Prognostic implications of six alternative definitions of schizophrenia. *Archives of General Psychiatry,* **36,** 25–31.

Kleist, K. (1960) Schizophrenic symptoms and cerebral pathology. *Journal of Mental Science,* **106,** 246–253.

Kraepelin, E. (1919) *Dementia Praecox* (trans. R. M. Barclay). Edinburgh: E. S. Livingstone.

Langfeldt, G. (1969) Schizophrenia: diagnosis and prognosis. *Behavioural Science,* **14,** 173–182.

Leonhard, K. (1961) The cycloid psychoses. *Journal of Mental Science,* **107,** 633–648.

McGlashan, T. H. (1984) Testing four diagnostic systems for schizophrenia. *Archives of General Psychiatry,* **41,** 141–144.

Mason, P., Harrison, G., Glazebrook, C., et al (1995) Characteristics of outcome in schizophrenia at 13 years. *British Journal of Psychiatry,* **167,** 596–603.

Pope, H. G. & Lipinski, J. F. (1978) Diagnosis in schizophrenia and manic depressive illness. A reassessment of the specificity of 'schizophrenic' symptoms in the light of current research. *Archives of General Psychiatry,* **35,** 811–828.

Robins, E. & Guze, S. B. (1970) Establishment of diagnostic validity in psychiatric illness: its implications to schizophrenia. *American Journal of Psychiatry,* **126,** 983–987.

Sartorius, N., Gulbinat, W., Harrison, G., et al (1996) Long term follow-up of schizophrenia in 16 countries. A description of the International Study of Schizophrenia conducted by the World Health Organization. *Social Psychiatry and Psychiatric Epidemiology,* **31,** 249–258.

Schneider, K. (1959) *Clinical Psychopathology* (trans. M.W. Hamilton & E.W. Anderson). New York: Grune & Stratton.

Stephens, J. H., Ota, K. Y., Carpenter, W. T., et al (1980) Diagnostic criteria for schizophrenia: prognostic implications and diagnostic overlap. *Psychiatry Research*, **2**, 1–12.

—, Astrup, C., Carpenter, W. T., et al (1982) A comparison of nine systems to diagnose schizophrenia. *Psychiatry Research*, **6**, 127–143.

Tsuang, M. T., Woolson, R. F., Winokur, G., et al (1981) Stability of psychiatric diagnosis. *Archives of General Psychiatry*, **38**, 535–539.

Wing, J. K., Cooper, J. E. & Sartorius, N. (1974) *The Measurement and Classification of Psychiatric Symptoms*. Cambridge: Cambridge University Press.

World Health Organization (1978a) *Mental Disorders: Glossary and Guide to their Classification in Accordance with the Ninth Revision of the International Classification of Diseases*. Geneva: WHO.

— (1978b) *Psychiatric and Personal History Schedule*. Geneva: WHO.

— (1979) *Schizophrenia: An International Follow-up Study*. New York: John Wiley.

— (1992a) *The ICD–10 Classification of Mental and Behavioural Disorders*. Geneva: WHO.

— (1992b) *Broad Rating Schedule*. Geneva: WHO.

— (1992c) *Life Chart Schedule*. Geneva: WHO.

Controlled trial of exposure and response prevention in obsessive–compulsive disorder

MERRAN LINDSAY, ROCCO CRINO and GAVIN ANDREWS

Rachman, Hodgson and Marks at the Maudsley Hospital in a different setting with a credible placebo; to examine the specific contribution of exposure and response prevention to outcome in OCD; and to examine the contribution of non-specific therapy factors, such as therapist supportiveness, to treatment outcome.

METHOD

Subjects

Eighteen subjects were recruited from a population of adult out-patients referred for treatment of OCD. All met DSM–IV diagnostic criteria for a primary diagnosis of OCD. The average duration of OCD was 11 years (range 1–26 years). Five subjects were taking clomipramine or fluoxetine and all had been on these medications for at least 12 months without improvement.

Assessment

The outcome measures used to assess the severity of obsessions, compulsions, anxiety and depression were:

The Padua Inventory

A 60-item self-report questionnaire (Sanavio, 1988) assessing the severity of obsessive–compulsive thoughts and behaviours. Each item is rated on a five-point scale (from 0 to 4), giving a maximum possible score of 240. The internal consistency is $\alpha=0.90$ for males ($n=489$), and $\alpha=0.94$ for females ($n=478$). Test–retest reliability correlations are $r=0.78$ (males) and $r=0.83$ (females), when retested after a 30-day interval.

The Maudsley Obsessional–Compulsive Inventory (MOCI)

A 30-item self-report questionnaire (Rachman & Hodgson, 1980) assessing the presence of common OCD symptoms. Each item is answered 'true' or 'false', giving a maximum possible score of 30. The MOCI has four subscales: checking, cleaning, slowness and doubting. Internal consistency estimates for these subscales range between $\alpha=0.7$ and $\alpha=0.8$. The test–retest reliability coefficient is 0.8 for an interval of one month. Significant correlations were obtained between change scores on this measure and therapist ratings of improvement ($r=0.67$ to $r=0.74$). (Rachman & Hodgson, 1980).

Background Exposure and response prevention is considered a treatment of choice for obsessive–compulsive disorder (OCD). Yet there have been very few randomised controlled trials employing credible placebo conditions. This study compares exposure and response prevention with a general anxiety management intervention.

Method Eighteen patients meeting DSM–IV criteria for OCD were randomly assigned to either exposure and response prevention or anxiety management. Both treatments involved approximately 15 hours of therapy over a three-week period.

Results There was a significant reduction in obsessive–compulsive symptoms following treatment with exposure and response prevention, while no change occurred in the control group. This was found to be statistically significant using a composite measure of OCD symptom severity, patient ratings of interference and therapist ratings of symptom severity.

Conclusions These findings suggest that the symptom reductions associated with behaviour therapy for OCD are a result of the specific techniques of exposure and response prevention, rather than non-specific aspects of the therapy process. General anxiety management techniques are not effective in the treatment of OCD.

Obsessive–compulsive disorder (OCD) is a complex and debilitating disorder with a lifetime prevalence of about 2% (Karno & Golding, 1991). It is not rare. Two treatments are effective: one is behaviour therapy using exposure and response prevention, the other is pharmacotherapy with selective serotonin reuptake inhibitors. The response of OCD to these drugs has prompted a large number of placebo-controlled treatment trials (Thoren et al, 1980; Insel et al, 1985; Crino, 1990). The largest placebo-controlled trial to date is the multi-centre clomipramine trial, which reported an average decrease in symptoms of around 40% (Clomipramine Collaborative Study Group, 1991), but half the patients showed no significant improvement. Similar findings have been obtained in controlled trials of fluoxetine, fluvoxamine and sertraline.

In a review of 273 OCD patients treated with behaviour therapy in open trials, Foa et al (1985) reported that 51% of patients were "cured" or "much improved" (i.e. greater than 70% symptom reduction), and at follow-up 76% of all patients had maintained a symptom reduction of at least 60%. There are, however, very few reports of randomised placebo-controlled trials of exposure and response prevention for OCD. The few controlled trials conducted to date have relied on progressive muscle relaxation training as a placebo condition against which to compare the active treatment (see Marks et al, 1975; Roper et al, 1975; Fals-Stewart et al, 1993). Marks et al (1988) used anti-exposure instructions as a control. While these trials have consistently shown exposure and response prevention to be superior to the control condition, the face validity of relaxation or anti-exposure as a treatment for OCD is questionable, particularly in the absence of an explicit rationale. None of the studies assessed therapist variables to ensure that these were constant across treatment and control conditions. The aims of the present study were threefold: to replicate the seminal work of

The Yale–Brown Obsessive–Compulsive Scale (Y–BOCS)

This is a clinician-rated scale (Goodman *et al*, 1989*a,b*) with 10 items. It was designed to assess severity of OCD symptoms independent of the type or number of obsessions or compulsions present. Severity is assessed in terms of time, interference, distress, resistance and control. Each item is rated on a five-point scale (0 to 4) giving a maximum possible score of 40. Interrater reliability correlations are very high for total Y–BOCS scores (lowest $r=0.98$), obsession and compulsion subtotals (lowest $r=0.95$) and individual items (lowest $r=0.80$). The mean internal consistency estimate is $\alpha=0.89$ (Goodman *et al*, 1989*a*). Scores on the Y–BOCS correlate strongly with the Clinical Global Impressions Scale of OCD Severity (CGI-OCS) ($r=0.74$), and moderately with the National Institute of Mental Health Global Obsessive Compulsive Severity Scale (NIMH-OC) ($r=0.67$) (Goodman *et al*, 1989*b*).

The State–Trait Anxiety Inventory (STAI; Spielberger *et al*, 1970) and the Beck Depression Inventory (BDI; Beck *et al*, 1961) were also used. They are scales with well established psychometric characteristics.

Interference rating scale

In addition to the above measures, each subject was asked to rate the extent to which OCD interfered with their life and activities. The scale was numbered 1 to 7, where 1 represented 'not at all', 3 represented 'a little', 5 represented 'a lot' and 7 represented 'totally'.

Therapist variables

In order to rule out the possibility that any observed differences in treatment outcome were due to differences in therapist variables, patients were contacted following treatment and asked to rate their therapist for two qualities: supportiveness and understanding. These interviews were conducted over the phone by an independent assessor. Ratings were made on a four-point scale, where 0=not at all, 1=somewhat, 2=moderately and 3=highly.

Treatment

Subjects were randomly assigned to one of two treatment conditions: exposure and response prevention or anxiety management (control). Both treatments involved approxi-mately 15 hours of face-to-face therapy over a three-week period with experienced clinical psychologists. All subjects received a treatment manual which outlined in detail a rationale for treatment and treatment guidelines.

Exposure and response prevention

Treatment consisted of graded exposure to situations previously associated with obsessional thoughts or impulses coupled with self-imposed prevention of compulsive rituals (for treatment manual see Andrews *et al*, 1994). Subjects were told that, with repeated exposure and response prevention, the anxiety and distress they experienced in response to obsessions would gradually decline, and the urge to ritualise would dissipate. In addition to attending out-patient therapy sessions in the clinic, these subjects were required to complete home-work exposure tasks each day.

Anxiety management

In the light of our views about the common neurotic syndrome (Andrews *et al*, 1994) general anxiety management techniques were seen to provide a credible and possibly effective placebo treatment condition. Treatment sessions focused on teaching the subjects anxiety management techniques, including breathing techniques for the management of hyperventilation, progressive muscle relaxation and structured problem-solving about non-OCD life stressors. The manual was derived from the GAD manual in Andrews *et al* (1994). Cognitive restructuring was not included, nor were any specific instructions given regarding exposure to triggers or prevention of rituals. As OCD patients frequently report a worsening of obsessional symptoms during periods of general life stress, patients in this group were told that by learning to control their anxiety and stress they would have the means to cope more effectively with the symptoms of their obsessive–compulsive disorder. They were also told that persistent practice of the anxiety management techniques would help to reduce their vulnerability to OCD. In addition to practice within sessions, subjects were required to practise these techniques at home each day during the three-week programme.

Treatment integrity

Treatment integrity was maintained by emphasising close adherence to the treat-ment guidelines provided in the treatment manuals. In addition, the structure and content of therapy sessions for both groups were agreed upon by all clinicians before the study began.

RESULTS

The demographic characteristics of patients allocated to each treatment group are provided in Table 1, along with the duration of OCD complaints.

Post-treatment ratings of therapists

Patients in both treatment groups rated their therapists as highly supportive and understanding. The same mean supportiveness rating was obtained for each group ($M=2.8$, s.d.$=0.5$), while the mean rating of understanding was 2.6 (s.d.$=0.5$) for the exposure and response prevention group, and 2.9 (s.d.$=0.4$) for the anxiety management group ($F(1,16)=1.27$, NS).

Pre-treatment dependent variables

Pre-treatment scores on all seven dependent variables were compared using a series of one-way ANOVAs (with Bonferroni adjustment). There was no significant difference between the groups on any of these measures (see Table 2). A high level of OCD symptomatology was present in both groups of patients.

Treatment effects

Scores on the different outcome measures were likely to be highly correlated, so treatment effects were examined using a principal components analysis of dependent variable scores followed by a two-way analysis of variance. Treatment effects were also examined on the seven outcome measures individually, giving a total of nine two-way ANOVAs with Bonferroni adjustment for multiple comparisons (critical value$=0.5/9=0.0056$).

Principal components analysis (with varimax rotation) yielded two components with an eigenvalue greater than one. The first of these components accounted for 62.6% of the variance in scores on individual measures. As can be seen in Table 3, this component provides a combined measure of OCD symptom severity, with high loadings for the Y–BOCS, MOCI, PADUA and the interference measure. The second component accounted for a further 16.7% of the variance, and appeared to be a more

Table 1 Demographic characteristics of patients

	Exposure and response prevention (n=9)	Anxiety management (n=9)
Gender		
Male	5	1
Female	4	8
Mean age (years) (s.d.)	31.6 (8.9)	34.0 (9.3)
Duration of complaints (years) (s.d.)	9.0 (8.7)	12.9 (8.9)
Marital status		
Single	44%	22%
Married or de facto	44%	78%
Divorced or widowed	11%	0%
Educational standard		
Low	22%	22%
Medium	33%	11%
High	45%	67%

Table 2 Group means (s.d.) pre- and post-treatment

	Exposure group		Control group	
	Pre	Post	Pre	Post
Interference	5.9 (0.93)	3.4 (0.88)	6.4 (0.88)	6.3 (0.87)*
Y–BOCS total	28.70 (4.56)	11.00 (3.81)	24.44 (6.98)	25.89 (5.80)*
Obsessions	14.11 (2.71)	6.33 (1.80)	11.56 (4.06)	12.89 (3.18)*
Compulsions	14.56 (2.12)	4.67 (2.35)	12.89 (3.22)	13.00 (2.83)*
MOCI total	17.00 (4.06)	9.56 (4.59)	20.33 (4.06)	17.89 (4.23)*
PADUA total	84.56 (28.36)	41.44 (22.54)	95.78 (39.44)	81.22 (35.15)*
STAI state	51.89 (12.18)	44.33 (8.97)	53.11 (11.38)	52.11 (13.77)
STAI trait	58.00 (10.08)	49.89 (8.71)	58.22 (12.03)	55.89 (12.89)
BDI total	21.33 (10.45)	13.11 (8.30)	19.22 (9.28)	18.33 (9.66)

Y–BOCS=Yale–Brown Obsessive–Compulsive Scale; MOCI=Maudsley Obsessional–Compulsive Inventory; PADUA=Padua Inventory; STAI=State–Trait Anxiety Inventory; BDI=Beck Depression Inventory.
*$P<0.05$ Exposure v. control at same time point

Table 3 Principal components: variable loadings and eigenvalues

Variable	Component 1 weight	Component 2 weight
Interference	0.897	0.176
Y–BOCS	0.808	0.196
MOCI	0.826	0.315
PADUA	0.716	0.509
STAI state	0.315	0.799
STAI trait	0.218	0.899
BDI depression	0.238	0.907
Eigenvalue	4.38	1.17
% Variance explained	62.6	16.7

Y–BOCS=Yale–Brown Obsessive–Compulsive Scale; MOCI=Maudsley Obsessional–Compulsive Inventory; PADUA=Padua Inventory; STAI=State–Trait Anxiety Inventory; BDI=Beck Depression Inventory.

general measure of anxiety and depression, with high loadings for both of the STAI measures and the BDI.

When scores on the first principal component were combined across groups, there was an overall reduction in scores following treatment ($F(1,32)=27.8$, $P<0.0056$). Likewise scores on this component were lower for the exposure and response prevention group than for the anxiety management group when combined across measurement occasions ($F(1,32)=35.0$, $P<0.0056$). However, there was also a significant interaction between component scores for each group over time, indicating that the reduction in obsessional symptoms following treatment was specific to patients in the exposure and response prevention group ($F(1,32)=20.3$, $P<0.0056$). There was no change in scores following treatment for patients in the anxiety management group.

By comparison, there were no significant differences between the groups ($F(1,32)=0.002$, NS) or following treatment ($F(1,32)=0.434$, NS) in scores on the second principal component, and no significant interaction effects ($F(1,32)=0.031$, NS). Analysis of variance in individual measures showed similar results. When scores for both groups were combined, there was a significant reduction from pre-treatment to post-treatment in scores on the Y–BOCS ($F(1,32)=20.1$, $P<0.0056$) and the MOCI ($F(1,32)=12.2$, $P<0.0056$), and in subjective ratings of the degree to which OCD interfered with life and activities ($F(1,32)=18.6$, $P<0.0056$). When pre-treatment and post-treatment scores were combined there were significant differences between the groups in scores on the MOCI ($F(1,32)=17.0$, $P<0.0056$) and in subjective ratings of interference ($F(1,32)=33.7$, $P<0.0056$). More importantly, the interactions between group scores over time were significant using the Y–BOCS ($F(1,32)=27.9$, $P<0.0056$), and subjective ratings of interference ($F(1,32)=15.5$, $P<0.0056$). These results show that the reduction in Y–BOCS and interference scores from pre-treatment to post-treatment was specific to the exposure and response prevention group, with no change in scores for the anxiety management group. This is illustrated using Y–BOCS scores in Fig. 1.

DISCUSSION

The results of the present study are consistent with those of previous placebo-

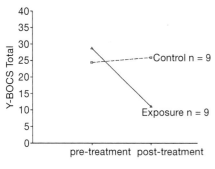

Fig. I Mean Y–BOCS total scores

CLINICAL IMPLICATIONS

- Exposure and response prevention is an effective treatment.

- Anxiety management was not effective.

- A good therapeutic relationship alone was not effective.

LIMITATIONS

- The small number of subjects.

- Random allocation did not equalise gender ratios.

- Credibility of control group was not assessed.

controlled trials of exposure and response prevention in the treatment of OCD (Marks *et al*, 1975; Fals-Stewart *et al*, 1993). However, the current study differs from previous studies in a number of ways. First, rather than controlling for non-specific aspects of therapy with a simple relaxation condition, we used a credible placebo condition in the form of a comprehensive anxiety management package which was designed to maximise face validity and was conducted by an experienced therapist. Second, the contribution of therapist variables was assessed and time spent in face-to-face therapy was held constant for the two groups. Finally, while a number of previous studies had used sequential treatment conditions in which patients were aware that exposure would follow relaxation, the present study used a randomisation procedure for allocation to one condition or the other.

The results of the present study provide considerable evidence for the specificity of change associated with exposure and response prevention techniques. The failure of the control group to show any significant changes in OCD symptoms following treatment with general anxiety management techniques is further evidence for the specific effects of exposure and response prevention in the reduction of obsessional symptoms. The absence of change in this group cannot be attributed to differences in treatment expectations since considerable effort was made to design a control treatment package which would have good face validity for patients. This is supported by the high compliance with monitoring tasks in the control group and the fact that no patients dropped out of treatment.

The different outcomes for each group cannot be attributed to differences in therapist variables either, since both groups rated their therapists as highly supportive and

understanding. The importance of a good patient–therapist relationship in the behavioural treatment of OCD was first noted by Marks *et al* (1975). Such relationships have been shown to predict better outcomes (Keijsers *et al*, 1994) and fewer drop-outs (Hansen *et al*, 1992). Similarly, Rabavilas *et al* (1979) found that patients whose illness had a better outcome rated their therapists as more respectful, understanding, interested and challenging. The results of the present study suggest that while therapist variables may be important in maximising treatment outcomes with behaviour therapy, they make little difference to obsessional symptoms in the absence of exposure and response prevention.

In summary, by evaluating the contribution of non-specific therapy factors to treatment outcomes with obsessional patients, the current investigation adds further evidence to the efficacy of exposure and response prevention in the treatment of OCD. The findings clearly show that the therapeutic benefits associated with exposure and response prevention are a function of the specific procedures involved. Supportive and understanding therapists offering face valid treatments with a comprehensive rationale make little difference to OCD in the absence of exposure-based treatment.

MERRAN LINDSAY, MPsychol(Clin), ROCCO CRINO, MPsychol(Clin), GAVIN ANDREWS, MD, Clinical Research Unit for Anxiety Disorders, School of Psychiatry, University of New South Wales at St Vincent's Hospital, Sydney, Australia

Correspondence: Rocco Crino, Clinical Research Unit for Anxiety Disorders, 299 Forbes Street, Darlinghurst, NSW 2010, Australia

(First received II September 1996, final revision 30 January 1997, accepted 7 February 1997)

REFERENCES

Andrews, G., Crino, R., Hunt, C., et al (1994) *The Treatment of Anxiety Disorders.* New York: Cambridge University Press.

Beck, A., Ward, C., Mendelson, M., et al (1961) An inventory for measuring depression. *Archives of General Psychiatry,* **4**, 561–571.

Clomipramine Collaborative Study Group (1991) Clomipramine in the treatment of patients with obsessive compulsive disorder. *Archives of General Psychiatry,* **48**, 730–738.

Crino, R. D. (1990) Serotonin and obsessive compulsive disorder. In *Anxiety* (eds N. McNaughton & G. Andrews), pp. 234–243. Dunedin: University of Otago Press.

Fals-Stewart, W., Marks, A. & Schafer, J. (1993) A comparison of behavioral group therapy and individual behavior therapy in treating obsessive–compulsive disorder. *Journal of Nervous and Mental Disease,* **181**, 189–193.

Foa, E. B., Steketee, G. S. & Ozarow, B. J. (1985) Behaviour therapy with obsessive–compulsives: from therapy to treatment. In *Obsessive Compulsive Disorder: Psychological and Pharmacological Treatments* (eds M. Mavissakalian, S. Turner & L. Michelsen). New York: Plenum Press.

Goodman, W., Price, L., Rasmussen, S., et al (1989a) The Yale–Brown obsessive compulsive scale: development, use and reliability. *Archives of General Psychiatry,* **46**, 1006–1011.

—, —, —, et al (1989b) The Yale–Brown obsessive compulsive scale: validity. *Archives of General Psychiatry,* **46**, 1012–1016.

Hansen, A., Hoogduin, C., Schaap, C., et al (1992) Do drop-outs differ from successfully treated obsessive–compulsives? *Behaviour Research and Therapy,* **30**, 547–550.

Insel, T. R., Mueller, E. A., Alterman, I., et al (1985) Obsessive compulsive disorder and serotonin: is there a connection? *Biological Psychiatry,* **20**, 1171–1188.

Karno, M. & Golding, J. (1991) Obsessive Compulsive Disorder. In *Psychiatric Disorders in America–The Epidemiological Catchment Area Study* (eds L. Robins & D. Regier), pp. 204–219. New York: Macmillan.

Keijsers, G., Hoogduin, C. & Schaap, C. (1994) Predictors of treatment outcome in the behavioral treatment of obsessive compulsive disorder. *British Journal of Psychiatry*, **165**, 781–786.

Marks, I., Hodgson, R. & Rachman, S. (1975) Treatment of chronic obsessive–compulsive neurosis by *in vivo* exposure: two year follow-up and issues in treatment. *British Journal of Psychiatry*, **127**, 349–364.

Marks, I., Lelliot, P., Basoglu, M., et al (1988) Clomipramine, self-exposure, and therapist-aided exposure for obsessive compulsive rituals. *British Journal of Psychiatry*, **152**, 522–534.

Rabavilas, A., Boulougouris, J. & Perissaki, C. (1979) Therapist qualities related to outcome with exposure *in vivo* in neurotic patients. *Journal of Behavior Therapy and Experimental Psychiatry*, **10**, 293–294.

Rachmans, S. & Hodgson, R. (1980) *Obsessions and Compulsions*. New Jersey: Prentice Hall.

Roper, G., Rachman, S. & Marks, I. (1975) Passive and participant modelling in exposure treatment of obsessive–compulsive neurotics. *Behavior Research and Therapy*, **13**, 271–279.

Sanavio, E. (1988) Obsessions and compulsions: the Padua inventory. *Behavior Research and Therapy*, **26**, 169–177.

Spielberger, C. D., Gorsuch, R. L. & Lushene, R. E. (1970) *STAI Manual for the State–Trait Anxiety Inventory*. Palo Alto, CA: Consulting Psychologists Press.

Thoren, P., Asberg, M., Bertilsson, L., et al (1980) Clomipramine treatment of obsessive compulsive disorder II: Biochemical aspects. *Archives of General Psychiatry*, **37**, 1289–1294.

Paroxetine in the treatment of panic disorder

A randomised, double-blind, placebo-controlled study

S. OEHRBERG, P. E. CHRISTIANSEN, K. BEHNKE, A. L. BORUP, B. SEVERIN,
J. SOEGAARD, H. CALBERG, R. JUDGE, J. K. OHRSTROM and P. M. MANNICHE

Background This study compared the efficacy and tolerability of paroxetine with placebo in the treatment of panic disorder.

Method After three weeks of placebo, patients received 12 weeks of treatment with paroxetine (20, 40, or 60 mg) or placebo, and finally two weeks of placebo. Dosages were adjusted according to efficacy and tolerability. Standardised cognitive therapy was given to all patients. The primary measure of outcome was reduction in the number of panic attacks.

Results Analysis of the results showed statistically significant differences in favour of paroxetine between the two treatment groups in two out of the three primary measures of outcome, i.e. 50% reduction in total number of panic attacks and number of panic attacks reduced to one or zero over the study period. For the third measure of outcome, the mean change in the total number of attacks from baseline, there was a positive trend in favour of paroxetine. The results of the primary measures of outcome were strongly supported by the results of the secondary efficacy measures of outcome. In addition, paroxetine, at all doses, was very well tolerated.

Conclusion Paroxetine plus cognitive therapy was significantly more effective than placebo plus cognitive therapy in the treatment of panic disorder.

In 1980, panic disorder was recognised as a distinct diagnostic entity by the DSM–III (American Psychiatric Association, 1980). It is a common disorder, with a lifetime prevalence of about 2%. Being female, divorced, or separated is associated with higher prevalence of panic disorder. The hazard rates for panic disorder appear to be highest between the ages of 25 and 34 years for women and between the ages of 30 and 44 years for men (Wittchen & Essau, 1993).

Studies of pharmacological and psychological treatments have shown their efficacy in panic disorder. Of the psychological treatments, cognitive therapy is of particular note (Beck *et al*, 1992; Chambless & Gillis, 1993).

Studies of pharmacological treatments have centred mainly on benzodiazepines and antidepressants. The standard benzodiazepines, diazepam and clonazepam, have been shown to be effective at higher doses (Kahn & van Praag, 1992) and alprazolam has, in several studies, shown efficacy and rapid onset of action (Rosenberg *et al*, 1991). However, the use of benzodiazepines is associated with several disadvantages, including sedation, reduced coordination, impaired cognition, and, most importantly, development of dependence with associated withdrawal symptoms (Salzman, 1993).

Studies with antidepressants include those with clomipramine, imipramine, and desipramine and, more recently, with selective serotonin reuptake inhibitors (SSRIs) such as fluvoxamine and fluoxetine (Schneier *et al*, 1990; Den Boer, 1988; Black *et al*, 1993), all of which show good efficacy in the treatment of panic disorder. However, the tricyclic agents are associated with significant anticholinergic side-effects which may be troublesome for some patients. No previous study has compared an SSRI with placebo when both groups received standardised cognitive therapy.

The efficacy of paroxetine as an antidepressant is well established (Feighner & Boyer, 1989). The purpose of the present study was to evaluate the efficacy and tolerability of the highly selective SSRI, paroxetine, in the treatment of patients with panic disorder.

METHOD

This study was a double-blind, placebo-controlled, parallel-group comparison. An initial three-week placebo period was followed by a 12-week treatment period with either paroxetine or placebo, after which patients underwent a two-week placebo period. Seven Danish centres participated in the study.

To be included in the study, patients of either sex had to be aged 18–70 years and have a diagnosis of panic disorder according to DSM–III–R (American Psychiatric Association, 1987), with or without agoraphobia, and have to have had at least three full panic attacks during the four weeks before entry in the study. A baseline score of 14 or less on the Hamilton Depression Scale (Hamilton, 1969), 17-item version, was also required.

Among the exclusion criteria were primary diagnosis of major depression (DSM–III–R) or generalised anxiety disorder (DSM–III–R), schizophrenia or dementia, organic brain disease, or alcohol or drug abuse, or concomitant treatment with psychotropics, monoamine oxidase inhibitors, anticoagulants, or benzodiazepines. In the case of benzodiazepines, patients were excluded if they were still receiving these drugs at entry to the three-week placebo period, or if there was an emergence of benzodiazepine-withdrawal symptoms in the placebo period.

All patients received placebo tablets in the first three weeks (placebo period), followed by random allocation to either paroxetine or placebo treatment. Regardless of the magnitude of improvement seen in the placebo period, patients could enter the active treatment period as long as they satisfied the inclusion criteria. In the first two weeks of study treatment, paroxetine doses were gradually increased from 10 to 20 mg/day ('low dose'). From week 3 onward, the dosage was flexible, either 20 mg/day ('low dose') or 40 mg/day ('medium dose'), and from week 4 onward dosage could be further increased to 60 mg daily ('high dose') according to efficacy and tolerability. In both treatment groups, all daily doses consisted of two visually identical tablets. Patient compliance was assessed at each visit by tablet counts. Urinalysis was done to determine whether patients had been taking concomitant benzodiazepines. In addition to pharmacological treatment, all patients received standardised psychotherapy according to the principles developed by Hawton *et al* (1989).

Patients were assessed at weekly intervals during the placebo period; at the end of weeks 1, 2, 3, 4, 6, 9, and 12, and at the end of the two-week placebo period. Throughout the study period, regular joint racing sessions with the participating psychiatrists were arranged to minimise interrater variability on the observer rating scales. Assessment of response was based on consecutive three-week intervals.

The principal measure of outcome was the reduction in the number of panic attacks, as recorded by the patient in a daily diary. A reduction equal to or more than 50% from baseline was considered to be beneficial. In addition, the percentage of patients who had their panic attacks reduced to zero, or one, in a three-week interval was determined, and the mean change in the number of panic attacks from baseline in each group was evaluated from the diary assessments. The daily diary card was used to document the severity of each panic attack, the duration of each attack, whether or not there were any precipitating factors, and the severity of agoraphobia, if present, for each attack.

Secondary measures of outcome included:

(a) a reduction in score equal to or greater than 50% on the Hamilton Anxiety Scale (HAM–A) (Hamilton, 1969)

(b) a response on the Clinical Global Impression (CGI) scale (Guy, 1976) where a response was defined as a score of 2 (borderline illness) or less at the assessments for patients whose baseline score was 3 (mildly ill) or more

(c) the mean reduction on the Zung Self-Rating Scale for Anxiety (Zung, 1971).

At each assessment, adverse events were noted. These were detected by observation or could be reported by the patient either spontaneously or in response to the open question, "Do you feel different in any way since starting the treatment or since the last visit?"

Safety assessments included vital signs, e.g., blood pressure, pulse and body weight and laboratory tests of haematology and clinical chemistry variables. Ethical considerations were all in accordance with the Helsinki Declaration.

The sample size was based upon the assumption that response rates in the paroxetine and the placebo groups would be 70% and 40%, respectively ($\alpha=0.05$, $1-\beta=0.80$). To allow for a 30% attrition rate, we considered it necessary to recruit 120 patients in total. Data analysis of the efficacy variables was based on the Cochran–Mantel–Haenszel χ^2 test, adjusting for centre, categorical data, the Breslow–Day test for homogeneity over centres, and analysis of variance with the factors treatment, centre, and treatment/centre interaction for continuous variables. In all cases, a two-tailed significance level of 5% was used to determine presence of statistical significance.

RESULTS

In the analysis of this study, two populations were considered – the intention to treat and the per protocol. Within these populations, the analyses used the observed cases data set, consisting of each patient's observations at each interval and the endpoint, which was generated from the observed cases data set by taking the last valid result between weeks 3 and 12. Results are presented for the intention to treat population (consisting of each patient's observations at each interval) only, as the other analyses yielded similar results.

Demographic data and patient history

A total of 129 patients were enrolled, nine patients dropped out during the placebo period, and the remaining 120 patients were equally allocated to receive either paroxetine or placebo. Thus, 60 patients in each group comprised the intention to treat analysis. The two treatment groups were comparable with respect to demographic variables. Eighty per cent of the paroxetine group and 72% of the placebo group were female, the mean ages being 37.7 years and 37.0 years for paroxetine and placebo, respectively; the age range was 21–69 years for the population. Familial disposition to panic disorder was seen in 33% of the paroxetine group and 25% of the placebo group. Almost all of the

patients had panic attacks which were rated as moderate or severe at baseline. Only seven patients in the paroxetine group and nine patients in the placebo group did not report any agoraphobic avoidance at baseline. Of those that did report agoraphobic avoidance, 66% and 63% reported the severity as moderate or severe in the paroxetine and placebo groups respectively.

Patient withdrawals

Of the 120 patients entering the 12-week treatment period, 55 (92%) paroxetine patients and 52 (87%) placebo patients completed the 12-week treatment period. Five patients on paroxetine were withdrawn, as compared with eight on placebo: one paroxetine patient was withdrawn for lack of efficacy plus adverse events, three were withdrawn because of adverse events, and one was withdrawn for lack of compliance. The adverse events leading to withdrawal in this group were abdominal pain, confusion, decreased appetite, depression, dizziness, headache, incoordination, decreased libido, nausea, and unintended pregnancy. Three placebo patients were withdrawn for lack of efficacy/relapse, one for lack of compliance, three for protocol violations, and one for uncertain diagnosis.

Concomitant medication

No concomitant medication was taken at baseline by 49 paroxetine patients (82%) and 53 placebo patients (88%). During the study, 16 (27%) paroxetine patients and six (10%) placebo patients were prescribed analgesic, anti-allergic, or other non-psychotropic drugs. Concomitant psychotropic medication was not permitted during the study.

Efficacy

The primary efficacy evaluations were based on measures of changes in the frequency of panic attacks occurring in three-week intervals. Comparisons between the groups were based on consecutive three-week intervals. The first three-week interval after the placebo run-in period was referred to as week 3, the second as week 6, the third as week 9, and the fourth as week 12.

The number of patients with at least 50% reduction from baseline in number of panic attacks (Fig. 1) was significantly greater in the paroxetine group at six

Fig. I Panic attack response rates. Percentage of patients with at least 50% reduction from baseline number of panic attacks per three-week period. Statistically significant differences in favour of paroxetine were seen at 6, 9, and 12 weeks (P=0.006, P=0.001, and P=0.001, respectively). ◆–◆: paroxetine; ■–■: placebo.

Fig. 3 Panic attack response rates – mean changes from baseline total number of panic attacks per three-week period. Differences were not statistically significant at any time point (P > 0.05). ◆–◆: paroxetine; ■–■: placebo.

weeks, at nine weeks (P=0.006 and P=0.001, respectively), and at 12 weeks (P=0.001) when 82% (n=42) of the paroxetine patients, as compared with 50% (n=25) of the placebo patients, had responded. Both treatment groups showed early onset of action, improvement being evident in the first three-week period.

Evaluation of the reduction in number of panic attacks to one or zero (Fig. 2) showed similar differences in favour of paroxetine, although statistical significance was not seen until week 12 when 36% (n=19) of the paroxetine patients, as compared with 16% (n=8) of the placebo patients, had responded (P=0.024).

The third measure, the mean change from baseline in the number of panic attacks (Fig. 3), showed at week 12 a mean reduction of 16.0 from a baseline mean of

21.2 in the paroxetine group, as compared with a mean reduction of 9.8, from a baseline mean of 26.4 in the placebo group (not statistically significant; P=0.084).

In the placebo group, all three measures reflected deterioration in the fourth three-week period, whereas such a pattern was not seen in the paroxetine group.

In the range of the secondary measures of outcome, the results all supported the response pattern seen on the primary measures of outcome. On the HAM–A and the CGI, the response rates were significantly higher in the paroxetine group

at 6 and 12 weeks, as compared with the placebo group (Table 1).

On the patient self-rated assessment, the Zung Self-Rating Scale, the effect of paroxetine, measured as the mean change from baseline score, was significantly superior to placebo at 6 and 12 weeks (Table 1).

As this study employed flexible dosing, it is not possible to determine a minimally effective dose. However, in the paroxetine group, most patients (75%) were treated with a 40 or 60 mg dose and 47% of patients received the 60 mg dose at some point in the study.

Adverse events

The number of patients reporting at least one adverse event was 46 (77%) in the paroxetine group and 33 (55%) in the placebo group: this difference between groups was statistically significant (P=0.012).

Emergent adverse events (i.e., any adverse events which started on or after the first day of study medication) reported by 10% or more of the patients in either treatment group were as follows: for paroxetine: nausea (23%), sweating (23%), headache (22%), dizziness (17%), asthenia (15%), decreased libido (12%), and dry mouth (10%); for placebo: nausea (12%), sweating (5%), headache (23%),

Fig. 2 Panic attack response rates – percentage of patients with number of panic attacks reduced to one or zero per three-week period. Statistically significant difference in favour of paroxetine was seen at 12 weeks (P=0.024). ◆–◆: paroxetine; ■–■: placebo.

Table I Secondary efficacy measures, Hamilton Anxiety Scale (HAM–A), Clinical Global Impression (CGI), and Zung Patient Self-Rating Scale for Anxiety (ZUNG): summary of statistically significant differences between treatment groups

HAM–A	Mean baseline score	Percentage of patients with at least 50% reduction from baseline score	
		Week 6	Week 12
Paroxetine	24.3	59%	85%
Placebo	23.5	38%	51%
P value	–	0.021	<0.001

CGI		Percentage of patients with severity of illness ≤2 (mildly ill)	
	Baseline	Week 6	Week 12
Paroxetine	0%	42%	71%
Placebo	0%	22%	40%
P value	–	0.023	0.003

ZUNG	Mean baseline score	Mean change from baseline score	
		Week 6	Week 12
Paroxetine	42.1	−6.0	−6.5
Placebo	41.6	−3.4	−4.3
P value	–	0.013	0.042

P values for mean changes from baseline in ZUNG rating scale were obtained with F-tests in analysis of variance adjusting for centre. All other P values were obtained with Cochran–Mantel–Haenszel χ^2 tests.

dizziness (7%), asthenia (3.3%), decreased libido (2%), and dry mouth (8%).

Anticholinergic events, particularly dry mouth, were observed with similar incidence in the two treatment groups. Overall, the side-effect profile for paroxetine was as expected of a drug of this class, and was not different from the side-effect profile seen in depressed patients treated with paroxetine.

Two patients in both treatment groups had serious emergent adverse events during the study. These comprised 'joint disorder' and 'pulmonary oedema' in the paroxetine groups, and 'anxiety' and 'surgical procedure' in the placebo group. None of these events were considered by the investigators to be related to treatment.

Since most psychotropic medications seem to have some effects on discontinuation of medication, an attempt was made to ascertain the extent to which these occurred after discontinuation of paroxetine.

In this study, all patients who completed 12 weeks of active treatment then received two weeks of placebo, thus enabling adverse events occurring after discontinuation of paroxetine or placebo to be compared. In this placebo period, only 19 patients out of 55 (34.5%) who had received paroxetine reported any adverse event on discontinuation, as compared with seven out of 52 (13.5%) patients who had received placebo. Most patients reported just one adverse event, most being rated as of mild or moderate severity. The adverse event which was reported with greatest excess over placebo was 'dizziness'. This was reported by four patients (7.3%) who had received paroxetine and one who had received placebo.

Overall, paroxetine was well tolerated and most patients were able to discontinue abruptly without ill effect, even from the higher doses (40 and 60 mg).

Safety data

No clinically significant changes in haematologic variables, clinical chemistry variables, or vital signs that were considered to be related to treatment were observed.

DISCUSSION

Significant improvement was seen in panic disorder (DSM–III–R) patients treated with paroxetine, as compared with placebo, for both the primary and secondary outcome measures. In the paroxetine group, clear improvement for the primary outcome measures was seen at three weeks, and statistical significance, as compared with placebo, was seen from week 6 onward. With regard to the primary outcome measures, the response in the paroxetine group increased and was maintained over the 12-week treatment period, while in the placebo group, deterioration, after initial improvement up until nine weeks, was seen during the last three-week period. Of particular clinical significance is the fact that from a baseline mean of 21.2 panic attacks in the paroxetine group, at week 12, 36% of these patients had become almost free of panic attacks in that their panic-attack frequency had been reduced to zero or one over the last three weeks of the study.

Placebo response rates can be quite high for panic disorder patients – up to 40% being reported in some studies (Maier et al, 1991; Rosenberg et al, 1991). The placebo response seen in this study was higher, but that was to be expected since both treatment groups received standardised cognitive therapy.

Generally, unspecific treatment factors are probably responsible for high response rates on placebo; for example, patients receive more attention and explanation. These factors are also an inherent part of behaviour/cognitive therapies.

As expected, more adverse events were recorded among paroxetine patients. The predominant adverse events noted were class-specific effects of the SSRIs, and the same pattern of adverse events has been noted for depressed patients in trials with paroxetine (Dunbar, 1989).

However, the more frequent occurrence of adverse events in the paroxetine group did not lead to a higher withdrawal rate: 92% of the paroxetine patients, as compared with 87% of the placebo patients, completed with 12-week treatment period. Thus paroxetine appeared to be well tolerated, even at higher doses (40 and 60 mg).

Symptoms occurring after discontinuation of paroxetine were minor, occurring in only a few patients, despite the fact that 75% of patients were discontinued from doses of paroxetine of 40 mg or greater.

Previous studies of antidepressants in panic disorder, particularly fluoxetine (Schneier et al, 1990; Humble & Wistedt, 1992), have shown that an increase of some adverse events such as agitation, restlessness, jitteriness ('jitteriness syndrome') (Schneier et al, 1990), diarrhoea, and insomnia may occur, particularly if the dose is initiated at too high a level or increased too rapidly. In this study, such an increase of adverse events constituting the 'jitteriness syndrome' was not seen; therefore, it would appear that the slow titration of dose in the first week of this study was a well-tolerated regimen.

This study was not designed for dose finding, but 47% of the paroxetine patients received the highest dose of 60 mg daily. However, this may overestimate the required dose of paroxetine, since the trial method confounded dose and time.

No analysis was done to attempt to ascertain which patients are more likely to benefit from paroxetine or placebo.

Panic disorder appears to be a chronic condition in most patients. Although a minority of patients have a short episode, the rest have either recurrent episodes of varying severity or chronic, persistent symptoms (Uhde et al, 1985). Thus long-term treatment appears to be indicated for many patients, and therefore a safe and well tolerated treatment regimen is essential. Such long-term studies are under way with paroxetine.

This study is the first comparison of an SSRI with placebo in which both groups received standardised cognitive therapy. A clear advantage for combination therapy, i.e. paroxetine plus cognitive therapy, in the treatment of panic disorder, was demonstrated.

ACKNOWLEDGEMENTS

We thank Vibeke Weinreich, CRA, and Dr Charles H. Black, medical adviser, Novo Nordisk A/S, for invaluable support in carrying out this study. We also thank Mr Niklas Morton for statistical support for this study.

REFERENCES

American Psychiatric Association (1980) *Diagnostic and Statistical Manual of Mental Disorders* (3rd edn) (DSM–III). Washington, DC: APA.

___ **(1987)** *Diagnostic and Statistical Manual of Mental Disorders* (3rd edn, revised) (DSM–III–R). Washington, DC: APA.

Beck, A. T., Sokol, I., Clark, D. A., et al (1992) A crossover study of focussed cognitive therapy for panic disorder. *American Journal of Psychiatry,* **149**, 6.

Black, D. W., Wesner, R., Bowers, W., et al (1993) A comparison of fluvoxamine, cognitive therapy and placebo in the treatment of panic disorder. *Archives of General Psychiatry,* **50**, 44–50.

Chambless, D. L. & Gillis, M. M. (1993) Cognitive therapy of anxiety disorders. *Journal of Consulting and Clinical Psychology,* **61**, 248–260.

den Boer, J. A. (1988) *Serotonergic Mechanisms in Anxiety Disorder.* Cip-Gegevens Koninklijke Bibliotheek, Den Haag.

Dunbar, G. C. (1989) An interim overview of safety and tolerability of paroxetine. *Acta Psychiatrica Scandinavica,* **80** (suppl. 350), 135–137.

Feighner, J. P. & Boyer, W. F. (1989) Paroxetine in the treatment of depression: a comparison with imipramine and placebo. *Acta Psychiatrica Scandinavica,* **80** (suppl.), 125–129.

Guy, W. (1976) *ECDEU Assessment Manual for Psychopharmacology.* US Department of Health, Education, and Welfare, Public Health Service, Alcohol, Drug Abuse, and Mental Health Administration.

Hamilton, M. (1969) Diagnosis and rating of anxiety. *British Journal of Psychiatry,* **3**, 76–79.

Hawton, K., Salkowski, P., Kirk, J., et al (1989) *Cognitive Behaviour Therapy for Psychiatric Problems.* Oxford: Oxford University Press.

Humble, M. & Wistedt, B. (1992) Serotonin, panic disorder and agoraphobia: short term and long term efficacy of citalopram in panic disorders. *International Clinical Psychopharmacology,* **6** (suppl. 5), 21–39.

Kahn, R. S. & van Praag, H. M. (1992) Panic disorder: a biological perspective. *European Neuropsychopharmacology,* **2**, 1–20.

Maier, W., Roth, M., Argyle, N., et al (1991) Avoidance behaviour: a predictor of the efficacy of pharmacotherapy in panic disorder. *European Archives of Psychiatry and Clinical Neuroscience,* **241**, 151–158.

Rosenberg, N. K., Andersch, S., Kullingslio, H., et al (1991) Efficacy and safety of alprazolam, imipramine and placebo in treating panic disorder. *Acta Psychiatrica Scandinavica,* (suppl. 365), 18–27.

Salzman, C. (1993) Benzodiazepine treatment of panic and agoraphobic symptoms: use, dependence, toxicity, abuse. *Journal of Psychiatric Research,* **27** (suppl. 1), 97–100.

Schneier, F. R., Liebowitz, M. R., Davies, S. O., et al (1990) Fluoxetine in panic disorder. *Journal of Clinical Psychopharmacology,* **10**, 119–121.

Uhde, T. W., Boulenger, J. P., Roy Byrne, P. P., et al (1985) Longitudinal course of panic disorder: clinical and biological considerations. *Progress in Neuropsychopharmacology and Biological Psychiatry,* **9**, 39–51.

Wittchen, H. U. & Essau, C. A. (1993) Epidemiology of panic disorder: progress and unresolved issues. *Journal of Psychiatric Research,* **27** (suppl.), 47–68.

Zung, W. W. K. (1971) A rating instrument for anxiety disorders. *Psychosomatics,* **12**, 371–379.

S. OEHRBERG, MD, Vor Frue Straede 4, DK-9000 Aalborg, Denmark; P. E. CHRISTIANSEN, MD, Rosenkrantzgade 2, DK-8000 Aarhus, Denmark; K. BEHNKE, MD, Falkoner Alle 112, DK-2000 Frederiksberg, Denmark; A. L. BORUP, MD, Radhusvej 12, DK-4180 Soroe, Denmark; B. SEVERIN, MD, Noerrebrogade, DK-2200 Copenhagen N, Denmark; J. SOEGAARD, MD, Algade 63C, DK-4000 Roskilde, Denmark; H. CALBERG, MD, Idraetsvej 101, DK-2650 Hvidovre, Denmark; J. K. OHRSTROM, MD, Novo Nordisk A/S, Krogshoejvej 41, DK-2800 Bagsvaerd, Denmark; R. JUDGE, MBChB, MRCPsych, Smith Kline Beecham, New Frontier Science Park South, Harlow, Essex; P. M. MANNICHE, MSc, Novo Nordisk A/S, Krogshoejvej 41, DK-2880 Bagsvaerd, Denmark

Correspondence: Dr R. Judge, CNS Therapeutic Unit, Smith Kline Beecham Pharmaceuticals, New Frontier Science Park South, Third Avenue, Harlow, Essex CM19 5AG

(First received 17 January 1994, final revision 29 November 1994, accepted 20 January 1995)

Discontinuation rates of SSRIs and tricyclic antidepressants: a meta-analysis and investigation of heterogeneity

MATTHEW HOTOPF, REBECCA HARDY and GLYN LEWIS

Background Previous meta-analyses suggest that individuals treated with serotonin-specific reuptake inhibitors (SSRIs) in randomised controlled trials (RCTs) are less likely to discontinue treatment than those on tricyclic antidepressants. This meta-analysis investigates whether this is due to the frequent use in RCTs of older reference tricyclics (imipramine and amitriptyline), which may have worse side-effects than more recent compounds.

Method A meta-analysis of RCTs comparing tricyclic and heterocyclic antidepressants with SSRIs in the treatment of depression.

Results The overall odds ratio of discontinuation on tricyclic/heterocyclic antidepressants compared with SSRIs was 0.86 (95% CI 0.78–0.94). The odds ratio for reference tricyclics was 0.82 95% CI 0.72–0.23), newer tricyclics 0.89 (95% CI 0.74–1.06), and heterocyclics 1.02 (95% CI 0.78–1.35). The pooled advantage of SSRIs over tricyclics was maintained whether the population studied consisted of younger adults or only the elderly. No differences in discontinuation rates were detected between the SSRIs.

Conclusions The lower rate of discontinuation in patients on SSRIs may be due to the use of old tricyclics (which have worse side-effects) as reference compounds. The SSRIs do not show a statistically significant difference in discontinuation rates when compared with newer tricyclics or heterocyclics.

The serotonin-specific reuptake inhibitors (SSRIs) and tricyclic or heterocyclic antidepressants have been compared in 105 randomised controlled trials (RCTs), but there is little consensus as to which class of drug should be given as first-line treatment in depression (Paykel, 1989; Effective Health Care, 1993). Drugs and Therapeutic Bulletin, 1993). It has been argued that the SSRIs are better tolerated and this is reflected in improved compliance (Boyer & Feighner, 1993; Jönsson & Bebbington, 1994; Le Pen et al, 1994), but SSRIs are very much more costly than tricyclics. Previous attempts to model costs (Boyer & Feighner, 1993; Jönsson & Bebbington, 1994; Le Pen et al, 1994) have been based on unsound assumptions (Hotopf et al, 1996).

Much of the present controversy has focused on the acceptability of SSRIs, assessed by discontinuation rates in RCTs. Song et al (1993) in a meta-analysis found no difference between SSRIs and tricyclic and heterocyclic antidepressants, although some of the latter are as expensive as the SSRIs. Montgomery et al (1994) excluded trials comparing heterocyclic antidepressants with SSRIs, and found lower discontinuation rates due to side-effects for SSRIs, although there was no significant difference in total discontinuation rates (Hotopf et al, 1996). Finally, Anderson & Tomenson (1995) used a larger group of studies to show a modest advantage of SSRIs compared with tricyclics in total discontinuation rates, which was explained by lower discontinuation rates for side-effects in patients on SSRIs. These meta-analyses suggest that those treated with SSRIs in RCTs have lower discontinuation rates than those treated with tricyclic antidepressants. However, tricyclics differ in their side-effect profiles and most RCTs have compared SSRIs with 'reference' antidepressants (i.e. imipramine and amitriptyline) which are said to have the worst side-effects (Henry & Martin, 1987). Some of the newer anti-

depressants are among the most commonly prescribed in the UK but cost little more than imipramine and amitriptyline. The present meta-analysis investigated whether the advantage in discontinuation rates of SSRIs was present when compared with newer tricyclics or heterocyclics.

METHOD

Literature search

All RCTs reported in the previous meta-analyses, where the SSRIs were fluoxetine, sertraline, paroxetine or fluvoxamine, were used. These studies are all relatively short-term comparisons of SSRIs with tricyclic or heterocyclic antidepressants in treatment of depression. Studies of these compounds for other indications have not been included. A MEDLINE search was performed checking all papers that used the drug name in the title, abstract or keywords. In addition, owing to the failure of electronic searches to detect all relevant references (Adams et al, 1994), two journals which contained a high proportion of the trials, *International Clinical Psychopharmacology* and *Acta Psychiatrica Scandinavica*, were searched manually. If studies did not produce full details of overall discontinuation rates, the first author was contacted and asked for details. The same duplicated studies were excluded as in Anderson & Tomenson (1995). This systematic review is part of an ongoing Cochrane Collaboration review.

Studies were classified according to three criteria:

(a) the SSRI used;

(b) the type of tricyclic or heterocyclic used: reference compounds (imiprimine and amitriptyline), newer tricyclics (dothiepin, nortriptyline, desipramine, clomipramine and doxepin) and heterocyclic antidepressants (bupropion, mianserin, trazodone, maprotiline, amineptine and nomifensine);

(c) whether or not the treated group was defined as elderly in the RCT (cut-off points varied from 60 to 70 years of age).

Data analysis

The odds ratio and relative risk were calculated for each study, together with the relevant standard errors. A fixed-effect meta-analysis method (Woolf, 1955) was used to obtain the estimate of overall effect in terms of the odds ratio (empirical logits were used since some studies had small or zero drop-outs). Heterogeneity of treatment

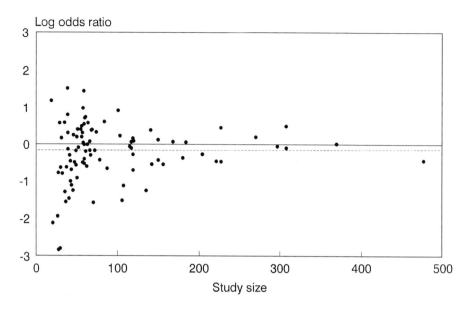

Log odds ratio

Study size

Fig. I Funnel plot of estimated logarithmic odds ratio against the size of the study. Broken horizontal line represents the overall estimate of the logarithmic odds ratio (− 0.l5).

effects between studies was formally tested using the Q statistic (Der Simonian & Laird, 1986). However, since the test is known to have low power (Berlin *et al*, 1989), possible sources of heterogeneity were considered and investigated with the aid of a Galbraith plot (Galbraith, 1988). A random-effects estimate, which takes account of any additional between-study variation, was calculated using a moment estimator of the between-study variance (Der Simonian & Laird, 1986) as a sensitivity check on the fixed-effect estimate. Since the data are sparse, and some RCTs report no drop-outs in at least one group, the methods described above may be unreliable as they are based on asymptotic assumptions. Hence, the analyses were checked using an approach based on the exact distribution of the 2×2 contingency tables, as described by van Houwelingen *et al* (1993), providing both fixed-effect and random-effects estimates of the overall odds ratio, as well as a likelihood ratio test of the null hypothesis of homogeneity of effects across studies. There was little difference between the results obtained from the two approaches, hence, the results from the simple weighted average method using empirical logits are presented here, although where results do differ a comment is made.

An overall estimate of the relative risk was also calculated, in order to compare results with previous papers and to express the difference as a percentage reduction in risk. A Mantel–Haenszel-type estimator

proposed by Nurminen (1981) and Kleinbaum *et al* (1982), which is suitable for sparse data, was used, together with the relevant confidence interval (CI; Greenland & Robins, 1985).

Finally, a separate meta-analysis, both in terms of odds ratio and relative risk, was carried out for each of the pre-defined tricyclic/heterocyclic groups compared with SSRIs.

RESULTS

A funnel plot (Fig. 1) (Wilson & Henry, 1992) showed no evidence of publication bias being a problem in the data collected. Table 1 summarises the odds ratios and 95% CIs for each study. Most estimates are close to one, with CIs including one. Three studies were omitted from the analysis as they had no drop-outs in either group and thus provide no information about a difference in effect.

The estimate of the overall odds ratio for drop-outs in the SSRI group compared with drop-outs in the tricyclic/heterocyclic group indicates significantly fewer drop-outs on SSRIs (odds ratio 0.86, 95% CI 0.78–0.94). The test statistic for heterogeneity indicated evidence of homogeneity (Q=113.62, d.f.=91, P=0.05) and the likelihood ratio test for heterogeneity gave a more significant value of P=0.033. Furthermore, the estimate of the between-study variance was greater than zero. Possible sources of heterogeneity were therefore investigated.

A Galbraith plot (Fig. 2) is a plot of the standardised effect (z statistic) of each study against the reciprocal of the standard error. The standardised effect is the logarithmic odds ratio for the study, divided by its standard error. The gradient of the plot is therefore equivalent to the treatment effect, and in this study the overall fixed-effect estimate of the logarithmic odds ratio may be represented by a line with gradient equal to − 0.15 [=ln(0.86)]. A negative z statistic indicates fewer drop-outs in the SSRI group, whereas a positive statistic indicates fewer drop-outs in the comparison tricyclic/heterocyclic group. Parallel lines at +2 and − 2 standard deviations either side of this line may be used as an aid to interpreting the heterogeneity within these data, since the further a study's estimate is away from this line the greater the contribution it makes to the test statistic for heterogeneity.

It is noticeable that four out of the five points with a z statistic of < − 2 units from the overall estimate are comparisons of SSRIs with older tricyclics, and the largest trial that is also highly negative on the plot is a comparison with an old tricyclic. On the other hand, two of the four with a z statistic of > +2 units from the overall estimate are comparisons with new tricyclics. This may suggest that the reference tricyclics perform less well compared with SSRIs than the newer ones, although the pattern within the limits is less clear.

Separate overall odds ratios were calculated for the three groups of trials with different types of comparison antidepressants (reference tricyclics, newer tricyclics and non-tricyclics). Table 2 shows that there is a significant difference in drop-out rates between SSRIs and reference tricyclics. However, there is also evidence of heterogeneity within this group of study estimates (Q=60.50, d.f.=50, P=0.05). The CIs of the random-effects estimates still did not include one (overall odds ratio 0.86, 95% CI 0.76–0.96). Conversely, the overall estimate of difference in drop-out rates for both the newer tricyclics and the heterocyclics do not suggest any significant differences. There is far less heterogeneity within these two subgroups (P=0.24 and 0.65 for the newer tricyclics and the heterocyclics, respectively). The relative risk estimates show a similar pattern (Table 2).

There were only 11 RCTs on elderly populations and the results of these did not appear to differ from the results of trials on younger populations. There appears to be some variation in the results for different

Table I Summary of trials used with odds ratios for SSRI drop-outs by tricyclic drop-outs.

Paper	Tricyclic or heterocyclic	SSRI	n randomised to tricyclics (drop-outs)	n randomised to SSRIs (drop-outs)	Odds ratio (95% CI)
Old tricyclics					
Altamura et al, 1989	amitriptyline	fluoxetine	14 (4)	14 (2)	0.47 (0.08–2.71)
Amore et al, 1989	amitriptyline	fluvoxamine	15 (5)	15 (0)	0.06 (0.003–1.20)
Bascara, 1989	amitriptyline	paroxetine	23 (3)	27 (2)	0.57 (0.10–3.19)
Battegay et al, 1985	amitriptyline	paroxetine	10 (8)	11 (3)	0.12 (0.02–0.79)
Beasley et al, 1993b	amitriptyline	fluoxetine	71 (24)	65 (8)	0.29 (0.12–0.68)
Bersani et al, 1994	amitriptyline	sertraline	34 (4)	34 (3)	0.75 (0.17–3.30)
Bignamini & Rapisardi, 1992	amitriptyline	paroxetine	153 (20)	156 (31)	1.64 (0.89–3.01)
Byrne, 1989	amitriptyline	paroxetine	35 (9)	35 (12)	1.49 (0.54–4.09)
Chouinard, 1985	amitriptyline	fluoxetine	28 (6)	23 (2)	0.40 (0.08–1.93)
Cohn et al, 1990	amitriptyline	sertraline	64 (41)	121 (79)	1.06 (0.56–1.99)
Fawcett et al, 1989	amitriptyline	fluoxetine	19 (10)	19 (7)	0.54 (0.15–1.91)
Feighner, 1985	amitriptyline	fluoxetine	22 (12)	22 (6)	0.33 (0.10–1.12)
Gasperini et al, 1992	amitriptyline	fluvoxamine	26 (1)	30 (2)	1.49 (0.18–12.09)
Harris et al, 1991	amitriptyline	fluvoxamine	34 (8)	35 (11)	1.47 (0.52–4.17)
Hutchinson et al, 1992	amitriptyline	paroxetine	32 (11)	56 (12)	0.53 (0.20–1.37)
Judd et al, 1993	amitriptyline	fluoxetine	28 (5)	30 (7)	1.37 (0.40–4.73)
Keegan et al, 1991	amitriptyline	fluoxetine	22 (3)	20 (2)	0.75 (0.13–4.29)
Kuhs & Rudolf, 1989	amitriptyline	paroxetine	20 (3)	20 (6)	2.22 (0.51–9.70)
Laursen et al, 1985	amitriptyline	paroxetine	23 (9)	21 (5)	0.51 (0.14–1.81)
Masco & Sheetz, 1985	amitriptyline	fluoxetine	21 (5)	20 (1)	0.20 (0.03–1.37)
Moller et al, 1993	amitriptyline	paroxetine	110 (48)	112 (37)	0.64 (0.37–1.10)
Remick et al, 1994	amitriptyline	fluvoxamine	17 (6)	16 (3)	0.46 (0.10–2.10)
Reimherr et al, 1990	amitriptyline	sertraline	149 (63)	149 (61)	0.94 (0.59–1.49)
Amin et al, 1984	imipramine	fluvoxamine	113 (64)	115 (52)	1.10 (0.76–1.58)
Arminen et al, 1994	imipramine	paroxetine	32 (15)	25 (13)	1.22 (0.44–3.41)
Beasley et al, 1993a	imipramine	fluoxetine	62 (38)	56 (33)	0.91 (0.55–1.51)
Bramanti et al, 1988	imipramine	fluvoxamine	30 (1)	30 (2)	1.72 (0.21–13.89)
Bremner, 1984	imipramine	fluoxetine	20 (3)	20 (4)	1.37 (0.29–6.46)
Bressa et al, 1989	imipramine	fluoxetine	15 (1)	15 (2)	1.79 (0.21–15.46)
Cohn & Wilcox, 1985	imipramine	fluoxetine	54 (34)	54 (19)	0.33 (0.15–0.72)
Cohn et al, 1989	imipramine	fluoxetine	30 (16)	30 (13)	0.68 (0.25–1.85)
Dominguez et al, 1985	imipramine	fluvoxamine	30 (11)	31 (17)	2.04 (0.74–5.59)
Feighner et al, 1989a	imipramine	fluoxetine	57 (28)	61 (31)	1.06 (0.52–2.17)
Feighner et al, 1989b	imipramine	fluvoxamine	36 (11)	31 (10)	1.09 (0.40–3.01)
Feighner et al, 1993	imipramine	paroxetine	237 (127)	240 (102)	0.64 (0.53–0.77)
Fontaine, 1991	imipramine	paroxetine	50 (23)	54 (28)	1.27 (0.59–2.72)
Gonella et al, 1990	imipramine	fluvoxamine	10 (0)	10 (1)	3.33 (0.12–92.00)
Guelfi et al, 1983	imipramine	fluvoxamine	77 (18)	74 (19)	1.14 (0.55–2.37)
Itil et al, 1983	imipramine	fluvoxamine	25 (12)	22 (12)	1.28 (0.42–3.94)
Lapierre et al, 1987	imipramine	fluvoxamine	21 (12)	22 (7)	0.37 (0.11–1.24)
Levine et al, 1987	imipramine	fluoxetine	30 (2)	30 (8)	4.35 (0.96–19.78)
Lydiard et al, 1989	imipramine	fluvoxamine	18 (4)	18 (1)	0.21 (0.03–1.51)
March et al, 1990	imipramine	fluvoxamine	18 (3)	18 (5)	1.81 (0.39–8.32)
Nielsen et al, 1991	imipramine	paroxetine	15 (9)	16 (7)	0.54 (0.14–2.15)
Nielsen et al, 1993	imipramine	fluoxetine	30 (8)	29 (8)	1.04 (0.34–3.19)
Norton et al, 1984	imipramine	fluvoxamine	59 (30)	62 (33)	1.10 (0.54–2.23)
Øhrberg et al, 1992	imipramine	paroxetine	77 (19)	74 (13)	0.66 (0.30–1.44)
Shrivastava et al, 1992	imipramine	paroxetine	38 (7)	33 (15)	0.21 (0.07–0.60)
					(continued)

Table I (continued)

Paper	Tricyclic or heterocyclic	SSRI	n randomised to tricyclics (drop-outs)	n randomised to SSRIs (drop-outs)	Odds ratio (95% CI)
Stark & Hardison, 1985	imipramine	fluoxetine	186 (87)	185 (87)	1.01 (0.67–1.52)
Stratta et al, 1991	Imipramine	fluoxetine	14 (5)	14 (0)	0.06 (0.003–1.22)
Newer tricyclics					
Danish University Group, 1990	clomipramine	paroxetine	58 (19)	62 (12)	0.50 (0.22–1.14)
De Wilde & Doogan, 1982	clomipramine	fluvoxamine	15 (0)	15 (0)	
De Wilde et al, 1983 (single dosing)	clomipramine	fluvoxamine	21 (0)	22 (0)	
De Wilde et al, 1983 (three-times dosing)	clomipramine	fluvoxamine	15 (0)	15 (0)	
Dick & Ferrero, 1983	clomipramine	fluvoxamine	15 (3)	17 (4)	1.19 (0.24–5.86)
Guillibert et al, 1989	clomipramine	paroxetine	39 (12)	40 (9)	0.66 (0.25–1.77)
Klok et al, 1981	clomipramine	fluvoxamine	18 (3)	18 (5)	1.81 (0.39–8.32)
Link & Dunbar, 1992	clomipramine	paroxetine	154 (28)	155 (26)	0.91 (0.52–1.59)
Link & Dunbar, 1992	clomipramine	paroxetine	56 (26)	60 (27)	0.94 (0.46–1.94)
Link & Dunbar, 1992	clomipramine	paroxetine	43 (9)	42 (14)	1.85 (0.71–4.82)
Moon et al, 1993	clomipramine	sertraline	55 (10)	51 (2)	0.22 (0.05–0.92)
Noguera et al, 1991	clomipramine	fluoxetine	60 (16)	60 (13)	0.77 (0.34–1.76)
Ropert, 1989	clomipramine	fluoxetine	72 (24)	71 (16)	0.59 (0.28–1.23)
Bowden et al, 1993	desipramine	fluoxetine	30 (8)	28 (5)	0.62 (0.18–2.10)
Nathan et al, 1990	desipramine	fluvoxamine	20 (2)	17 (0)	0.21 (0.01–4.69)
Remick et al, 1993	desipramine	fluoxetine	20 (5)	26 (2)	0.29 (0.06–1.47)
Roth et al, 1990	desipramine	fluvoxamine	30 (9)	30 (6)	0.60 (0.19–1.90)
Corne & Hall, 1990	dothiepin	fluoxetine	53 (7)	49 (14)	2.56 (0.96–6.85)
Mullin et al, 1994	dothiepin	fluvoxamine	36 (12)	37 (11)	0.85 (0.32–2.24)
Rahman et al, 1991	dothiepin	fluvoxamine	26 (5)	26 (7)	1.49 (0.42–5.25)
South Wales Group, 1988	dothiepin	fluoxetine	28 (7)	31 (15)	2.70 (0.91–7.97)
Thompson, 1991	dothiepin	paroxetine	93 (9)	88 (6)	0.70 (0.25–1.99)
Dunner et al, 1992	doxepin	paroxetine	135 (39)	136 (45)	1.22 (0.73–2.04)
Feighner & Cohn, 1985	doxepin	fluvoxamine	79 (48)	78 (37)	0.59 (0.31–1.11)
Remick et al, 1989	doxepin	fluoxetine	37 (10)	38 (13)	1.39 (0.53–3.67)
Tammimen & Lehtinen, 1989	doxepin	fluoxetine	25 (4)	26 (5)	1.22 (0.31–4.86)
Fabre et al, 1991	nortriptyline	fluoxetine	102 (45)	103 (39)	0.78 (0.45–1.36)
Heterocyclic antidepressants					
Dalery et al, 1992	amineptine	fluoxetine	87 (14)	82 (14)	1.08 (0.49–2.40)
Ferreri, 1989	amineptine	fluoxetine	32 (7)	31 (4)	0.56 (0.15–2.03)
Feighner et al, 1991	bupropion	fluoxetine	60 (16)	60 (18)	1.18 (0.54–2.59)
De Jonghe et al, 1991a	maprotiline	fluoxetine	34 (3)	28 (5)	2.13 (0.50–9.01)
De Jonghe et al, 1991b	maprotiline	fluvoxamine	24 (6)	24 (4)	0.63 (0.16–2.43)
Poelinger & Haber, 1989	maprotiline	fluoxetine	69 (8)	73 (12)	1.47 (0.57–3.76)
Besançon et al, 1993	mianserin	fluoxetine	33 (9)	32 (13)	1.79 (0.64–4.97)
Dorman, 1992	mianserin	paroxetine	28 (3)	29 (5)	1.64 (0.38–6.99)
Mertens & Pintens, 1988	mianserin	paroxetine	31 (3)	36 (3)	0.85 (0.18–4.06)
Moon & Jesinger, 1991	mianserin	fluvoxamine	31 (7)	31 (6)	0.83 (0.25–2.72)
Muijen et al, 1988	mianserin	fluoxetine	27 (13)	26 (12)	0.93 (0.32–2.67)
Perez & Ashford, 1990	mianserin	fluvoxamine	30 (8)	30 (8)	1.00 (0.33–3.05)
Phanjoo et al, 1991	mianserin	fluvoxamine	25 (10)	25 (9)	0.85 (0.28–2.60)
Taneri & Kohler, 1989	nomifensine	fluoxetine	20 (1)	20 (5)	4.55 (0.66–31.18)
Debus et al, 1988	trazodone	fluoxetine	21 (10)	22 (8)	0.64 (0.19–2.10)
Falk et al, 1989	trazodone	fluoxetine	13 (9)	14 (3)	0.14 (0.03–0.72)
Perry et al, 1989	trazodone	fluoxetine	19 (4)	21 (4)	0.88 (0.20–3.85)

1. Odds ratios and 95% confidence intervals calculated as empirical logits (odds ratios of less than one favour SSRIs).

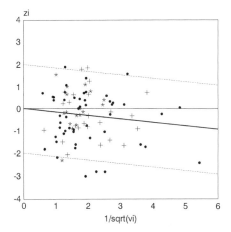

Fig. 2 Galbraith plot. Solid inclined line represents the fixed-effect estimate, bounded by plus and minus two units (broken inclined lines). ●, old tricyclics; +, newer tricylcics; *, non-tricyclic antidepressants.

SSRIs, with fluvoxamine producing a more homogeneous set of results than either fluoxetine or paroxetine. Furthermore, the overall estimate for fluvoxamine is closer to one than those for either fluoxetine or paroxetine. There are only six studies using sertraline, so any conclusions regarding this drug are tentative. Hence, the type of SSRI used does not explain much of the heterogeneity present in these data, but it appears that the drugs that produce the greatest overall effect are also those with the greatest variation in individual effect estimates across studies. Furthermore, within each comparison group (older tricyclics, newer tricyclics and heterocyclics) each SSRI (excluding sertraline) is represented reasonably consistently. Hence, it is not the case that each comparison group is compared with one particular SSRI.

Summary of main findings

This meta-analysis shows slightly lower discontinuation rates for the SSRIs compared with tricyclic and heterocyclic antidepressants when these compounds are pooled. When SSRIs are compared with the three subgroups of compounds classified above, it was only against the older compounds (amitriptyline and imipramine) that SSRIs showed a significant advantage (at the 5% level). These results are consistent with the view that the previously reported advantage of SSRIs over tricyclics is due to the high drop-out rates of subjects on older tricyclics.

DISCUSSION

The estimate of effect for the heterocyclics compared with SSRIs is very close to one, with no evidence of heterogeneity between the estimates from the different trials. The CI is wider than for the other comparisons because of the smaller number of trials (17) included, and suggests that the increase in risk of using SSRIs versus heterocyclics could be as much as 25%, or the decrease in risk could be 17%. Further information, preferably in terms of a large clinical trial, is required before a definite conclusion can be made. The inclusion of these compounds in Song et al's (1993) meta-analysis may have led to their negative result.

Methodological concerns

There are reasons for interpreting these results with caution. First, we have not been able to show results for efficacy of the two groups of compound when measured on the Hamilton Rating Scale for Depression (HRSD; Hamilton, 1960). It could be that one group is slightly more efficacious than the other, but the inadequacy of the reporting of the RCTs prevents these data from being used. We have misgivings over the usefulness of discontinuation rates as a measure of clinical acceptability. Trials are stringently regulated, and patients entered on trials do so voluntarily and are assured that they are able to withdraw consent at any time. It is likely that discontinuing treatment in clinical practice is determined by different factors than in RCTs.

Second, most RCTs were small. The median sample size per group was 30 subjects, so few would be powerful enough in themselves to detect any meaningful differences between the two treatments. The combined effect of all the trials was very small. If a single trial were to detect a relative risk of 0.9 with 80% power and 95% confidence, it would require 3620 subjects in each group, assuming a drop-

out rate of 30%. This problem of the need for a large sample size is reflected in the CIs reported here: there is still considerable room for error in our estimates of effect size.

Finally, subgroup analyses in meta-analysis should be interpreted carefully, especially if such investigations are *post hoc* (Thompson & Pocock, 1991). However, in the case considered here, the possible differences in effect between the three different types of comparison drug were proposed in advance.

Implications of the meta-analysis

These findings have three main implications. First, they cast doubt on previous economic models of cost-effectiveness (Boyer & Feighner, 1993; Jönsson & Bebbington, 1994; Le Pen et al, 1994), which assumed a considerably greater difference in risk of attrition. These studies used selected RCTs to estimate risk of drop-out in those treated on tricyclics to be 8–12% higher than for patients on SSRIs. If we use the same approach as Anderson & Tomenson (1995), then the total discontinuation rate for this meta-analysis is 31% and the relative risk is 0.90. Hence 31 out of 100 will drop out using tricyclics, compared with 28 out of 100 on SSRIs. In other words, the drop-out rate of those on tricyclics is 3% higher. These findings are in agreement with Anderson & Tomenson (1995). This suggests that the economic models overestimated attrition on tricyclics by a factor of 2.7–4.0. If these findings are translated to a clinical situation, a physician would need to treat 33 patients to prevent one drop-out and in any case, if someone did drop out of treatment due to tricyclic side-effects, the physician would still have the option of changing them to an alternative compound.

Second, these findings suggest that the oldest tricyclics are not necessarily the best comparison for new treatments. Although using amitriptyline and imipramine in trials respects a tradition that upholds these as

Table 2 Fixed-effect meta-analysis results using odds and risk ratios as outcome measurements

Meta-analysis (number of studies)	Odds ratio (95% CI)	Risk ratio (95% CI)	Test statistic for heterogeneity (P)
Overall (92)	0.86 (0.78–0.94)	0.91 (0.86–0.96)	113.62 (0.05)
Old tricyclics (51)	0.82 (0.72–0.92)	0.88 (0.82–0.94)	70.50 (0.03)
Newer tricyclics (24)	0.89 (0.74–1.06)	0.92 (0.81–1.03)	27.48 (0.24)
Heterocyclics (17)	1.02 (0.78–1.35)	1.02 (0.83–1.25)	13.35 (0.65)

reference compounds for efficacy, it may be unreasonable to generalise acceptability from these compounds to all tricyclics. Newer tricyclics are widely used but only marginally more expensive. These compounds might be a more realistic comparison for future study. The evidence from this meta-analysis and elsewhere indicates that older tricyclics have higher drop-out rates than SSRIs. There is less certainty regarding the newer tricyclics and this issue is worth investigating further to provide a clear conclusion.

The smaller number of studies (24 trials) for the comparison between SSRIs and newer tricyclics, and their generally small size means there is less power to detect any difference in drop-out rates, if one exists. The point estimates of both odds ratio and relative risk suggest that there is a still greater risk of drop-out on the tricyclics than SSRIs. However, the homogeneous nature of the estimates of effect in this group of trials means that the estimate and CIs obtained from fixed-effect methods will be valid. Hence, it must be concluded that with the present data there is no statistical evidence of a benefit for SSRIs versus newer tricyclics or heterocyclics. Together with the small effect, these data support the use of tricyclics as first-line treatment for depression.

ACKNOWLEDGEMENTS

Dr Hotopf is funded by a Medical Research Council Clinical Training Fellowship. We are grateful to Professor van Houwelingen for providing the program to carry out the Mantel–Haenszel-type meta-analysis. We thank Nick Freemantle for providing information on RCTs where drop-out information was not available in the original paper.

REFERENCES

Adams, C. E., Power, A., Frederick, K., et al (1994) An investigation of the adequacy of MEDLINE searches for randomized controlled trials (RCTs) of the effects of mental health care. Psychological Medicine, 24, 741–748.

Altamura, A. C., De Novellis, F., Guercetti, G., et al (1989) Fluoxetine compared with amitriptyline in elderly depression: a controlled clinical trial. International Journal of Clinical Pharmacology Research, 9, 391–396.

Amin, M. M., Ananth, J. V., Coleman, B. S., et al (1984) Fluvoxamine: antidepressant effects confirmed in a placebo-controlled international study. Clinical Neuropharmaoclogy, 7(suppl. 1), 580–581.

Amore, B., Bellini, M., Berardi, D., et al (1989) Double blind comparison of fluvoxamine and imipramine in depressed patients. Current Therapeutic Research, 46, 815–820.

Anderson, I. M. & Tomenson, B. M. (1995) Treatment discontinuation with selective serotonin reputake inhibitors compared with tricyclic antidepressants: a meta-analysis. British Medical Journal, 310, 1433–1438.

Arminen, S. L., Ikonen, U., Pulkkinen, P., et al (1994) A 12-233k double-blind multi-centre study of paroxetine and imipramine in hospitalized depressed patients. Acta Psychiatrica Scandinavica, 89, 382–389.

Bascara, B. (1989) A double blind study to compare the effectiveness and tolerability of paroxetine and amitriptyline in depressed patients. Acta Psychiatrica Scandinavica, 80(suppl. 350), 141–142.

Battegay, R., Hager, M. & Rauchfleisch, U. (1985) Double-blind comparative study of paroxetine and amitriptyline in depressed patients of a university psychiatric outpatient clinic. Neuropsychobiology, 13, 31–37.

Beasley, C. M., Holman, S. L. & Potvin, J. H. (1993a) Fluoxetine compared with imipramine in the treatment of inpatient depression: a multicentre trial. Annals of Clinical Psychiatry, 5, 199–208.

—, Sayler, M. E. & Potvin, J. H. (1993b) Fluoxetine versus amitriptyline in the treatment of major depression: a multicenter trial. International Clinical Psychopharmacology, 8, 143–149.

Berlin, J. A., Laird, N. M., Sacks, H. S., et al (1989) A comparison of statistical methods for combining event rates from clinical trials. Statistics in Medicine, 8, 141–151.

Bersani, G., Rapisarda, V., Ciani, N., et al (1994) A double-blind comparative study of sertraline and amitriptyline in outpatients with major depressive episodes. Human Psychopharmacology, 9, 63–68.

Besançon, G., Cousin, R., Guitton, B., et al (1993) Étude en double aveugle de la mianserine et de la fluoxetine chez des patients déprimes traites en ambulatoire. L'Encéphale, 19, 341–345.

Bignamini, A. & Rapisarda, V. (1992) A double-blind multicentre study of paroxetine and amitriptyline in depressed outpatients. International Clinical Psychopharmacology, 6(suppl 4), 37–41.

Bowden, C. L., Schatzberg, A. F., Rosenbaum, A., et al (1993) Fluoxetine and desipramine in major depressive disorder. Journal of Clinical Psychopharmacology, 13, 305–311.

Boyer, W. F. & Feighner, J. P. (1993) The financial implications of starting treatment with a selective serotonin reuptake inhibitor or tricyclic antidepressant in drug-naive depressed patients. In Health Economics of Depression (eds B. Johnsson & J. Rosenbaum), pp 65–75. London: John Wiley & Sons.

Bramanti, P., Ricci, R. M., Roncari, R., et al (1988) An Italian multicenter experience with fluvoxamine, a new antidepressant drug, versus imipramine. Current Therapeutic Research, 43, 718–724.

Bremner, J. D. (1984) Fluoxetine in depressed patients: a comparison with imipramine. Journal of Clinical Psychiatry, 45, 414–419.

Bressa, G. M., Brugnoli, R. & Pancheri, P. (1989) A double blind study of fluoxetine and imipramine in major depression. International Clinical Psychopharmacology, 4(supppl 1), 69–73.

Byrne, M. M. (1989) Meta-analysis of early phase II studies with paroxetine in hospitalized depressed patients. Acta Psychiatrica Scandinavica, 80(suppl. 350), 138–139.

Chouinard, G. (1985) A double-blind controlled trial of fluoxetine and amitriptyline in the treatment of outpatients with major depression. Journal of Clinical Psychiatry, 46, 32–37.

Cohn, J. B. & Wilcox, C. (1985) A comparison of fluoxetine, imipramine and placebo in patients with major depressive disorder. Journal of Clinical Psychiatry, 46, 26–31.

—, Collins, G., Ashbrook, E., et al (1989) A comparison of fluoxetine imipramine and placebo in patients with bipolar depressive disorder. International Clinical Psychopharmacology, 4, 313–322.

—, Shrivastava, R., Mendels, J., et al (1990) Double-blind, multicenter comparison of sertraline and amitriptyline in elderly depressed patients. Journal of Clinical Psychiatry, 51(suppl B), 28–33.

Corne, S. J. & Hall, J. R. (1990) A double-blind comparative study of fluoxetine and dothiepin in the treatment of depression in general practice. International Clinical Psychopharmacology, 4, 245–254.

Dalery, J., Rochat, C., Peyron, E., et al (1992) Étude comparative de l'efficacité et de l'acceptabilité de l'amineptine et de la fluoxetine chez de patients dépressifs majeurs. L'Encéphale, 18, 257–262.

Danish University Antidepressant Group (1990) Paroxetine: selective serotonin reuptake inhibitor showing better tolerance, but weaker antidepressant effect than clomipramine in a controlled multicenter study. Journal of Affective Disorders, 18, 289–299.

De Jonghe, F., Ravelli, D. P. & Tuynman-Qua, H. (1991a) Randomized double-blind study of fluoxetine and maprotiline in the treatment of major depression. Pharmacopsychiatry, 24, 62–67.

—, Swinkel, H. & Tuynman-Qua, H. (1991b) A randomized, double blind study of fluvoxamine and maprotiline in treatment of depression. Pharmacopsychiatry, 24, 21–27.

De Wilde, J. E. M. & Doogan, D. P. (1982) Fluvoxamine and chlorimipramine in endogenous depression. Journal of Affective Disorders, 4, 249–259.

—, Mertens, C. & Wakelin, J. S. (1983) Clinical trials of fluvoxamine vs clomipramine with single and three times dosing. British Journal of Clinical Pharmacology, 15(suppl 3), 427–431.

Debus, J. R., Rush, A. J., Himmel, C., et al (1988) Fluoxetine versus trazodone in the treatment of outpatients with major depression. Journal of Clinical Psychiatry, 49, 422–426.

Der Simonian, R. & Laird, N. (1986) Meta-analysis in clinical trials. Controlled Clinical Trials, 7, 177–188.

Dick, P. & Ferrero, E. (1983) A double-blind comparative study on the efficacy of fluvoxamine and clomipramine. British Journal of Clinical Pharmacology, 15, 419–425.

Dominguez, R. A., Goldstein, B. J., Jacobson, A. F., et al (1985) A double-blind, placebo controlled study of fluvoxamine and imipramine in depression. Journal of Clinical Psychiatry, 46, 84–87.

Dorman, T. (1992) Sleep and paroxetine: a comparison with mianserin in elderly depressed patients. International Clinical Psychopharmacology, 6(suppl. 4), 53–58.

Drugs and Therapeutic Bulletin (1993) Selective serotonin reuptake inhibitors for depression. Drugs and Therapeutic Bulletin, 31, 57–58.

Dunner, D. L., Cohn, J. B., Walshe, T., et al (1992) Two combined, multicenter double-blind studies of paroxetine and doxepin in geriatric patients with major depression. Journal of Clinical Psychiatry, 53(suppl. 2), 57–60.

Effective Health Care (1993) The treatment of depression in primary care. Effective Health Care Bulletin, 5, 1–12.

Fabre, L. F., Scharf, M. B. & Itil, T. M. (1991) Comparative efficacy and safety of nortriptyline and fluoxetine in the treatment of major depression: a clinical study. Journal of Clinical Psychiatry, 52(suppl. 6), 62–67.

Falk, W. E., Rosenbaum, J. F., Otto, M. W., et al (1989) Fluoxetine versus trazodone in depressed geriatric patients. Journal of Geriatric Psychiatry and Neurology, 2, 208–214.

Fawcett, J., Zajecka, J. & Kravitz, H. (1989) Fluoxetine vs amitriptyline in adult inpatients with major depression. Current Therapeutic Research, 45, 821–832.

Feighner, J. P. (1985) A comparative trial of fluoxetine and amitriptyline in patients with major depressive disorder. *Journal of Clinical Psychiatry*, **46**, 369–372.

___ & Cohn, J. B. (1985) Double-blind comparative study of fluoxetine and doxepin in geriatric patients with major depressive disorder. *Journal of Clinical Psychiatry*, **46**, 20–25.

___ , Boyer, W. F., Meredith, C. H., et al (1989a) A double-blind comparison of fluoxetine, imipramine and placebo in outpatients with major depression. *International Clinical Psychopharmacology*, **4**, 127–134.

___ , ___ , ___ , et al (1989b) A placebo-controlled inpatient comparison of fluvoxamine maleate and imipramine in major depression. *International Clinical Psychopharmacology*, **4**, 239–244.

___ , Gardner, E. A., Johnston, J. A., et al (1991) Double-blind comparison of bupropion and fluoxetine in depressed outpatients. *Journal of Clinical Psychiatry*, **52**, 229–235.

___ , Cohn, J. B., Fabre, L. F., et al (1993) A study comparing paroxetine placebo and imipramine in depressed patients. *Journal of Affective Disorders*, **28**, 71–79.

Ferreri, M. (1989) Fluoxetine versus amipentine in the treatment of outpatients with major depressive disorder. *International Clinical Psychopharmacology*, **4**(suppl. 1), 97–101.

Fontaine, R. (1991) The efficacy of sertraline versus imipramine in outpatients with major depression: a six month double-blind, parallel multicenter study. *European Neuropsychopharmacology*, **1**, 447.

Galbraith, R. F. (1988) A note on graphical presentation of estimated odds ratios from several clinical trials. *Statistics in Medicine*, **7**, 889–894.

Gasperini, M., Gatti, F., Bellini, L., et al (1992) Perspectives in clinical psychopharmacology of amitriptyline and fluvoxamine. *Neuropsychobiology*, **26**, 186–192.

Gonella, G., Baignoli, G. & Ecari, U. (1990) Fluvoxamine and imipramine in the treatment of depressive patients. *Current Medical Research Opinions*, **12**, 177–184.

Greenland, S. & Robins, J. M. (1985) Estimation of a common effect parameter from sparse follow-up data. *Biometrics*, **41**, 55–68.

Guelfi, J. D., Dreyfus, J. F., Pichot, P., et al (1983) A double-blind controlled clinical trial comparing fluvoxamine with imipramine. *British Journal of Clinical Pharmacology*, **15**(suppl. 3), 411–417.

Guillibert, E. Pelicier, Y., Archambaul, J. C., et al (1989) A double-blind, multicentre study of paroxetine versus clomipramine in depressed elderly patients. *Acta Psychiatrica Scandinavica*, **80**(suppl. 350), 132–134.

Hamilton, M. (1960) A rating scale for depression. *Journal of Neurology, Neurosurgery and Psychiatry*, **23**, 56–62.

Harris, B., Szujelecka, T. K. & Anstee, J. A. (1991) Fluvoxamine versus amitriptyline on depressed hospital out-patients: a multicentre double blind comparative trial. *British Journal of Clinical Research*, **2**, 89–99.

Henry, J. A. & Martin, A. J. (1987) The risk–benefit assessment of antidepressant drugs. *Medical Toxicology*, **2**, 445–462.

Hotopf, M., Lewis, G. & Normand, C. (1996) Are SSRIs a cost-effective alternative to tricyclics? *British Journal of Psychiatry*, **168**, 404–409.

Hutchinson, D. R., Tong, S., Moon, C. A., et al (1992) Paroxetine in the treatment of elderly depressed patients in general practice: a double-blind comparison with amitriptyline. *International Clinical Psychopharmacology*, **6**(suppl. 4), 43–51.

Itil, T. M., Shrivastava, R., Mukherjee, S., et al (1983) A double-blind placebo-controlled study of fluvoxamine and imipramine in outpatients with primary depression. *British Journal of Clinical Pharmacology*, **15**, 433–438.

Jönsson, B. & Bebbington, P. E. (1994) What price depression? The cost of depression and the cost-effectiveness of pharmacological treatment. *British Journal of Psychiatry*, **164**, 665–673.

Judd, F. K., Moore, K., Norman, T. R., et al (1993) A multicentre double blind trial of fluoxetine versus amitriptyline in the treatment of depressive illness. *Australian and New Zealand Journal of Psychiatry*, **27**, 49–55.

Keegan, D., Bowen, R. C., Blackshaw, S., et al (1991) A comparison of fluoxetine and amitriptyline in the treatment of major depression. *International Clinical Psychopharmacology*, **6**, 117–124.

Kleinbaum, D. G., Kupper, L. L. & Morgenstern, H. (1982) *Epidemiologic Research: Principles and Quantitative Methods*. Belmont, CA: Lifetime Learning Publications.

Klok, C. J., Brouwer, G. J., van Praag, H. M., et al (1981) Fluvoxamine and clomipramine in depressed patients. *Acta Psychiatrica Scandinavica*, **64**, 1–11.

Kuhs, H. & Rudolf, G. A. E. (1989) A double-blind study of the comparative antidepressant effect of paroxetine and amitriptyline. *Acta Psychiatrica Scandinavica*, **80**(suppl. 350), 145–146.

Lapierre, Y. D., Browne, M., Horn, E., et al (1987) Treatment of major affective disorder with fluvoxamine. *Journal of Clinical Psychiatry*, **48**, 65–68.

Laursen, A, L., Mikkelsen, P. L. & le Fievre Honore, P. (1985) Paroxetine in the treatment of depression – a randomized comparison with amitriptyline. *Acta Psychiatrica Scandinavica*, **71**, 249–255.

Le Pen, C., Levy, E., Ravily, V., et al (1994) The cost of treatment dropout in depression. A cost benefit analysis of fluoxetine vs tricyclics. *Journal of Affective Disorders*, **31**, 1–18.

Levine, S., Deo, R. & Mahadevan, K. (1987) A comparative trial of a new antidepressant fluoxetine. *British Journal of Psychiatry*, **150**, 653–655.

Link, C. & Dunbar, G. (1992) An overview of studies comparing the efficacy, safety, and tolerability of paroxetine and clomipramine. *Nordic Journal of Psychiatry*, **46**(suppl. 7), 17–22.

Lydiard, R. B., Laird, L. K., Morton, A. W., et al (1989) Fluvoxamine, imipramine and placebo in the treatment of depressed outpatients: effects on depression. *Psychopharmacology Bulletin*, **25**, 68–70.

March, J. S., Kobak, K. A., Jefferson, J. W., et al (1990) A double blind, placebo-controlled study of fluvoxamine versus imipramine in outpatients with major depression. *Journal of Clinical Psychiatry*, **51**, 200–202.

Masco, H. L. & Sheetz, M. S. (1985) Double-blind comparison of fluoxetine and amitriptyline in the treatment of major depressive illness. *Advances in Therapy*, **2**, 275–283.

Mertens, C. & Pintens, H. (1988) Paroxetine in the treatment of depression. A double blind multicentre study versus mianserin. *Acta Psychiatrica Scandinavica*, **77**, 683–688.

Moller, H. J., Berzewski, H., Eckmann, F., et al (1993) Double-blind multicenter study of paroxetine and amitriptyline in depressed patients. *Pharmacopsychiatry*, **26**, 75–78.

Montgomery, S. A., Henry, J., McDonald, G., et al (1994) Selective serotonin reuptake inhibitors: meta-analysis of discontinuation rates. *International Clinical Psychopharmacology*, **9**, 47–53.

Moon, C. A. L. & Jesinger, D. K. (1991) The effects of psychomotor performance of fluvoxamine versus mianserin in depressed patients in general practice. *British Journal of Clinical Practice*, **45**, 259–262.

___ , Jago, L. W., Wood, K., et al (1994) A double-blind comparison of sertraline and clomipramine in the treatment of major depressive disorder and associated anxiety in general practice. *Journal of Psychopharmacology*, **8**, 171–176.

Muijen, M., Roy, D., Silverston, T., et al (1988) A comparative clinical trial of fluoxetine, mianserin and placebo in depressed outpatients. *Acta Psychiatrica Scandinavica*, **78**, 384–390.

Mullin, J. M., Pandita-Gunawardena, V. R. & Whitehead, A. M. (1994) A double-blind comparison of fluvoxamine and dothiepin in the treatment of major affective disorder. *British Journal of Clinical Practice*, **42**, 51–55.

Nathan, R. S., Perel, J. M., Pollock, B. G., et al (1990) The role of neuropharmacologic selectivity in antidepressant action: fluvoxamine versus desipramine. *Journal of Clinical Psychiatry*, **51**, 367–372.

Nielsen, O. A., Morsing, I., Peterson, J. S., et al (1991) Paroxetine and imipramine treatment of depressive patients in a controlled multicentre study with plasma amino acid measurements. *Acta Psychiatrica Scandinavica*, **84**, 233–241.

___ , Behnke, K., Arup, P., et al (1993) A comparison of fluoxetine and imipramine treatment of depressive patients in a controlled multicentre study with plasma amino acid measurements. *Acta Psychiatrica Scandinavica*, **84**, 233–241.

Noguera, R., Altuna, R., Alvarez, E., et al (1991) Fluoxetine vs clomipramine in depressed patients: a controlled multi-centre trial. *Journal of Affective Disorders*, **22**, 119–124.

Norton, K. R. W., Sireling, L. I., Bhat, A. V., et al (1984) A double blind comparison of fluvoxamine, imipramine and placebo in depressed patients. *Journal of Affective Disorders*, **7**, 297–308.

Nurminen, M. (1981) Asymptotic efficiency of general noniterative estimators of common relative risk. *Biometrika*, **68**, 525–530.

Øhrberg, S., Christiansen, P. E., Severin, B., et al (1992) Paroxetine and imipramine in the treatment of depressive patients in psychiatric practice. *Acta Psychiatrica Scandinavica*, **86**, 437–444.

Paykel, E. (1989) The background: extent and nature of the disorder. In *Depression: An Integrative Approach* (eds. K. Herbst & E. Paykel), pp. 3–17. Oxford: Heinemann.

Perez, A. & Ashford, J. J. (1990) A double-blind, randomized comparison of fluvoxamine with mianserin in depressive illness. *Current Medical Research Opinions*, **12**, 234–241.

Perry, P. J., Garvey, M. J., Kelly, M. W., et al (1989) A comparative trial of fluoxetine versus trazodone in outpatients with major depression. *Journal of Clinical Psychiatry*, **50**, 290–294.

Phanjoo A., Wonnacott, S. & Hodgson, A. (1991) Double-blind comparative multicentre study of fluvoxamine and mianserin in the treatment of major depressive episode in elderly people. *Acta Psychiatrica Scandinavica*, **83**, 476–479.

Poelinger, W. & Haber, H. (1989) Fluoxetine 40 mg vs maprotiline 75 mg in the treatment of outpatients with depressive disorders. *International Clinical Psychopharmacology*, **4**(suppl 1), 47–50.

Rahman, M. K., Akhtar, M. J., Salva, N. C., et al (1991) A double-blind, randomised comparison of fluvoxamine with dothiepin in the treatment of depression in elderly patients. *British Journal of Clinical Practice*, **45**, 255–258.

Reimherr, F. W., Chouinard, G., Cohn, C. K., et al (1990) Antidepressant efficacy of sertraline: a double blind, placebo- and amitriptyline-controlled, multicenter comparison study in outpatients with major depression. *Journal of Clinical Psychiatry*, **51**(suppl B), 18–27.

Remick, R. A., Keller, F. D., Gibson, R. E., et al (1989) A comparison between fluoxetine and doxepin in depressed patients. *Current Therapeutic Research*, **46**, 842–848.

___ , Claman, J., Reesal, R., et al (1993) Comparison of fluoxetine and desipramine in depressed outpatients. *Current Therapeutic Research*, **53**, 457–465.

___ , Reesal, R., Oakander, M., et al (1994) Comparison of fluvoxamine and amitriptyline in depressed outpatients. Current Therapeutic Research, 55, 243–250.

Ropert, R. (1989) Fluoxetine versus clomipramine in major depressive disorders. International Clinical Psychopharmacology, 4(suppl. 1), 89–95.

Roth, D., Mattes, J., Sheehan, K. H., et al (1990) A double-blind comparison of fluvoxamine, desipramine and placebo in outpatients with depression. Progress in Neuropsychopharmacology and Biological Psychiatry, 14, 929–939.

Shrivastava, R., Patel Shrivastava, S. H., Overweg, N., et al (1992) A double blind comparison of paroxetine, imipramine and placebo in major depression. Journal of Clinical Psychiatry, 53(suppl. 2), 48–51.

Song, F., Freemantle, N., Sheldon, T. A., et al (1993) Selective serotonin reuptake inhibitors: meta-analysis of efficacy and acceptability. British Medical Journal, 306, 683–687.

South Wales Antidepressant Drug Trial Group (1988) A double-blind multi-centre trial of fluoxetine and dothiepin in major depressive illness. International Clinical Psychopharmacology, 3, 75–81.

Stark, P. & Hardison, D. (1985) A review of multicenter controlled studies of fluoxetine vs imipramine and placebo in outpatients with major depressive disorder. Journal of Clinical Psychiatry, 46, 53–58.

Stratta, P., Bolino, F., Cupillari, M., et al (1991) A double blind parallel study comparing fluoxetine with imipramine in the treatment of atypical depression. International Clinical Psychopharmacology, 6, 193–196.

Tamminen, T. T. A. & Lehtinen, V. V. (1989) A double-blind parallel study to compare fluoxetine with doxepin in the treatment of major depressive disorders. International Clinical Psychopharmacology, 4(suppl. 1), 51–56.

Taneri, Z. & Kohler, R. (1989) Fluoxetine versus nomifensine in outpatients with neurotic or reactive depressive disorder. International Clinical Psychopharmacology, 4(suppl. 1), 57–61.

Thompson, C. (1991) Setraline in a primary care setting. In Biological Psychiatry (ed. Anonymous), pp. 863–865. Amsterdam: Elsevier.

Thompson, S. G. & Pocock, S. J. (1991) Can meta-analysis be trusted? Lancet, 338, 1127–1130.

van Houwelingen, H. C., Zwinderman, K. H. & Stijnen, T. (1993) A bivariate approach to meta-analysis. Statistics in Medicine, 12, 2273–2284.

Wilson, A. & Henry, D. A. (1992) Meta-analysis. Part 2. Assessing the quality of published meta-analyses. Medical Journal of Australia, 156, 173–187.

Woolf, B. (1955) On estimating the relation between blood group and disease. Annals of Human Genetics, 19, 251–253.

Young, J. P. R., Coleman, A. & Lader, M. H. (1987) A controlled comparison of fluoxetine and amitriptyline in depressed out-patients. British Journal of Psychiatry, 151, 337–340.

CLINICAL IMPLICATIONS

■ On the whole, tricyclic and heterocyclic antidepressants are less well tolerated than SSRIs.

■ This appears to be due to the predominance of randomised controlled trials which have used imipramine and amitriptyline. Newer TCAs and heterocyclics are as well tolerated as the SSRIs.

■ Previous cost-effectiveness studies have grossly overestimated the benefit of SSRIs expressed as differential drop-out rates.

LIMITATIONS

■ The use of drop-out rates from randomised controlled trials is only a crude proxy for clinical tolerability.

■ The statistical power to detect a difference in drop-out rates for the newer TCAs is limited by the smaller number of trials in this group.

■ Clinical efficacy in terms of response to treatment was not considered in this meta-analysis.

MATTHEW HOTOPF, MRCPsych, Department of Psychological Medicine, King's College School of Medicine and Dentistry and Institute of Psychiatry; REBECCA HARDY, PhD, Department of Epidemiology and Public Health, University College London Medical School, 119 Torrington Place, London WC1E 6BT; GLYN LEWIS, PhD, Division of Psychological Medicine, University of Wales College of Medicine, Heath Park, Cardiff CF4 4XN, Wales

Correspondence: Dr Matthew Hotopf, Department of Psychological Medicine, King's College School of Medicine and Dentistry and Institute of Psychiatry, 103 Denmark Hill, London SE5 8AZ

(First received 16 April 1996, final revision 28 August 1996, accepted 29 August 1996)

Brief physician advice for problem alcohol drinkers

A randomised controlled trial in community-based primary care practices

MICHAEL F. FLEMING, MD, MPH; KRISTEN LAWTON BARRY, PhD; LINDA BAIER MANWELL; KRISTEN JOHNSON, MA; and RICHARD LONDON, MD

Objective   Project TrEAT (Trial for Early Alcohol Treatment) was designed to test the efficacy of brief physician advice in reducing alcohol use and health care utilization in problem drinkers.

Design   Randomized controlled clinical trial with 12-month follow-up.

Setting   A total of 17 community-based primary care practices (64 physicians) located in 10 Wisconsin counties.

Participants   Of the 17 695 patients screened for problem drinking, 482 men and 292 women met inclusion criteria and were randomized into a control (n=382) or an experimental (n=392) group. A total of 723 subjects (93%) participated in the 12-month follow-up procedures.

Intervention   The intervention consisted of two 10- to 15-minute counseling visits delivered by physicians using a scripted workbook that included advice, education, and contracting information.

Main outcome measures   Alcohol use measures, emergency department visits, and hospital days.

Results   There were no significant differences between groups at baseline on alcohol use, age, socioeconomic status, smoking status, rates of depression or anxiety, frequency of conduct disorders, lifetime drug use, or health care utilization. At the time of the 12-month follow-up, there were significant reductions in 7-day alcohol use (mean number of drinks in previous 7 days decreased from 19.1 at baseline to 11.5 at 12 months for the experimental group vs 18.9 at baseline to 15.5 at 12 months for controls; $t=4.33$; $P<.001$), episodes of binge drinking (mean number of binge drinking episodes during previous 30 days decreased from 5.7 at baseline to 3.1 at 12 months for the experimental group vs 5.3 at baseline to 4.2 at 12 months for controls; $t=2.81$; $P<.001$), and frequency of excessive drinking (percentage drinking excessively in previous 7 days decreased from 47.5% at baseline to 17.8% at 12 months for the experimental group vs 48.1% at baseline to 32.5% at 12 months for controls; $t=4.53$; $P<.001$). The χ^2 test of independence revealed a significant relationship between group status and length of hospitalisation over the study period for men ($P<.01$).

Conclusions   This study provides the first direct evidence that physician intervention with problem drinkers decreases alcohol use and health resource utilization in the US health care system.

JAMA 1997, **277**, 1039–1045

From the Department of Family Medicine (Dr Fleming and Ms Johnson) and the Center for Addiction Research and Education (Dr Fleming and Ms Manwell), University of Wisconsin Medical School, Madison; Department of Veterans Affairs, Serious Mental Illness Treatment Research and Evaluation Center, and the Department of Psychiatry, University of Michigan, Ann Arbor (Dr Barry); and the Family Health Plan Cooperative, Milwaukee, Wis (Dr London).
Reprints: Michael Fleming, MD, MPH, 777 S Mills St, Madison, WI 53715.

Alcohol use disorders are an important public health problem. Alcohol use is associated with a number of adverse health and economic effects.[1] Problem drinking is associated with increased mortality rates and with premature mortality. Estimates indicate that 9 to 22 years of life are lost for an individual death from alcoholic liver disease compared with 2 years for cancer and 4 years for heart disease.[2] Fetal alcohol effects occur in 1 in 1000 live births,[3] and the total cost of alcohol-related deaths exceeds $75 billion per year in the United States.[4] As a result of these findings, the testing of effective alcohol abuse prevention strategies has become an important national research priority.

One method of prevention is to use brief intervention techniques in clinical settings to reduce alcohol use in nondependent problem drinkers. These clinically based interventions include assessment and direct feedback, contracting and goal setting, behavioral modification techniques, and using written materials such as self-help manuals.[6-7] A number of trials, conducted primarily in Europe, have examined the efficacy of brief advice in reducing alcohol use.

Kristenson et al[8] reported the results of a trial conducted in Malmö, Sweden, in the late 1970s. The subjects, advised to reduce their alcohol use in a series of visits, subsequently demonstrated significant reductions in γ-glutamyl transferase levels and health care utilisation for up to 5 years after the brief interventions. The Medical Research Council (MRC) trial, conducted in 47 general practitioners' offices in Great Britain,[9] found significant reductions in alcohol use by the intervention group compared with the control group 12 months following the intervention. The World Health Organization Trial, conducted in 10 countries, found similar differences in alcohol use between the control and intervention groups.[10] Meta-analyses conducted by Bien et al[11] and Kahan et al[12] found an effect size of 20% to 30% in studies conducted in health care settings.

This article presents the results from Project TrEAT (Trial for Early Alcohol Treatment), the first large US clinical trial conducted in community-based primary care practices to test the efficacy of brief physician advice in reducing alcohol use by problem drinkers. This randomized controlled trial reports 1-year outcome data. The research procedures and measures were similar to those used in the MRC trial.[9]

METHODS

Protocol

Physician–Clinic Site Recruitment. – Physicians were recruited in 1992 through the Wisconsin Research Network, Madison, local community hospitals, managed care organisations, and personal contacts. Physicians who participated in the trial met the following criteria: (1) trained in family medicine or internal medicine; (2) practicing medicine at least 50% time; (3) based in a community primary care clinic outside a university or Department of Veterans Affairs medical center; (4) amenable to participating in a training program; and (5) amenable to following the research protocol. Physicians or their practices were paid $300 for participation in the trial.

A total of 64 family physicians and general internists participated in the trial. The 17 clinics, located in rural and urban areas in south central and south-eastern Wisconsin, varied from solo sites to large health maintenance organisation (HMO) groups. The 46 male physicians and 18 female physicians had a mean age of 46 years with an average of 13 years in practice. All physicians were board eligible or board certified in family medicine or internal medicine. A total of 34 physicians (53%) had received prior training in alcohol use disorders in medical school and residency. Of the physicians, 22 practiced in a staff-model HMO in Milwaukee County; 15 practiced in 3 preferred provider organisation models located in Dane County; and the remaining 27 physicians were in private practices located in small rural communities.

Study Population. – All adult patients aged 18 to 65 years were asked to complete a health screening survey by reception personnel as they arrived for regularly scheduled appointments to see their primary care physicians. The rate of patient refusal varied by clinic with a range of 2% to 30% and a weighted mean of 13% for an 87% response rate. All patients who screened positive and who had signed a consent form were contacted by telephone by 1 of 10 researchers and invited to participate in a face-to-face interview to determine their eligibility for the trial. The characteristics of the sample are reported in Table 1.

Inclusion Criteria. – Problem drinkers were defined as men who drank more than 14 drinks a week (168 g of alcohol) and women who drank more than 11 drinks a week (132 g of alcohol). Patients were ex-

Table I Demographic characteristics and health status by group and sex*

Characteristics	No. (%)			
	Men		Women	
	Treatment (n=244)	Control (n=238)	Treatment (n=148)	Control (n=144)
Age, years				
18–30	49 (20.2)	61 (26.0)	64 (43.5)	51 (35.7)
31–40	66 (27.2)	59 (25.1)	38 (25.9)	51 (35.7)
41–50	58 (23.9)	50 (21.3)	23 (15.6)	26 (18.2)
51–65	70 (28.8)	65 (27.7)	22 (15.0)	15 (10.5)
Ethnicity				
White	221 (94.4)	213 (92.6)	126 (88.1)	123 (88.5)
Hispanic	3 (1.3)	3 (1.3)	3 (2.1)	1 (0.7)
African American	6 (2.6)	6 (2.6)	9 (6.3)	10 (7.2)
Other	4 (1.7)	8 (3.5)	5 (3.5)	5 (3.6)
Marital status				
Never married	40 (16.6)	52 (22.4)	41 (28.9)	43 (30.1)
Widowed, divorced, separated	28 (11.6)	24 (10.3)	23 (16.2)	30 (21.0)
Married, living with partner	173 (71.8)	156 (67.2)	78 (54.9)	70 (49.0)
Education				
High school or less	86 (36.3)	89 (39.0)	68 (47.6)	60 (42.6)
Some college	95 (40.1)	93 (40.8)	50 (35.0)	61 (43.3)
College degree or more	56 (23.6)	46 (20.2)	25 (17.5)	20 (14.2)
Occupation				
Professional	72 (30.9)	57 (25.4)	32 (22.7)	34 (24.5)
Technical/mechanical	57 (24.5)	49 (21.9)	6 (4.3)	2 (1.4)
Student	1 (0.4)	8 (3.6)	14 (9.9)	10 (7.2)
Labor/machine	44 (18.9)	49 (21.9)	16 (11.3)	22 (15.8)
Retired	27 (11.6)	31 (13.8)	6 (4.3)	2 (1.4)
Farm	1 (0.4)	2 (0.9)	0	1 (0.7)
Sales-services	25 (10.7)	21 (9.4)	20 (14.2)	20 (14.4)
Homemaker	1 (0.4)	3 (1.3)	32 (22.7)	27 (19.4)
Unemployed	5 (2.1)	4 (1.8)	1 (0.7)	6 (4.3)
Mental health[†]				
Depression in lifetime	68 (28.0)	68 (28.9)	69 (47.3)	75 (52.8)
Depression in last 30 days	29 (12.0)	18 (7.6)	31 (21.1)	30 (21.4)
Childhood conduct disorder	28 (11.5)	35 (14.7)	16 (10.9)	9 (6.3)
Antisocial personality disorder	25 (10.3)	28 (11.8)	11 (7.5)	7 (4.9)
Family health				
Parents with alcohol/drug problem	76 (31.1)	88 (37.0)	55 (37.2)	67 (46.5)
Siblings with alcohol/drug problem	65 (26.6)	59 (24.8)	55 (37.2)	58 (40.3)
Health behaviors				
Exercised in last 6 months	177 (72.8)	184 (77.6)	100 (67.6)	91 (63.6)
Smoked in last 6 months	133 (54.5)	120 (50.4)	89 (60.1)	80 (55.6)
Used mood altering drugs in last 6 months	60 (24.6)	71 (29.8)	54 (37.0)	48 (33.3)
Used marijuana in last 6 months	38 (15.6)	51 (21.4)	32 (21.9)	33 (22.9)
Used cocaine in last 6 months	7 (2.9)	9 (3.8)	9 (6.1)	9 (6.3)

*Sample totals vary slightly across variables. Percentages are based on numbers shown in parentheses relative to other data points for that variable.
[†] Percentage reflects the patients in whom symptoms were present.

cluded from participation in the study if they were pregnant, younger than 18 years or older than 65 years, had attended an alcohol treatment program in the previous year, reported symptoms of alcohol withdrawal in the last 12 months, received advice from their physician in the previous 3 months to change their alcohol use, drank more than 50 drinks per week, or reported symptoms of suicide. Patients were paid a total of $50 if they completed the required procedures. Informed consent was obtained from patients prior to the face-to-face interview. The research protocol was reviewed and approved by the University of Wisconsin Human Subjects Committee.

Intervention Protocol. – The brief intervention protocol consisted of a workbook that contained feedback regarding current health behaviors, a review of the prevalence of problem drinking, a list of the adverse effects of alcohol, a worksheet on drinking cues, a drinking agreement in the form of a prescription, and drinking diary cards. The intervention was based on protocols developed for the MRC trial. Two 15-minute visits with the physician were scheduled 1 month apart (brief intervention and reinforcement session). Each patient received a follow-up telephone call from the clinic nurse 2 weeks after each meeting with the physician.

Outcome Variables. – The primary outcome variables of interest were changes in alcohol use (previous 7-day use, binge drinking, excessive drinking), health care utilization (hospital days and emergency department visits), and changes in health status measures (smoking status, depression, motor vehicle crashes, and unintentional injuries). The variables were selected a priori and were based on the findings of previous trials.[8–10] Biological measures such as γ-glutamyl transferase were not included owing to low sensitivity in this population.[2]

Research Procedures. – All patients aged 18 to 65 years with regularly scheduled appointments between April 1, 1992, and April 1, 1994, were asked to complete the health screening survey. The survey was designed as a general lifestyle questionnaire in order to increase patient acceptance of the research procedures and to minimize the intervention effect of the alcohol questions.[13] The survey contained 4 sets of parallel questions on exercise, smoking, weight, and alcohol use.[14] Subjects who screened positive for problem drinking were invited to participate in a research interview.

The face-to-face 30-minute research interview took place in each patient's primary care clinic and was conducted by 1 of 10 trained researchers. This assessment interview, the Research Lifestyle Interview, included a 7-day timeline follow-back procedure,[15] number of episodes of binge drinking in the past 28 days using the timeline procedures, number of weeks of abstinence in the past 3 months, symptoms of alcohol withdrawal (lifetime and previous year), and treatment for alcohol problems (lifetime and previous year). Additional questions included the frequency of licit and illicit drug use, injuries, emergency department visits, hospitalizations, limitations of daily activities, health status,[16] and family function.[17] The Diagnostic Interview Schedule[18] for current and lifetime depression, childhood conduct disorder, and antisocial personality disorder was administered along with the SCL–90 anxiety scale[19] and a family history schedule developed by Andreasen et al.[20]

Subjects assigned to the control group received a health booklet on general health issues and were followed up at 6 and 12 months. They were instructed to address any health concerns in their usual manner. Patients in the experimental group were given the same booklet and scheduled to see their personal physician for the brief intervention treatment.

Physicians were trained to administer the intervention protocol through role playing and general skills techniques in educational programs at each of the 17 clinics. The physicians also received additional training in booster sessions that occurred at least twice during the trial, as subjects were randomized into the trial over a 9-month period. Physicians were asked to complete a form following each intervention visit to document that the patient had received the protocol and had contracted to reduce his or her alcohol use.

Follow-up procedures included a telephone interview at 6 and 12 months by one of the researchers not assigned to the subject's clinic. Family members were contacted at 12 months to corroborate patient self-report. Medical record reviews were completed after the 12-month follow-up telephone interview.

Analysis. – Statistical analyses of the data were conducted to investigate alcohol consumption and health care utilization among study participants. The analyses examined changes in behavior over time by comparing outcome measures at the base-

line survey and at the 6-month and 12-month follow-up reports. The t tests of difference between means and the χ^2 tests of independence provided estimates of significant differences in outcome measures between the experimental and control groups. A logistic regression model was estimated to examine the independent effect of treatment status on alcohol use after controlling for other variables. Analyses were conducted separately for men and women and by group status (experimental, control).

Assignment

The unit of randomization was the individual patient. Randomization of subjects to the experimental and control groups was carried out separately for men and women in each physician's practice using a computer-generated allocation method. Each physician had both control and experimental patients in his or her practice. The goal of the trial was to have 6 to 8 control patients and 6 to 8 experimental patients for each physician in the study.

Masking (blinding)

One of the goals of the trial was to blind subjects assigned to the control groups to minimize the intervention effect of the research procedures. The subjects randomized into the control group were told the trial focused on health behaviors including alcohol. All research procedures including the follow-up patient and family member interviews asked parallel questions on smoking, exercise, weight, and alcohol use.

The physicians and their staff were not told which of their patients were randomized into the control group. While it could be expected that the physicians in the trial would identify alcohol problems in the control subjects as a result of their brief intervention training, only 50 control subjects (13%) reported a physician intervention in the 12 months following randomization. To avoid interviewer bias at the 6- and 12-month follow-up interviews, researchers were rotated for the telephone interviews so that they did not interview any patients from the clinics to which they were assigned.

Medical record audit showed that 4 patients in the control group (3 men and 1 woman), 1 man in the experimental group, and 1 man in the failed experimental group (those assigned to treatment but who did not follow up with the intervention visit to the physician, $n=6$) received formal

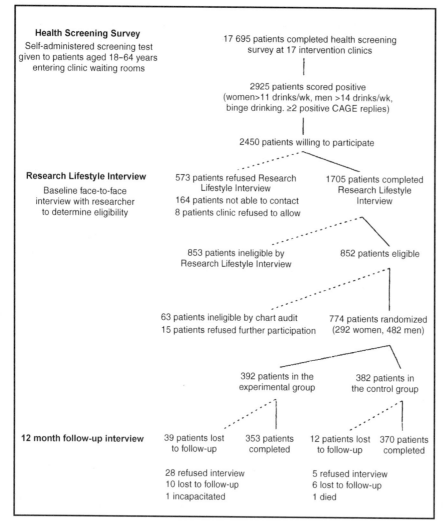

Health Screening Survey
Self-administered screening test given to patients aged 18–64 years entering clinic waiting rooms

17 695 patients completed health screening survey at 17 intervention clinics

2925 patients scored positive (women>11 drinks/wk, men >14 drinks/wk, binge drinking. ≥2 positive CAGE replies)

2450 patients willing to participate

Research Lifestyle Interview
Baseline face-to-face interview with researcher to determine eligibility

573 patients refused Research Lifestyle Interview
164 patients not able to contact
8 patients clinic refused to allow

1705 patients completed Research Lifestyle Interview

853 patients ineligible by Research Lifestyle Interview

852 patients eligible

63 patients ineligible by chart audit
15 patients refused further participation

774 patients randomized (292 women, 482 men)

392 patients in the experimental group

382 patients in the control group

12 month follow-up interview

39 patients lost to follow-up

353 patients completed

12 patients lost to follow-up

370 patients completed

28 refused interview
10 lost to follow-up
1 incapacitated

5 refused interview
6 lost to follow-up
1 died

Fig. I. Trial profile.

treatment in an alcohol treatment program during the 1-year follow-up period. There was no mention of referral to Alcoholics Anonymous.

RESULTS

Participation Flow and Follow-up

A total of 17 695 subjects from 17 clinics completed the health screening survey (Figure). Of those, 2450 subjects screened positive (more than 14 drinks per week for men, more than 11 drinks per week for women, more than 5 drinks 4 or more times in previous 30 days, and 2 or more positive answers to the 4 questions from a standard screening instrument used to assess the possibility of a drinking problem called CAGE[21]) and were invited to participate in a face-to-face interview at their physicians' offices. A total of 1705 patients completed the Research Lifestyle Interview with 16.6% meeting current criteria for

alcohol dependence based on criteria from the *Diagnostic and Statistical Manual of Mental Disorders, Third Edition, Revised (DSM–III–R).*[22]

A total of 774 subjects met all inclusion criteria and were randomized into an experimental group (n=392) and a control group (n=382). Most of the subjects who did not meet inclusion criteria did so because their alcohol use in the previous 7 days was below the selected cutoff limit. The timeline follow-back procedure was used in the Research Lifestyle Interview to assess daily alcohol use in the previous 7 days and provided more accurate information than the health screening survey. Other reasons for exclusion included recent suicide ideation, symptoms of alcohol dependence, alcohol treatment in the previous year, and severe medical problems.

A total of 307 subjects completed the intervention protocol; 9 received only 1 physician visit. A total of 85 persons

randomized to the experimental group failed to keep their appointment with the physician and did not receive the physician intervention. These subjects were scheduled at least 3 times by the researchers. Primary reasons given by these patients for not following through with the scheduled intervention included lack of time, family illness, transportation problems, and inability to take time off from work. This group was not statistically different at baseline from the persons who completed the intervention on age, sex, alcohol use, health services utilization, employment status, marital status, education, or frequency of mental illness. Of the 85 subjects who did not receive the intervention, 77 participated in the 12-month follow-up interview. All persons initially randomized to the experimental group (n=392) remained in this group for the analysis.

Of the 774 subjects enrolled in the trial, 723 completed the 12-month follow-up procedures. Of the 51 subjects who did not complete the 12-month follow-up interview, 33 refused the interview, 16 were lost to follow-up, 1 died, and 1 had a stroke. The greater number of persons in the experimental group who refused the 12-month follow-up interview may be related to their resistance to change their alcohol use.

Family member interviews were conducted in order to corroborate subjects' self-report. Of family members 612 (79%) completed the 12-month interview. Family members of subjects in both the control and experimental groups consistently reported lower amounts of alcohol use than the subjects.

Analysis

Patient Characteristics. – Minimal differences were found between the experimental and control groups on a number of potential confounding variables (Table 1). The sample consisted of 482 males and 292 females. The race/ethnicity distribution of the sample is similar to the distribution for primary care patients throughout Wisconsin. The age distribution was similar for each decade. The population was well educated the majority of the sample had attended college. Only 2% reported unemployed. A family history of alcohol problems was more commonly reported in the female sample.

Over half of the sample (n=422) reported tobacco use at baseline. The category "used

Table 2 Alcohol consumption at baseline and follow-up by treatment status*

Status	All patients				Men				Women			
	Treatment (n=392)	Control (n=382)	t	P	Treatment (n=244)	Control (n=238)	t	P	Treatment (n=148)	Control (n=144)	t	P
	No. of drinks in previous 7 days											
	Mean (s.d.)	Mean (s.d.)			Mean (s.d.)	Mean (s.d.)			Mean (s.d.)	Mean (s.d.)		
Baseline	19.14 (12.26)	18.94 (11.84)	0.22	...	21.67 (12.85)	21.95 (12.39)	0.60	...	15.05 (10.02)	15.69 (10.13)	0.52	...
6 months	11.57 (10.94)	14.98 (11.12)	4.10	<0.001	13.84 (11.99)	17.12 (12.51)	2.78	<0.005	7.91 (7.73)	11.54 (7.23)	3.99	<0.001
12 months	11.48 (11.31)	15.46 (12.93)	4.33	<0.001	13.62 (12.39)	16.86 (13.49)	2.6	<0.005	8.03 (8.26)	13.20 (11.67)	4.16	<0.001
% Reduction												
Base to 6 months	39.54	20.88	...	...	36.12	22.02	...	...	47.48	26.45	...	...
Base to 12 months	40.02	18.35	...	...	37.16	23.17	...	...	46.65	15.89	...	...
	No. of binge drinking episodes in previous 30 days											
	Mean (s.d.)	Mean (s.d)			Mean (s.d)	Mean (s.d.)			Mean (s.d.)	Mean (s.d.)		
Baseline	5.65 (5.95)	5.34 (5.03)	0.76	...	6.13 (6.58)	5.40 (4.98)	1.30	...	4.88 (4.70)	5.23 (5.13)	0.57	...
6 months	2.88 (4.86)	3.93 (4.80)	2.90	<0.005	3.33 (5.35)	4.37 (5.29)	2.04	<0.025	2.14 (3.94)	3.22 (3.80)	2.29	<0.02
12 months	3.07 (5.23)	4.21 (5.52)	2.81	<0.005	3.43 (5.52)	4.48 (5.66)	1.95	<0.05	2.50 (4.70)	3.79 (5.27)	2.11	<0.02
% Reduction												
Base to 6 months	49.13	26.32	...	...	45.65	19.08	...	...	56.19	38.39	...	...
Base to 12 months	45.67	21.05	...	...	44.08	17.12	...	...	48.89	27.60	...	...
	Binge drinking in the previous 30 days											
	n (%)	n (%)			n (%)	n (%)			n (%)	n (%)		
Baseline	288 (85.46)	317 (86.61)	0.44	...	177 (85.10)	197 (87.17)	0.62	...	111 (86.05)	120 (85.71)	0.08	...
6 months	200 (59.35)	266 (72.68)	3.77	<0.001	133 (63.94)	168 (74.34)	2.36	<0.005	67 (51.94)	98 (70.0)	3.08	<0.005
12 months	188 (55.79)	261 (71.31)	4.33	<0.001	118 (56.73)	167 (73.89)	3.82	<0.001	70 (54.26)	94 (67.14)	2.17	<0.025
% Reduction, mean												
Base to 6 months	30.56	16.09	...	...	24.86	14.72	...	...	39.64	18.33	...	...
Base to 12 months	34.72	17.67	...	...	33.33	15.23	...	...	36.94	21.67	...	...
	Drinking excessively in the previous 7 days											
	n (%)	n (%)			n (%)	n (%)			n (%)	n (%)		
Baseline	160 (47.48)	176 (48.09)	0.16	...	95 (45.67)	101 (44.69)	0.21	...	65 (50.39)	75 (53.57)	0.52	...
6 months	67 (19.88)	115 (31.42)	3.52	<0.001	46 (22.12)	65 (28.76)	1.59	...	21 (16.28)	50 (35.71)	3.69	<0.001
12 months	60 (17.80)	119 (32.51)	4.53	<0.001	38 (18.27)	70 (30.97)	3.08	<0.005	22 (17.05)	49 (35.00)	3.39	<0.001
% Reduction, mean												
Base to 6 months	58.13	34.66	...	...	51.58	35.64	...	...	67.69	33.33	...	...
Base to 12 months	62.50	32.39	...	...	60.00	30.69	...	...	66.15	34.67	...	...

*Excessive drinking was defined as having more than 20 drinks per week for men and more than 13 drinks per week for women; binge drinking is defined as having more than 4 drinks for women and 5 drinks for men in 1 occasion. Ellipses indicate not applicable.

mood altering drugs in the last 6 months" included marijuana, cocaine, amphetamines, LSD, illicit narcotics, and prescription drugs such as alprazolam (Xanax), chlordiazepoxide hydrochloride (Librium), diazepam (Valium), and opioids. Higher total rates of drug use in women are related to increased use of prescribed benzodiazepines. The rates of self-report marijuana and cocaine use in the last 6 months were higher than general population samples and may reflect higher rates in primary care clinical samples. Rates of major depression (based on Diagnostic Interview Schedule a DSM–III–R criteria) were higher in women.

Alcohol Use Outcome Measures. The major alcohol use outcome variables were average drinks per week, binge drinking, and excessive drinking. The average drinks per week, the total number of drinks in the last 7 days, was determined by timeline follow-back procedures.[15] As shown in Table 2, there were large decreases in all alcohol use variables in all groups at 6 and 12 months. Reductions in drinking over time were significant within each group, but the experimental

Physician advice for problem drinkers – Fleming *et al*

Table 3 Logistic regression model of 20% or more reduction in drinking*

Characteristics	Adjusted odds ratio (95% CI)
Women	1.08 (0.77–1.51)
Smoking in last 6 months	0.73† (0.53–1.01)
Age, years	
18–30	1.07 (0.83–1.39)
31–40	0.94 (0.73–1.22)
41–50	0.88 (0.66–1.17)
51–65	1.12 (0.83–1.51)
Depressed in last 30 days	0.73 (0.49–1.09)
Experimental	2.15‡ (1.58–2.93)
Child conduct disorder	1.30 (0.87–1.94)
Adult antisocial personality	1.18 (0.67–2.06)

*Overall predictive power, 60%.
†$P \leqslant 0.06$.
‡$P \leqslant 0.001$.

Table 4 Health care utilization by group and sex

Status	All patients		Men		Women	
	Treatment ($n=392$)	Control ($n=382$)	Treatment ($n=244$)	Control ($n=238$)	Treatment ($n=148$)	Control ($n=144$)
Self-reported number of emergency department visits (No. of patients) in last 6 months						
Baseline	75 (58)	80 (65)	49 (38)	47 (47)	26 (20)	32 (24)
6-months follow-up	47 (40)	70 (56)	29 (25)	46 (37)	18 (15)	24 (19)
12-months follow-up	60 (47)	62 (50)	33 (28)	39 (34)	27 (19)	23 (16)
	$\chi^2=2.45$ ($P>.10$)		$\chi^2=2.60$ ($P>.10$)		$\chi^2=1.48$ ($P>.10$)	
Self-reported number of days of hospitalization (No. of patients) in last 6 months						
Baseline	93 (18)	42 (17)	84 (13)	37 (13)	9 (5)	5 (4)
6-months follow-up	35 (8)	164 (21)	29 (5)	159 (14)	6 (3)	21 (7)
12-months follow-up	91 (22)	146 (17)	65 (13)	118 (13)	26 (9)	16 (4)
	$\chi^2=89.53$ ($P<.001$)		$\chi^2=93.01$ ($P<.001$)		$\chi^2=11.85$ ($P<.01$)	

group reduced their alcohol use more than the control group.

The greatest reduction in alcohol consumption over time occurred among women in the experimental group. These women decreased their alcohol use by almost one half, drank to excess and binge drank in far fewer numbers, and significantly decreased their average number of binge episodes per month. At baseline, women in the experimental group drank 15 drinks per week, but this figure was reduced by 47% to 8 drinks per week after 12 months. Two thirds fewer women drank to excess at the time of the 12-month survey. While women in the control group also decreased their use, the relative difference between the groups varied from 16% to 35% and was statistically significant ($P<0.05$) at both follow-up points.

Men in the experimental group reduced their alcohol consumption slightly less than their female counterparts, but decreases were reported across all alcohol use measures. Twelve months after the baseline survey, men in the experimental group demonstrated a 37% reduction in 7-day alcohol use, a 60% decrease in the number who drank to excess, and a 44% decline in the frequency of binge drinking. On average, men in the experimental group reduced their weekly alcohol consumption by 8 drinks (from 21.67 to 13.62) and decreased the frequency of binge episodes from 6 per

month to 3 per month. Reductions in alcohol consumption were consistently greater among men in the experimental group. These changes were statistically significant ($P<0.01$) at all but 1 point of measurement (percentage drinking to excess at 6 months).

The results from a logistic regression model (Table 3) show that other demographic characteristics and health behaviors do not account for differences in alcohol consumption between the groups; the only variable significantly predicting a 20% or greater reduction in drinking was exposure to the physician intervention. Smoking, age, depression, conduct disorder, and adult antisocial personality disorder did not significantly affect a reduction in drinking. Individuals in the experimental group were 2 times more likely to reduce their drinking by 20% or more (odds ratio, 2.15; 95% confidence interval, 1.58–2.93). In contrast, other variables examined did not make individuals any more (or less) likely to reduce their alcohol consumption by 20%.

Health Care Utilization. – Table 4 examines patterns of health care utilization by sex and group status. In interviews at baseline and at 6 and 12 months, study participants were asked to report the length of any hospitalizations and the number of visits to an emergency department during the previous 6 months. Neither men nor women reported significantly different numbers of visits to the emergency department during the course of the study; the

numbers of visits deviate only slightly from each other at all time points, and there were no significant associations between group status and emergency department use.

Utilization of health care facilities differs significantly between the experimental and control groups for days of hospitalization (Table 4). Men in the control group experienced substantially longer hospitalizations during the study period than those in the experimental group (314 vs 178 days). Although an assessment of whether physician intervention significantly reduces hospitalization over time awaits analysis of long-term follow-up surveys, χ^2 tests indicate that hospital utilization is significantly related to group status. Additional analyses performed after temporarily removing 4 individuals with hospital stays longer than 6 weeks – more than 1 month longer than any other reported hospitalization – were not appreciably changed. Another potential factor influencing higher rates of hospital days in the control group are primary care visits. A preliminary analysis of outpatient visits showed no significant difference by group status.

The number of women hospitalized in the sample was small, and the numbers were not stable. Many of the hospital days in women were related to obstetrical care. While the sample excluded women who were pregnant at the beginning of the trial, 10 women became pregnant after randomization.

Health Status Measures. – Other outcome variables showed no significant changes in general health rating, mean number of cigarettes smoked, or number of depressive symptoms after 12 months for men or women in either group.

COMMENT

Project TrEAT found significant reductions in alcohol use and health care utilization in men drinking more than 14 drinks per week and women drinking more than 11 drinks per week. After 12 months there was a 14% reduction of alcohol use by men in the experimental group and a 31% reduction by women in the experimental group. There were also significant reductions in the proportion of male and female subjects who were drinking excessively. Men in the experimental group experienced lower rates of binge drinking than control group men. As expected, large reductions in use occurred at the 6-month point after intervention. These changes were maintained at the 12-month follow-up. With the exception of a larger reduction in 7-day alcohol use in the female sample, these findings are consistent with the findings of the MRC trial.[9] The changes in health care utilization were significant and suggest a treatment effect. The men in the experimental group experienced a greater than 2-fold difference in the total number of hospital days in the 12 months following the intervention when compared with the control group.

This trial has a number of strengths. Project TrEAT is the first large-scale alcohol trial with a diverse sample of community-based, primary care practices in rural and urban settings in the United States. The involvement of 4 managed care organizations with physicians in community-based practices makes the study unique. As a result of using community-based physicians who traditionally provide more than 90% of the care in the United States, the findings may be applicable to primary care practices throughout the United States. The patient sample represents an employed population of adults in a state with a strong economy and a high rate of alcohol use. Wisconsin is third only to Alaska and the District of Columbia in total per capita alcohol consumption.

Project TrEAT is the third largest brief intervention trial reported in the world literature. The WHO[10] and the MRC[9] trials had samples of 1655 and 909 subjects, respectively. The number of women in our study (n=292) was similar to the number of women in the WHO (n=299) and MRC (n=268) studies. We had a high physician retention and a patient follow-up rate of 93% at 12 months, the highest rate of all brief intervention alcohol trials. Corroborative family member interviews suggest patient self-report was a valid estimate of alcohol use. Control procedures were maintained throughout the trial with only 13% of the control subjects receiving alcohol consumption advice from their physicians during the 12-month follow-up period.

A number of methodological issues that are potential limitations to the study should be considered when interpreting our results. Reliance on self-report of alcohol consumption as one of the primary outcome measures is an important consideration. Research conducted by a number of investigation indicates that self-reported alcohol consumption is more reliable than other methods of inquiry or testing.[22–25] Methods used in this trial to minimize self-report bias included: (1) informing patients that the researchers administering the follow-up interviews were from the University of Wisconsin; (2) reassuring subjects that the information provided to the researchers was confidential; (3) using follow-up questionnaires containing parallel questions regarding weight, exercise, sleeping patterns, alcohol use, and smoking to lessen the impact of the alcohol questions; and (4) using multiple measures of alcohol use.

Another methodological issue is the concern that persons who received the physician intervention may have wanted to "please their physicians" by subsequently reporting lower rates of alcohol use. In the absence of the use of a biological measure to assess recent alcohol use, family member interviews were conducted at 12 months with 79% of the sample to corroborate subject self-report. The family member interviews did not reveal any systematic differences from subject self-report by group status. This finding suggests that patient responses were not significantly affected by a desire to please the physician.

The use of self-report data for changes in health care utilization is another potential limitation of the study. Traditionally, at least 3 sources can be used to assess changes in utilization including claims data, medical record reviews and self-report. The trial was not able to use claims data due to access and cost restraints. We estimate that the subjects in the trial had over 20 different health care insurance carriers. When we examined medical record data to estimate changes in utilization, we found that patients reported greater numbers of emergency department visits and hospital days than those recorded in the medical records. Patients reported 33% more emergency department visits and 40% more hospital days. The κ statistic comparing self-report with medical records was 0.536 for emergency department visits and 0.44 for hospital visits. The Yules Y for emergency department visits was 0.54 and 0.60 for hospital visits. The reason for this visit discrepancy may be related to a lack of routine reporting from emergency departments and hospitals to primary care physicians' offices. Also, some patients may have gone to out-of-area hospitals or emergency departments to prevent their physicians, insurance companies, or employers from being notified.

A limitation of studies conducted in community-based clinical settings is the follow-through of subjects in receiving the intervention protocol. Nearly 22% of the subjects randomized to the experimental group did not receive a physician intervention. This is a common finding in alcohol and mental health intervention trials[11,26] and is related to time issues, illness, travel distance, and loss of interest in participating in the research trial. It is important to note that 77 of the 85 subjects who did not receive the intervention participated in the follow-up interviews. The inclusion of this group in the analysis provides a more conservative estimate that strengthens confidence in the results of the trial.

The generalizability of the results is limited to those populations included in the study. The results of brief intervention techniques may not apply to people treated for an alcohol use disorder in the past year, people with suicidal ideation, or those who drink on average more than 50 drinks per week. The trial specifically excluded patients with alcoholism, and the effectiveness of brief intervention was not tested among this population. Current standards of care require more intensive, specialized treatment for persons who meet *Diagnostic and Statistical Manual of Mental Disorders, Fourth Edition,*[27] criteria for alcohol dependence. The effectiveness of the brief intervention technique may also differ for minority populations. Although the race/ethnicity of the sample matched the population of Wisconsin and the Mid-west in general, African Americans, Asians, and Hispanic Americans were underrepresented.

Intervention protocols may need to be adapted according to cultural beliefs and expectations.

The 20% reduction in alcohol use in the control groups was interesting. A majority of the other trials have similar reductions in alcohol use.[11,12] The reason for this change is not known but may be related to regression to the mean, historical changes in alcohol use, and the intervention effect of the research procedures. It is our impression that research procedures can have a significant intervention effect. Each control subject was asked about his or her

alcohol use 4 times over the 12-month period.

This trial indicates that brief advice protocols can provide a successful strategy for changing drinking behavior and improving health outcomes for at-risk and problem drinkers in primary care settings. Since 70% of people in the United States visit their physician at least once every 2 years, brief physician advice could have enormous implications for the US health care system. This trial supports the implementation of screening assessment, and brief intervention for all patients who seek health

care services in primary care community-based settings.[28]

This work was supported by grant AA 08512-01A from the National Institutes of Health, National Institute on Alcohol Abuse and Alcoholism, and was assisted by the Wisconsin Research Network, Madison, and the Wisconsin Institute of Family Medicine, Milwaukee.

The authors would like to thank John Beasley, MD, Director of the Wisconsin Research Network; Michael French, PhD, health economist at Research Triangle Institute, Research Triangle Park, NC, and the University of Miami, Miami, Fla; and the 64 primary care physicians who participated in the trial.

REFERENCES

1. Holder HD, Blose JO. The reduction of health care costs associated with alcoholism treatment. J Stud Alcohol. 1992;53:293–302.
2. US Dept of Health and Human Services. Eighth Special Report to the US Congress on Alcohol and Health From the Secretary of Health and Human Services, September 1993. Washington, DC: US Dept of Health and Human Services, Public Health Service, National Institutes of Health, National Institute on Alcohol Abuse and Alcoholism; 1993. Publication ADM-281-91-0003.
3. Institute of Medicine. Committee to Study Fetal Alcohol Syndrome. Washington, DC: National Academy Press; 1996.
4. Rice DP, Rosenberg HM, Curtin LR, Hodgson TA. Changing mortality patterns, health services utilization and health care expenditures. Vital Health Stat. 3, 1983;23:1–35.
5. Babor TF. Brief intervention strategies for harmful drinkers: new directions for medical education. Can Med Assoc J. 1990;143:1070–1076.
6. Heather N, Campion PD, Neville RG, MacCabe O. Evaluation of a controlled drinking minimal intervention for problem drinkers in general practice. J R Coll Gen Pract. 1987;37:358–363.
7. Miller WR. Techniques to modify hazardous drinking patterns. Recent Dev Alcohol 1987;5:425–438.
8. Kristenson H, Ohlin H, Hulten-Nosslin M, Trell C, Hood B. Identification and intervention of heavy drinking in middle-aged men. Alcohol Clin Exp Res. 1983;7:203–209.

9. Wallace P, Cutler S, Haines A. Randomized controlled trial of general practitioner intervention in patients with excessive alcohol consumption. BMJ 1988;297:663–668.
10. World Health Organization Brief Intervention Study Group. Across national trial of brief intervention with heavy drinkers. Am J Pub Health 1996;86:948–955.
11. Bien TH, Miller WR, Tonigan JS. Brief interventions for alcohol problems: a review. Addiction 1993;88:315–335.
12. Kahan M, Wilson L, Becker L. Effectiveness of physician-based interventions with problem drinkers: a review. Can Med Assoc J. 1995;152:851–859.
13. Fleming M, Barry K. A three-sample test of a masked alcohol screening questionnaire. Alcohol Alcohol. 1991;26:81–91.
14. Wallace P, Haines A. The use of a questionnaire in general practice to increase the recognition of patients with excessive alcohol consumption. BMJ 1985;290:1949–1953.
15. Sobell LC, Sobell MB. Self-report issues in alcohol abuse. Behav Assess. 1990;12:77–90.
16. Stewart AL, Hays RD, Ware JE Jr. The MOS short-form general health survey. Med Care. 1988;26:724–735.
17. Moos R, Moos B. Family Environment Scale Manual. 2nd ed. Palo Alto, Calif: Consulting Psychology Press; 1986.
18. Robins IN, Helzer JE, Croughan JL, Ratcliff KS. National Institute of Mental Health Diagnostic Interview Schedule: its history, characteristics, and validity. Arch Gen Psychiatry. 1981;38:381–389.
19. Derogatis LR, Lipman RS, Covi L. SCL–90: an

outpatient psychiatric rating scale – preliminary report. Psychopharmacol Bull. 1973;9:13–28.
20. Andreasen NC, Endicott J, Spitzer R, Winokur G. The family history method using diagnostic criteria. Arch Gen Psychiatry. 1977;34:1229–1235.
21. Ewing JA. Detecting alcoholism: the CAGE questionnaire. JAMA 1984;252:1905–1907.
22. American Psychiatric Association. Diagnostic and Statistical Manual of Mental Disorders, Third Edition, Revised. Washington, DC: American Psychiatric Association; 1987.
23. Babor TF, Stephens RS, Marlatt GA. Verbal report methods in clinical research on alcoholism. J Stud Alcohol. 1987;48:410–424.
24. Maisto SA, McKay JR, Connors JJ. Self-report issues in substance abuse: state of the art and future directions. Behav Assess. 1990;12:117–134.
25. Midanik LT. Validity of self-reported alcohol use. Br J Addict. 1988;83:1019–1030.
26. Chick J. Early intervention for hazardous drinking in the general hospital setting. Alcohol Alcohol. 1991;1:477–479.
27. American Psychiatric Association. Diagnostic and Statistical Manual of Mental Disorders. Fourth Edition. Washington, DC: American Psychiatric Association; 1994.
28. National Institute on Alcohol Abuse and Alcoholism. The Physicians' Guide to Helping Patients With Alcohol Problems. Washington, DC: US Dept of Health and Human Services, Public Health Service, National Institutes of Health, National Institute of Alcohol Abuse and Alcoholism; 1995, NIH publication 95-3769.

Characteristics of Outcome in Schizophrenia at 13 Years

PETER MASON, GLYNN HARRISON, CRISTINE GLAZEBROOK,
IAN MEDLEY, TIM DALKIN and TIM CROUDACE

Background   This paper describes the 13-year outcome of an epidemiologically defined and representative cohort of patients selected when they were experiencing their first episode of schizophrenia.

Method   In a 13-year follow-up study of a cohort identified in Nottingham in 1978–80, the outcome (symptoms, disability, residence and treatment) was assessed using standardised instruments

Results   Four of the original 67 patients with ICD–9 schizophrenia were lost to follow-up and five were dead: 52% were without psychotic symptoms in the last two years of follow-up, 52% were without negative symptoms and 55% showed good/ fair social functioning. However, only 17% were alive at follow-up, without symptoms and disability, and receiving no treatment.

Conclusion   The findings reported are similar to those of other long-term follow-up studies of schizophrenia and also to 5-year follow-up studies. Kraepelin's emphasis on the longitudinal implications of a diagnosis of schizophrenia are supported, but may be over-pessimistic.

There have been numerous follow-up studies of schizophrenia. Hegarty *et al* (1994) identified 821 such studies between 1895 and 1992. It is difficult to generalise from their findings, however, because the methods used differed considerably (Harrison & Mason, 1993), with different diagnostic criteria, different concepts of outcome, sampling biases, different lengths of follow-up and completeness of follow-up. Nevertheless, recent short-term outcome studies in schizophrenia have demonstrated a fairly consistent clinical picture. After 2 years, MacMillan *et al* reported that 60% of their subjects had relapsed and the Scottish Schizophrenia Research Group found 37% with a good clinical outcome (MacMillan *et al*, 1986; Scottish Schizophrenia Research Group, 1989). At 5 years, approximately 50% show considerable improvement in symptoms (Prudo & Blum, 1987; Shepherd *et al*, 1989; Scottish Schizophrenia Research Group, 1992). Five-year outcome findings in the International Pilot Study of Schizophrenia showed marked differences in outcome between developed and developing countries: over 60% of patients in Aarhus were actively psychotic at the outcome date, whereas two-thirds of the patients in both Agra and Ibadan were asymptomatic (Leff *et al*, 1992). In contrast to the number of studies on short-term outcome, there have been relatively few studies of the medium to longer term (10–25 years) outcome. Nevertheless, several European authors (e.g. Bleuler, 1978; Huber *et al*, 1980; Ciompi, 1980) have reported data suggesting that the long-term outcome is better than previously believed. Since we don't know a great deal about the longer-term outcome in schizophrenia, and since many previous studies had problems with methods, we carried out a 13-year follow-up study of an epidemiologically defined and representative cohort of patients selected when they experienced their first episode of schizophrenia. This cohort was part of the International Study of Schizophrenia, a transcultural investigation

in 20 centres in 15 countries coordinated by the World Health Organization. It was designed to explain findings of previous WHO studies in this area, to identify patterns of long-term course and outcome of severe mental disorders in different cultures, to further develop methods for the study of characteristics of mental disorders and their course in different settings, and to strengthen the scientific basis for future international multidisciplinary research on schizophrenia and other psychiatric disorders seen in a public health perspective. The cohort described in this paper was first identified in the World Health Organization's Determinants of Outcome of Severe Mental Disorder Study (1978–80), for which Nottingham was the UK field centre (Cooper *et al*, 1987; Jablensky *et al*, 1992). Data on residence at the 13-year follow-up for this sample have already been reported (Harrison *et al*, 1994). The present paper presents cross-sectional outcome data at 13 years, with particular reference to symptoms and social disability, employment and treatment status. These data are then compared with those for shorter (2–5 years) follow-up periods, in addition to those reported from other longer term follow-up studies.

METHOD

The methods used in the International Study of Schizophrenia (ISoS) have been described in detail elsewhere (Sartorius *et al*, 1995).

Sample (1978–1980)

This was an incidence cohort of 67 patients assigned a project ICD–9 diagnosis of schizophrenia, who made their first contact with psychiatric services in Nottingham between 1 August 1978 and 31 July 1980. It was derived from the 99 patients identified by the screening schedule used in the WHO Determinants of Outcome of Severe Mental Disorder Study (Jablensky *et al*, 1992). The method of identifying this cohort was based upon a careful case-finding design described by Cooper *et al* (1987) and Jablensky *et al* (1992). It consisted of all patients (ages 15–54) with psychotic symptoms making their first-ever contact with psychiatric services in Nottingham (population 390000) between the dates mentioned. Ascertained cases included not only inpatients but patients making every type of contact with services. The screening schedule was deliberately overinclusive and was based on symptoms rather than diagnosis. Patients with a clear organic cause for their symptoms and those with severe mental retardation were not included in the study.

Initial assessments

All patients were interviewed by a project psychiatrist using the Present State Examination (PSE; Wing *et al*, 1974) and the Psychological Impairments Rating Scale (PIRS; Jablensky, 1978). Other schedules covering the psychiatric, personal, family, and social background (PPHS) and social disability (DAS) were completed by a different interviewer with a close relative of the patient or other informant (Jablensky *et al*, 1992). When all the schedules had been completed, at least two project psychiatrists, together with the PPHS and DAS interviewer, discussed all available information about the patient to make a consensus project ICD–9 diagnosis. The diagnostic exercise conducted in Nottingham identified 67 patients who met ICD–9 criteria for schizophrenia (Cooper *et al*, 1987).

Leakage study

The initial investigators checked the Nottingham Case Register and contacted private practitioners and private hospitals near Nottingham for patients who should have been included in the sample but were not. This turned up only nine; one of these missing cases was later excluded, as she was found to have been receiving treatment for schizophrenia many years before the inclusion dates of this study. Of the remaining eight patients, only three were judged to fall into certain' or very likely' categories of schizophrenia (Cooper *et al*, 1987).

Follow-up study

Tracing exercise

We took considerable trouble to trace the cases for the present 13-year follow-up. Most were traced using the Nottingham Case Register and the Medical Records Department at Mapperley Hospital, Nottingham. Others were found using the Electoral Register and the Registrar for Births, Deaths and Marriages. In addition we used the National Health Service Central Register and various Family Health Services Authorities throughout the country. Patients who were still in contact with the psychiatric services were approached for interview via their consultant or key worker. Those patients who were out of contact with the

services were only approached for an assessment after first checking with their general practitioner.

Follow-up assessments

Lengthy assessments were carried out using both patients and a key informant for each, and further information was elicited from general practice records and hospital records. For the purposes of this paper, information from the following instruments was used:

(a) Present State Examination: the PSE at entry to the study and at 13-year follow-up. The CATEGO Diagnostic Program (Wing *et al*, 1974) was used to determine the number of subjects who met the restrictive definition of schizophrenia (CATEGO Class S+), at entry and at follow-up.

(b) Scale for the Assessment of Negative Symptoms (SANS) (Andreasen, 1982). The SANS was used to determine the number of patients who had 'negative symptoms' in the month before follow-up. 'Negative symptoms' means a 'summary score' greater than 2. The summary score is derived by adding the scores of the five global ratings of affective flattening, alogia, avolition–apathy, anhedonia–asociality and attentional impairment.

(c) Life Chart Schedule (LCS) (Sartorius *et al*, 1995). This schedule codes symptoms, treatment, residency and employment history for the most recent 2 years and for the entire follow-up period. Ratings are made on the basis of information obtained from the patient, informant and case notes. For the present paper, information was taken from the last 2 years' section of the LCS. The information used included the course of the illness, over the last 2 years (for types of course, see Table 1), and presence/absence of negative symptoms. For subjects whose illness followed the Neither Episodic nor Continuous' type of course, there is nowhere in the LCS to record negative symptoms, and so this information was recorded separately. In addition, in- formation on psychiatric admissions over the last 2 years was used, together with information on the use of neuroleptics and other medications for psychiatric problems. The sections concerning employment and residence were also used.

(d) Broad Rating Schedule (BRS) (Sartorius *et al*, 1995). The scales used from the BRS included the scale derived from Bleuler's (1978) four categories on the severity of psychotic symptoms in the past month (severe, moderate, mild and recovered). In

addition, the Global Assessment of Functioning (GAF) scales for symptoms and disability, derived from the Global Assessment Scale (Endicott *et al*, 1976), were used. These scales rate the severity of symptoms and the severity of disability in the last month on a scale from 1 (most severe) to 90 (no symptoms). Scores of 61 and above are generally taken to represent a favourable outcome. These scales have been incorporated in the DSM–III–R and were modified by the WHO (Sartorius *et al*, 1995).

(e) Disability Assessment Schedule (DAS) (Jablensky *et al*, 1992). The information used from this scale included the adjusted score for Dysfunctional Overall Behaviour (derived from scores for social withdrawal and self-care), the adjusted score for Dysfunction in Social Roles (derived from: scores for participation in household activities; affective and sexual marital roles; parental roles; sexual roles other than marriage; social contacts; work performance or interest in getting a job; and interests/ information) and a global evaluation for disability over the last month.

(f) Additional information regarding treatment contacts was obtained by the follow-up investigators (particularly PM), from the narrative accounts kept on each subject in the study.

For the subjects from the leakage study, only information on residence and contact with psychiatric services was recorded. These patients were not re-interviewed because of the inadequacy of baseline data.

Reliability exercise

All but four of the assessments were carried out by one of the investigators (PM). An inter-rater reliability exercise was carried out between the investigators (PM & GH and PM & IM) for the PSE, SANS, LCS and BRS (GAF, symptoms and disability). This was completed before the study began, on 10 subjects with long histories of psychotic disorders, but who were not part of the cohort under investigation. An inter-rater reliability exercise was also conducted on another 10 subjects during the phase of data collection, to ensure that reliability was maintained. Pairwise agreements (PAR) were calculated for categorical data, and grouped PARS were calculated for ordinal data with a narrow range of scores. Intra-class correlation coefficients (ICC) were calculated for the GAF symptoms and disability. Reliability was considered satisfactory if PAR was 0.7 or greater.

RESULTS

The sample

At entry to the study, 22 women and 45 men were assigned a project ICD–9 diagnosis of schizophrenia. Their mean age was then 29 years (range 15–54). The social class distribution (Registrar General's classification) showed that 35 (53%) were unemployed in the 6 months before entry. Two (3%) subjects were in social class 1/2, 16 (24%) in class 3 and 13 (20%) in class 4/5.

Tracing exercise

Sixty-three (94%) of the original 67 patients were traced. Of these, five (8%) had died. One had died of natural causes, three had committed suicide and one died in suspicious circumstances suggestive of suicide. Of the remaining 58 patients, face-to-face interviews were conducted with 48 (83%) and telephone interviews with two (3%). One patient was impossible to interview due to a cerebrovascular accident which left her with aphasia and a dense right hemiplegia. High-quality information was available on the remaining seven subjects from records and informants. Information was also available on one of the patients who was lost to follow-up up to July 1987. Face-to-face contact or high-quality collateral information was therefore available on 94% of those subjects still alive at the 13-year follow-up.

Comparisons were made between those subjects completing the follow-up (58) and those lost to follow-up (4) and those deceased at point of follow-up (5) for the following variables: age, sex, marital status, type of onset and proportion CATEGO S+, to see if they differed in any way. The groups were remarkably similar on each of these variables and there were no significant differences.

The leakage study turned up three patients who were likely to have met ICD–9 criteria for schizophrenia. All three were traced. One had died of natural causes, one was still in contact with psychiatric services and the other had only been followed up by psychiatric services for a few months. All were living independently in the community.

Reliability exercise

Pre-study reliability was satisfactory for 100% of PSE items, 99% of PIRS items, 79% of SANS items, 100% of DAS items and 96% of LCS items. The ICC for the GAF symptoms and disability scales were

0.85 and 0.94 respectively. Maintenance reliability was satisfactory for 100% of PSE items, 100% for PIRS items, 92% of SANS items, 86% of DAS items and 99% of LCS items. ICC for the GAF symptoms and disability scales were 0.96 and 0.89 respectively.

Assessments

Measures of positive symptoms

1. Present State Examination. A PSE and/or PSE Syndrome Checklist was carried out for 67 patients at entry and 57 patients at follow-up. Using the CATEGO program, at entry 47 (70%) patients were classified as S+ and at follow-up 11 (19%) were classified as S+.

2. Bleuler's Scale. The severity of psychotic symptoms in the last month was recorded for all the subjects except those lost to follow-up, those who had died and the one who had suffered the cerebrovascular accident. Thirty-two (56%) subjects were judged to be recovered on this scale, seven (12%) suffered mild symptoms, 15 (26%) moderate symptoms and only three (5%) were rated as having severe symptoms.

3. Life Chart Schedule. The course of the illness over the last 2 years is recorded in Table 1. Twenty-eight (48%) of the 58

subjects on whom information was available were psychotic at some point during the last 2 years; 20 (71%) of these had continuous psychotic symptoms.

Measures of negative symptoms

1. Life Chart Schedule. Table 1a gives information on the presence of negative symptoms during the last 2 years of follow-up. Twenty-seven (47%) of these 58 subjects had displayed negative symptoms at some stage in the last 2 years.

2. Scale for the Assessment of Negative Symptoms. Table 1b shows the global ratings from the five sections of the SANS. The mean summary score for the sample on the SANS was 3.9 (range 0–17). Twenty-three (48%) of the 48 patients on whom a SANS was possible had a summary score greater than 2, i.e. showed negative symptoms.

Measures of comorbidity

1. Life Chart Schedule. Seventeen (30%) of the sample reported non-psychotic episodes of mental disorder in the last 2 years of follow-up: 10 subjects with episodes of low mood, four with anxiety symptoms, two were alcohol-dependent and one was amphetamine-dependent.

Table I Symptoms after 13 years

(a) Type of course, and negative symptoms over last 2 years (LCS)

Course type	n (%)	Negative symptoms (%)
Episodic	6 (10)	3 (50)
Continuous	20 (34)	16 (80)
Neither episodic nor continuous	2 (3)	2 (100)
Never psychotic	30 (52)	6 (20)
Total	58[†]	

(b) Negative symptoms over last month (SANS)

Global rating	n (%)
Affective flattening	7 (15)
Alogia	3 (6)
Avolition/apathy	23 (48)
Anhedonia/asociality	24 (50)
Attention	4 (8)
Summary score >2	23 (48)
Total	48[2]

1. 9 cases missing: 4 lost to follow-up, 4 dead, I CVA.
2. 19 cases missing: 4 lost to follow-up, 5 dead, I CVA, 2 telephone interviews and 7 refused interview.

261

Global symptom measures

Global Assessment of Functioning Scale: Symptoms. The mean score on this scale was 58.7 (range 22–90). Twenty-eight (49%) of the 57 subjects on whom this schedule could be completed had absent/mild symptoms (score 61 or above).

Measures of disability

1. Disability Assessment Schedule (DAS). Twenty-four (44%) of the 55 subjects for whom information was available showed no dysfunction in their overall behaviour and 23 (43%) of the 54 subjects on whom information was available showed no dysfunction in their social roles. On the global scores, over the last month of follow-up 18 (31%) subjects rated at least good' with respect to disability, 14 (24%) rated fair' and 26 (45%) rated 'poor'.

2. Global Assessment of Functioning Scale: Disability. The mean score on this scale was 60.3 (range 15–90). Twenty-nine (50%) of the 58 subjects on whom this schedule could be completed had absent/mild disability (score 61 or above).

Associations

Table 2 shows the relationships between psychotic and negative symptoms, and between symptoms and disability. There is a correlation between psychotic and negative symptoms at the 13-year outcome, particularly in those patients with continuous psychotic symptoms. In addition, there is a strong association between disability and negative symptoms.

Residence and employment

Fifty-seven (97%) of the 59 subjects for whom information was available had spent most of the last two years in independent community living. Of these, 16 (28%) were living alone. More detailed information on residence has been published elsewhere (Harrison *et al*, 1994).

Only 22 (37%) of the 59 subjects available for follow-up had been employed over the last 2 years (19 were in full-time employment). Of these, six were rated as working below the level one might expect from someone with the same socioeconomic origin and educational background, but who is not mentally ill; 26 (44%) of the sample were receiving disability benefit for a mental condition and two (3%) were receiving disability benefit for a physical condition. Only one subject had reached

Table 2 Relationships between negative and positive symptoms, and between symptoms and disability, at 13 years

(a) Negative symptoms (SANS) and psychotic (LCS) symptoms

Psychotic symptoms	Negative symptoms		Total	Odds ratio (95% CI)	χ^2 (P)
	Present	Absent			
Present	17	8	225	6.02	6.84
Absent	6	17	23	(1.47–26.18)	(P<0.01)
Total	23	25	48[1]		

(b) Negative symptoms (SANS) and continuous psychotic (LCS) symptoms

Continuously psychotic	Negative symptoms		Total	Odds ratio (95% CI)	χ^2 (P)
	Present	Absent			
Yes	16	5	21	9.14	10.03
No	7	20	27	(2.07–43.94)	(P<0.01)
Total	23	25	48[1]		

(c) Disability (GAF) and global symptoms (GAF)

Symptoms	Disability		Total	Odds ratio (95% CI)	χ^2 (P)
	Nil/mild	Mod/severe			
Nil/mild	25	3	28	52.1	29.5
Moderate	4	25	29	(8.76–387.5)	(P<0.001)
Total	29	28	57[2]		

(d) Disability (DAS global adjustment score) and psychotic symptoms (LCS)

Psychotic symptoms	Disability		Total	Odds ratio (95% CI)	χ^2 (P)
	Poor	Fair/good			
Present	23	9	32	6.57	9.15
Absent	7	18	25	(1.79–25.37)	(P<0.01)
Total	30	27	57[2]		

(e) Disability (DAS global adjustment score) and negative symptoms (SANS)

Psychotic symptoms	Disability		Total	Odds ratio (95% CI)	χ^2 (P)
	Poor	Fair/good			
Present	22	1	23	253	33.39
Absent	2	23	25	(17.26–1652.83)	(P<0.001)
Total	24	24	48[1]		

1. 19 cases missing: 4 lost to follow-up, 5 dead, 1 CVA, 2 telephone interviews and 7 refused interview.
2. 9 cases missing: 4 lost to follow-up, 4 dead, 1 CVA.

retirement age and none were in full-time education.

Treatment status

Table 3 summarises some of the information collected on treatment at point of follow-up and over the 2 years up to the point of follow-up. Most (76%) of this sample were still receiving treatment for a psychiatric disorder, and most (59%) were utilising their local psychiatric services. Ten subjects were receiving their psychiatric care solely from their general practitioner. Neuroleptic medication was being used for a large proportion (64%) of the sample and half of the sample were receiving neuroleptics in depot form. The majority (80%) of the subjects, however, had not been hospitalised for psychiatric disorder in the 2 years prior to follow-up.

Complete recovery

If one defines complete recovery' as meaning that the subject is alive at follow-up with no symptoms, no disability and on no treatment, then only 11 (17%) of the sample available for follow-up had recovered completely at 13 years.

DISCUSSION

Methodology

These findings describe the state, after 13 years, of an epidemiologically defined cohort of patients at the same stage of their illness. Baseline assessments and diagnoses were applied prospectively using standardised instruments. Comparable follow-up assessments were carried out after reliability had been established. The 94% trace rate for residency, and the excellent information available for seven patients who refused to participate, suggest that selection biases have not seriously compromised these findings. The gender distribution is somewhat unusual, with more than twice as many men as women: this excess is most apparent in the younger age groups (Cooper *et al*, 1987; Jablensky *et al*, 1992).

The sample is small compared to those in the long-term studies of Bleuler (1978), Huber *et al* (1980) and Ciompi (1980), who followed up cohorts of 208, 502 and 289 respectively. The assessment rates in those studies were, however, considerably lower: Ciompi achieved only 18%.

Table 3 Treatment contacts and hospitalisation

	n	%
Receiving treatment for a psychiatric disorder at point of follow-up	45	76
In contact with psychiatric services at point of follow-up	35	59
Treatment with neuroleptics over the last 2 years		
never	17	24
sometimes	4	7
most of the time	38	64
On depot neuroleptics at point of follow-up	30	51
Number of admissions over the last 2 years		
none	47	80
one	9	15
more than one	3	5
		(range 2–7)
Total duration of hospitalisation over the last 2 years		
nil	47	80
up to 1 month	7	12
more than 1 month	5	8
		(range 2–13)

1. Sample size=59; 4 lost to follow-up and 4 dead (1 extra patient was dead at point of follow-up but was included here as he died only 1 month before follow-up).

Comparisons with other follow-up studies

In the present study, 49% of patients had no, or only mild, symptoms (GAF symptoms score of 61 or above) at the 13-year follow-up. Studies with shorter follow-ups report similar findings. For example, the Scottish Schizophrenia Research Group (1992) reported 5-year outcomes for a prospective cohort of 44 schizophrenic patients. Of 39 subjects reassessed after 5 years, 46% had no active symptoms. This is similar to the data of Shepherd *et al* (1989) who reported that 57% of the first admissions with schizophrenia whom they studied had no, or minimal, impairment after 5 years. In the 5-year outcome report on the London cohort of the International Pilot Study of Schizophrenia, Prudo & Blum (1987) reported considerable improvement in symptoms in 49%. Five-year outcomes reported from developing countries, however (Leff *et al*, 1992), show that outcomes appear to be consistently better than in industrialised centres.

Our 13-year data for the Nottingham cohort are compared with the long-term studies of Bleuler (1978) and Ciompi (1980) in Fig. 1, using Bleuler's criteria (psychotic symptoms present over the last month only). If one stratifies outcome in terms of the proportion of cases which are mild or

recovered, then the results are remarkably similar. However, it is clear that patients in Nottingham achieve better outcome overall, with a greater proportion of recoveries and fewer severe cases.

Few studies publish data for negative symptoms over the longer term course of the illness. In the month before follow-up, 48% of our sample showed negative symptoms. This is higher than the figure of Johnstone *et al* (1992), who found negative symptoms in 22.6% of their schizophrenic subjects after $2\frac{1}{2}$years, and higher also than the results of the Scottish Schizophrenia Research Group (1992), who reported 31% at the 5-year follow-up. It is possible that our data represent accrued morbidity for negative symptoms over longer periods of follow-up, although comparisons are not strictly valid because a different instrument, which rates only two negative symptoms (Krawiecka *et al*, 1977) was used in the investigations of Johnstone *et al* and the Scottish Schizophrenia Research Group. The present finding that psychotic symptoms are associated with the presence of negative symptoms at the 13-year outcome is in keeping with previous studies (Scottish Schizophrenia Research Group, 1992), and the higher relative risk of negative symptoms in patients with continuous psychotic symptoms has also been shown before (Fenton & McGlashan, 1991).

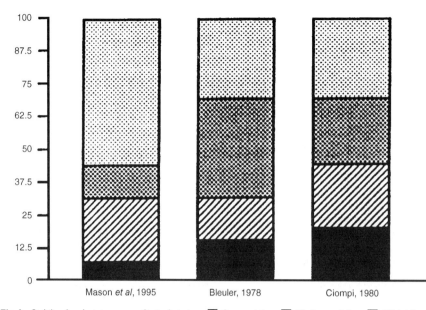

Fig. I Stabilised end-states among first admissions. ■, Severe defect; ▨, Moderate defect; ▨, Mild defect; ▨, Recovered.

Comorbidity

Few studies reported have investigated comorbidity over longer periods of follow-up. Shepherd *et al* (1989) reported that 22% of their patients with a first admission for schizophrenia had symptoms of depression after 5 years, and Harrow *et al* (1994) found full depressive syndromes in 30% of their schizophrenia patients after 4 years. This is higher than the present figure of 17.5%, which in itself suggests that there are significant levels of non-psychotic morbidity in the long-term outcome of schizophrenia. The comparatively low comorbidity for drug and alcohol use is notable, however (see Mueser *et al*, 1990 for a review).

Social disability

The status of symptoms may have little relevance to everyday social functioning, and it is important to keep these dimensions separate when reporting schizophrenia outcomes. For example, one man had had continuous auditory hallucinations throughout the entire follow-up period and yet he was able to work full-time as a surveyor. Another subject who suffered continuous auditory hallucinations and persecutory delusions was successfully caring for her son who was severely disabled by his schizophrenia. The results from the DAS suggest that nearly 55% had good/fair outcome. Other studies utilising the DAS include the 3–13-year follow-up of Leary *et*

al (1991), the 3-year follow-up study of De Jong *et al* (1985) and the 2-year follow-up of Schubart *et al* (1986). These all showed slightly better outcomes (good/fair outcome in 73.1%, 63% and 65%, respectively) than our study; this probably reflects shorter follow-up duration and different methods of case selection. In the present study, the risk of severe social disability in patients with persisting negative symptoms underlines the disabling impact of the deficit syndrome over the longer term evolution of the illness.

It is surprising that 97% of those subjects traced alive were living independently in the community, and we have previously reported remarkably low levels of imprisonment and homelessness (Harrison *et al*, 1994). There were, however, six subjects (11% of those in independent community living) who were felt to be a severe burden of care on their relatives and who would have been incapable of independent living were it not for the intensive support of their families, Social Services and Community Psychiatric Nurses; these included one person disabled by a cerebrovascular accident, one with florid delusions of persecution, and four with severe negative symptoms.

The full-time employment rate of 32% compares favourably with the findings of Leary *et al* (1991), 22.5% of whose sample were in full-time employment at 3–13-year follow-up. Carone *et al* (1991) reported that

33% of their sample were employed at 5-year follow-up. Employment rates partly reflect the availability of work and different styles of work available in different cultures. For example, Bland *et al* (1976) reported that 51.1% of their sample were normal with respect to economic productivity', but they note that their study was conducted at a time of relative wealth and easy employability in Alberta, Canada.

Conclusions

Thirteen years after the onset of illness 83% of the sample were either dead, showed some degree of symptomatic or social disability, or continued in some form of psychiatric treatment. This suggests that only 17% of patients who receive psychiatric care and who are assigned an ICD–9 diagnosis of schizophrenia achieve complete recovery' over the longer term.

These findings support Kraepelin's (1919) emphasis on the longitudinal implications of a diagnosis of schizophrenia. However, with 44% of patients achieving a mild/recovered treated outcome at 13 years, the suggestion made by many of his interpreters that the condition is inevitably chronic proves to be far too pessimistic.

Acknowledgements

This paper is based on the data and experience obtained during the participation of the authors in the WHO project on Long-term Course and Outcome of Schizophrenia, sponsored by the World Health Organization and funded by the World Health Organization, the Laureate Foundation (USA) and the participating field research centres. The chief collaborating investigators in the 20 field research centres of this study are: Aarhus, A. Bertelsen; Agra, K. C. Dube; Beijing, Shen Yucun; Cali, C. Leon; Chandigarh, V. Varma; Dublin, D. Walsh; Groningen, R. Giel; Hong Kong, P. Lee; Honolulu, A. J. Marsella; Ibadan, M. Olatawura; Khartoum, T. Baasher; Madras, D. Thara; Mannheim, H. Hafner; Moscow, S. J. Tsirkin; Nagasaki, Y. Nakane; Nottingham, G. Harrison; Orangeburg, E. Laska; Prague, S. Skoda; Rochester, NY, L. Wynne; Sofia, K. Ganev. At WHO Headquarters, Geneva, the study was coordinated by N. Sartorius until August 1993, and now by W. Gulbinat. We thank Professor J. E. Cooper for allowing access to these data and for help with this project, and also thank Sarah Doherty for her work in tracing of subjects and data processing. This follow-up study was supported by a grant provided by the Mental Health Foundation.

REFERENCES

Andreasen, N. C. (1982) Negative symptoms in schizophrenia, definition and reliability. *Archives of General Psychiatry,* **39**, 784–788.

Bland, R. C., Parker, J. H. & Orn, H. (1976) Prognosis in schizophrenia. A ten year follow-up of first admissions. *Archives of General Psychiatry*, **33**, 949–954.

Bleuler, M. (1978) *The Schizophrenic Disorders: Long-term Patient and Family Studies* (trans. S. M. Clemens). New Haven, CT: Yale University Press.

Carone, B. J., Harrow, M. & Westermeyer, J. F. (1991) Posthospital course and outcome in schizophrenia. *Archives of General Psychiatry*, **48**, 247–253.

Ciompi, L. (1980) Catamnestic long-term study on the course of life and aging of schizophrenics. *Schizophrenia Bulletin*, **6**, 606–618.

Cooper, J. E., Goodhead T, D., Craig, T., et al (1987) The incidence of schizophrenia in Nottingham. *British Journal of Psychiatry*, **151**, 619–626.

De Jong, A., Giel, R., Slooff, C. J., et al (1985) Social disability and outcome in schizophrenic patients. *British Journal of Psychiatry*, **147**, 631–636.

Endicott, J., Spitzer, R. L., Fleiss, J. L., et al (1976) The Global Assessment Scale. A procedure for measuring overall severity of psychiatric disturbance. *Archives of General Psychiatry*, **33**, 766–771.

Fenton, W. S. & McGlashan, T. H. (1991) Natural history of schizophrenia subtypes. II. Positive and negative symptoms and long-term course. *Archives of General Psychiatry*, **48**, 978–986.

Harrison, G. & Mason, P. (1993) Schizophrenia–falling incidence and better outcome? *British Journal of Psychiatry*, **163**, 535–541.

___ , ___ , Glazebrook, C., et al (1994) Residence of an incident cohort of psychotic patients after 13 years of follow-up. *British Medical Journal*, **308**, 813–816.

Harrow, M., Yonan, C. A., Sands, J. R., et al (1994) Depression in schizophrenia: are neuroleptics, akinesia, or anhedonia involved? *Schizophrenia Bulletin*, **20**, 327–338.

Hegarty, J. D., Baldessarini, R. J., Tohen, M., et al (1994) One hundred years of schizophrenia: a meta-analysis of the outcome literature. *American Journal of Psychiatry*, **151**, 1409–1416.

Huber, G., Gross, G., Schuttler, R., et al (1980) Longitudinal studies of schizophrenic patients. *Schizophrenia Bulletin*, **6**, 592–605.

Jablensky, A. (1978) *Psychological Impairments Rating Schedule.* Geneva: WHO.

—, Sartorius, N., Ernberg, E., et al (1992) *Schizophrenia: manifestations, incidence and course in different cultures. A World Health Organization Ten-Country Study.* Psychological Medicine, Monograph Supplement 20. Cambridge: Cambridge University Press.

Johnstone, E. C., Frith, C. D., Crow, T. J., et al (1992) 'The Northwick Park Functional' Psychosis Study: diagnosis and outcome. *Psychological Medicine*, **22**, 331–346.

Kraepelin, E. (1919) *Dementia Praecox* (trans. ed. R. M. Barclay). Edinburgh: E. S. Livingstone.

Krawiecka, M., Goldberg, D. & Vaughn, M. (1977) A standardised psychiatric assessment scale for rating psychotic patients. *Acta Psychiatrica Scandinavica*, **55**, 299–308.

Leary, J., Johnstone, E. C. & Owens, D. G. C. (1991) Disabilities and circumstances of schizophrenic patients–a follow-up study. II. Social outcome. *British Journal of Psychiatry*, **159** (suppl. 13), 13–20.

Leff, J., Sartorius, N., Jablensky, A., et al (1992) The International Pilot Study of Schizophrenia: five-year follow-up findings. *Psychological Medicine*, **22**, 131–145.

MacMillan, J. F., Crow T, T. J., Johnson, A. L., et al (1986) The Northwick Park Study of first episodes of schizophrenia. III. Short-term outcome in trial entrants and trial eligible patients. *British Journal of Psychiatry*, **136**, 384–395.

Mueser, K. T., Yarnold, P. R., Levinson, D. F., et al (1990) Prevalence of substance abuse in schizophrenia: demographic and clinical correlates. *Schizophrenia Bulletin*, **16**, 31–56.

Prudo, R. & Blum, H. M. (1987) Five-year outcome and prognosis in schizophrenia: A report from the London Field Research Centre of the International Pilot Study of Schizophrenia. *British Journal of Psychiatry*, **150**, 345–354.

Sartorius, N., Gulbina, W., Harrison, G., et al (1995) Long-term follow-up study of schizophrenia in ten countries. *Journal of Social Psychiatry and Epidemiology*, (in press).

Schubart, C., Krumm, B., Biehl, H., et al (1986) Measurement of social disability in a schizophrenic patient group. *Social Psychiatry*, **21**, 1–9.

Scottish Schizophrenia Research Group (1989) The Scottish first episode schizophrenia study. VII. Two-year follow-up. *Acta Psychiatrica Scandinavica*, **80**, 597–602.

___ (1992) The Scottish first episode schizophrenia study. VIII. Five-year follow-up: clinical and psychosocial findings. *British Journal of Psychiatry*, **161**, 496–500.

Shepherd, M., Watt, D., Falloon T, I., et al (1989) *The natural history of schizophrenia: a five-year follow-up study of outcome and prediction in a representative sample of schizophrenics.* Psychological Medicine Monograph Supplement 15. Cambridge: Cambridge University Press.

Wing, J. K., Cooper T, J. E. & Sartorius, N. (1974) *The Measurement and Classification of Psychiatric Symptoms. Cambridge: Cambridge University Press.*

P. MASON, MRCPsych, G. Harrison, MRCPsych, C. GLAZEBROOK, PhD, T. DALKIN, MRCPsych, Department of Psychiatry, University Hospital, Nottingham; I. Medley, MRCPsych, Mandala Centre, Nottingham; T. GOUDACE, BSc, Department of Psychology, University of Nottingham

Correspondence: Dr Mason, Department of Psychiatry, University Hospital, Nottingham NG7 2UH

(First received 1 November 1994, final revision 28 February 1995, accepted 18 April 1995)

Cross sectional study of symptom attribution and recognition of depression and anxiety in primary care

DAVID KESSLER, KEITH LLOYD, GLYN LEWIS and DENNIS PEREIRA GRAY

Abstract

Objectives   To examine the effect of patients' causal attributions of common somatic symptoms on recognition by general practitioners of cases of depression and anxiety and to test the hypothesis that normalising attributions make recognition less likely.

Design   Cross sectional survey.

Setting   One general practice of eight doctors in Bristol.

Subjects   305 general practice attenders.

Main outcome measure   The rate of detection by general practitioners of cases of depression and anxiety as defined by the general health questionnaire.

Results   Consecutive attenders completed the general health questionnaire and the symptom interpretation questionnaire, which scores style of symptom attribution along the dimensions of psychologising, somatising, and normalising. General practitioners detected depression or anxiety in 56 (36%; 95% confidence interval 28% to 44%) of the 157 patients who scored highly on the general health questionnaire. Subjects with a normalising attributional style were less likely to be detected as cases; doctors did not make any psychological diagnosis in 46 (85%; 73% to 93%) of 54 patients who had high questionnaire and high normalising scores. Those with a psychologising style were more likely to be detected; doctors did not detect 21 (38%; 25% to 52%) of 55 patients who had high questionnaire and high psychologising scores. The somatisation scale was not associated with low detection rates. This pattern of results persisted after adjustment for age, sex, general health questionnaire score, and general practitioner.

Conclusions   Normalising attributions minimise symptoms and are non-pathological in character. The normalising attributional style is predominant in general practice attenders and is an important cause of low rates of detection of depression and anxiety.

INTRODUCTION

Recognition of depression and anxiety is a key issue in general practice. If these disorders are not recognised they cannot be treated. There are a number of treatments of proved efficacy[1,2] and some evidence to show that recognition improves outcome[3,4], though this has been questioned[5].

Most episodes of depression and anxiety – the 'common mental disorders' – are contained and managed in primary care[6]. Yet less than half of these episodes are identified in the consultation[7]. Why is recognition of depression and anxiety such a problem in general practice? Doctors' skills and attitudes play a part. Certain key skills in the consultation have been identified that are both teachable and associated with increased rate of recognition[8]. Teaching better consultation skills, however, leads to only a modest increase in detection rates.

Most consultations in primary care are initiated by the patient. The content of the typical primary care consultation and its outcome will be influenced by what the patient chooses to present and how he or she chooses to present it[9]. Common somatic symptoms are the currency of general practice; they are also concomitants of anxiety and depression[10]. Numerous studies have categorised this combination of mood disorder and somatic symptomatology as 'somatisation' and have shown it reduces general practitioners' ability to identify mental disorder[10,11]. But this use of the term somatisation has certain disadvantages in the context of primary care. It associates a common mode of presentation with the much rarer, more serious, chronic, and treatment resistant 'somatisation disorder'[12]. It also implies that patients who present with psychological disorders and common bodily symptoms tend to think of themselves as physically ill. Attempts to redefine somatisation for primary care have led to a confusion of multiple and at times complex definitions[10,11,13]. One way to simplify the issue is to ask patients themselves for their causal attributions for common somatic symptoms.

Patients' beliefs about their symptoms are powerful influences on their decision to consult a doctor and how they present their problem when they do consult[14]. In other words, do we think our fatigue is caused by emotional exhaustion? Is it due to anaemia? Or could it be because we have been overdoing it or not doing enough exercise? In the example given above three types of explanation or attribution have been offered for a common somatic symptom, fatigue. The first, the idea that it is due to emotional exhaustion, can be called a psychologising attribution. The second, that it is caused by anaemia, is a somatising attribution. In the third explanation the experience of fatigue is thought to be related to overexertion or not exercising enough. This type of attribution has been called normalising[15].

Until now most studies that have looked at patients' beliefs about their symptoms have focused on the dichotomy between somatising and psychologising. These are, in effect, 'illness beliefs'. Normalising attributions are qualitatively different in that they are non-pathological. They are the most prevalent attribution in primary care attenders as well as in the population as a whole[15]. This study asks whether such attributions have any effect on the general practitioner's ability to make a diagnosis of depression or anxiety. In particular it tests the hypothesis that normalising attributions reduce the likelihood of the detection of such disorders.

METHODS

The study took place in an eight partner urban practice which serves 12 800 patients and has a slightly larger than average population of patients aged over 75. Surgeries were selected to ensure that both morning and evening attenders were represented and that all doctors were covered by the study. Consecutive attenders aged over 16 years were given two questionnaire before seeing their general practitioner. Twenty-four questionnaires were incomplete, and 26 patients declined to participate.

The 12 item general health questionnaire has been widely used to detect psychiatric disorder in primary care[16] and validated in comparison with more detailed assessments. In a recent study it was compared with a more detailed psychiatric assessment and the optimal threshold for 'caseness' found to be a score of 3 or more[17]. We have adopted this definition of a case of psychological disorder.

The symptom interpretation questionnaire is a self report questionnaire consisting of a list of 13 common bodily symptoms or sensations[15]. Attached to each symptom are three possible explanations, each one corresponding to one of the three styles of attribution: psychologising, somatising, or normalising. The patients were asked to choose one explanation for each symptom, giving each subject a numerical score from 0–13 along the three attributional dimensions. The sum of all three scales was therefore 13. Subjects were classified as predominantly normalisers, psychologisers, or somatisers if they scored 7 or more on that scale. Validation research has shown that these scores remain reasonably consistent over time, supporting the theory that they may reflect underlying health beliefs[15].

General practitioners, who were blind to the results of the questionnaires, were asked to report any diagnoses of depression or anxiety they made and to note whether this was a new diagnosis or if the patient was already under treatment. The proportion of patients diagnosed as anxious or depressed was calculated according to scores on the normalising, psychologising, and somatising scales of the symptom interpretation questionnaire. For presentation purposes the scores were divided into four categories, but the scales were also examined as continuous variables. Logistic regression was used to estimate odds ratios for the detection of psychiatric disorder and to adjust for the confounding variables of age, sex, general health questionnaire score, and general practitioner consulted (as a categorical variable). Results were unchanged when data from the subjects who were 'false positives' on the general health questionnaire were excluded. Statistical analysis was done with STATA[18]. Ethical approval was obtained from the local research ethics committee.

RESULTS

There were 225 women and 80 men in the study, a ratio of 2.8:1. The mean (range) age was 44 (16–90) years. The men were significantly older than the women (mean age 49.2, v 42.0 years; $P < 0.003$). On the general health questionnaire 157 (52%; 95% confidence interval 46% to 57%) of all the attenders scored 3 or more. The general practitioners made a diagnosis of depression in 57 (19%; 15% to 24%) patients and anxiety in 14 (5%; 3% to 8%). Measured against the general health questionnaire threshold of 3 or more the general practitioners showed a specificity of 80% (69% to 89%) and a sensitivity of 57% (50% to 63%). There were 14 false positive results: patients who were diagnosed as depressed or anxious by the general practitioner but scored less than 3 on the general health questionnaire. Of these, seven had already been diagnosed with depression by a general practitioner and were receiving treatment.

In the symptom interpretation questionnaire the normalising attribution was most often selected, with 146 out of 305 (48%) choosing seven or more normalising explanations out of a possible 13. Seventy-one patients (23%) selected seven or more psychologising explanations, and only 16 patients (5%) chose seven or more somatising attributions (Table 1). This pattern of distribution was also found in the initial validation studies[15]. High scorers on the somatisation scale were older, normalisers younger ($F_{3,301} = 7.54$; $P < 0.0001$). Psychologisers were more likely to be female and normalisers and somatisers to be male (likelihood ratio $\chi^2 = 11.2$; df=3; $P < 0.01$).

Symptom interpretation questionnaire and general practitioner diagnosis of anxiety and depression

Table 2 shows that the higher the patient's score on the normalising dimension of the symptom interpretation questionnaire the less likely the general practitioner was to diagnose depression or anxiety ($P < 0.0001$) and that the higher the patient's score on the psychologising dimension the more likely was the general practitioner to diagnose depression or anxiety ($P < 0.0001$). For normalising and psychologising the relation was still present after adjustment for age, sex, general health questionnaire score, and which doctor the patient saw. There was no evidence of an association between detection by the general practitioner and the patient's somatising score (Table 2). This lack of relation was confirmed by using somatisation as a continuous variable (likelihood ratio $\chi^2 = 0.19$; df=1; $P = 0.7$).

Recognition of anxiety and depression in general health questionnaire cases with different symptom attributional styles

General practitioners did not diagnose depression or anxiety in 21 (38%; 25% to 52%) of the 55 patients who were cases according to the general health questionnaire and had a predominantly psychologising style of symptom attribution. In contrast depression or anxiety went undetected in 46 (85%; 73% to 93%) of the 54 patients who were cases according to the general health questionnaire but had a predominantly normalising style of symptom attribution (see Table 1). There was no evidence that the association between normalising style and low rates of detection was influenced by score on the general health questionnaire (test for interaction, likelihood ratio $\chi^2 = 0.19$, df=1, $P = 0.66$). Patients

Table 1 Detection by general practitioner of anxiety and depression in 305 patients with different styles of symptom attribution

Attributional category	No of patients (no of women)	Mean age (years)	GHQ cases	
			No (%)	No (%; 95% CI) not detected*
Psychologising score ≥7	71 (61)	43.4	55 (77)	21 (38; 25 to 52)
Normalising score ≥7	146 (99)	40.4	54 (37)	45 (85; 73 to 93)
Somatising score ≥7	16 (9)	58.6	5 (38)	5 (83; 36 to 100)
No predominant score	72 (56)	48.8	42 (58)	29 (69; 53 to 82)

GHQ=general health questionnaire.
*Patients classified as depressed according to general health questionnaire but not diagnosed as such by general practitioner.

with a normalising style were less likely to be detected even when the analysis was restricted to those with a score of 7 or more.

DISCUSSION

We found that different styles of symptom attribution are strongly associated with different rates of detection of depression and anxiety. Patients who make psychologising attributions are more likely to get a psychological diagnosis; the stronger their tendency to make such attributions the more likely such a diagnosis becomes. A normalising style of attribution has the opposite effect, and the stronger a patient's tendency to normalise or minimise his or her symptoms the less likely he or she is to be seen as depressed or anxious by the general practitioner. Somatising attributions, which are the least common, had no measurable effect on diagnostic rates, though this may have been because of lack of statistical power.

Normalising attributions are the most common both in studies of populations and primary care attenders[15]. Even among those with a high general health questionnaire score there are large numbers of 'normalisers'. It is in this group, who tend to be younger and male, that general practitioners particularly did not detect depression and anxiety. Only eight out of 54 patients with a normalising attributional style and a high general health questionnaire score were diagnosed as being depressed or anxious. Forty-six of the 101 (45.5%; 35.6% to 55.8%) undetected cases had a predominantly normalising style of attribution. Does this strong association between a normalising style of attribution and low rates of detection of mental disorder represent a causal relation? Our study suggests that it does. The association is robust and remains strong even after adjustment for which general practitioner the patient saw, general health questionnaire score, age, and sex. One limitation of the study is that we were not able to adjust for presenting symptom, but we might expect this to be influenced by causal attributional style.

Table 2 Detection by general practitioner (GP) of anxiety and depression in 305 patients with different degrees of normalising, psychologising, and somatising symptoms

SIQ score*	No in category	No (%) detected by GP	Odds ratio (95% CI)	Adjusted odds ratio[†] (95% CI)
Normalising				
0–3	51	27 (53)	1	1
4–6	108	29 (27)	0.33 (0.16 to 0.65)	0.26 (0.11 to 0.62)
7–10	110	10 (9)	0.09 (0.04 to 0.21)	0.10 (0.04 to 0.29)
11–13	36	4 (11)	0.11 (0.03 to 0.36)	0.20 (0.05 to 0.82)
Psychologising				
0–3	136	16 (12)	1	1
4–6	96	16 (17)	1.32 (0.72 to 3.12)	1 (0.42 to 2.36)
7–10	61	29 (48)	6.91 (3.35 to 14.25)	4.05 (1.66 to 9.87)
11–13	10	9 (90)	68.8 (8.15 to 577)	31.6 (3.06 to 3.27)
Somatising				
0–3	228	52 (23)	1	1
4–6	61	14 (23)	1.00 (0.51 to 1.97)	1.45 (0.63 to 3.37)
7–10	16	4 (25)	1.13 (0.35 to 3.65)	1.86 (0.45 to 7.66)

*Symptom interpretation questionnaire; subjects classified as predominantly normalisers, psychologisers, or somatisers, if they scored 7 or more on that scale.
[†]Adjusted for age, sex, general health questionnaire score, and doctor consulted.

Key messages

- Many patients with psychological disorders present to their general practitioners with common somatic symptoms. This combination has been referred to as 'somatisation' and is associated with lower rates of diagnosis of depression and anxiety

- When questioned directly about the cause of their symptoms most patients choose 'normalising' attributions, which tend to minimise the importance of the symptoms; somatising attributions are uncommon

- The more normalising attributions patients choose, the less likely are general practitioners to diagnose depression or anxiety; the association remain after adjustment for age, sex, general health questionnaire score, and which doctor the patient saw

- The normalising attributional style makes a considerable contribution to the non-detection of depression and anxiety. A better understanding of how depressed patients view their symptoms may be the key to understanding low diagnostic rates

The normalising style arises out of the 'discounting principle'[19]. This is the idea that symptoms are often 'explained away' as being caused by a minor environmental irritant or as the result of 'overdoing it'. Such explanations propose a non-pathological cause for the symptoms. In other words 'normalisers' play down the significance of their symptoms. For the general practitioner to respond to the patient's own attribution of his or her symptoms is an expression of empathy and an important part of the negotiation between patient and doctor in moving towards a diagnosis. Such negotiations are the cornerstone of the doctor–patient relationship in general practice. Thus a psychological style of attribution is likely to elicit questions from the doctor about mental wellbeing and mood state and would favour a psychological formulation for the problem. In contrast, a normalising attribution, with its powerful 'commonsensical' overtones, may influence the doctor to join with the patient in minimising and even dismissing the symptoms.

It is easy to understand why people who make a somatising attribution for their symptoms would seek the advice of their general practitioner. It is also clear that the general practitioner is the first port of call for many in psychological distress. But when 'normalising' attributions are concerned there seems to be a paradox. Why should someone who is making a normalising attribution seek a doctor's advice? The answer may lie in a need to check the normalising style of attribution and to be reassured that it is the correct one. If this is so, then the implicit question that the normaliser asks the physician is 'there's nothing really wrong with me, is there?' In the same way that we respond to somatisers and psychologisers by accepting their attribution, so we may respond to the normalisers by agreeing with them. This collusion could result in a tendency to neglect symptoms of depression and anxiety.

The rate of apparent underdiagnosis of psychological disorder in primary care remains stubbornly high. Patients with such disorders may often present with somatic symptoms but are rarely committed 'somatisers'. Instead they are more likely to be normalising their symptoms and giving them a non-pathological attribution. The question of whether such patients would benefit from detection could be examined by a comparison of outcomes for detected and undetected depressed patients with different attributional styles.

ACKNOWLEDGEMENTS

With thanks to the patients, doctors, and staff at Horfield Health Centre, Bristol.

Contributors: DK had the original idea for the study, which was developed in discussions with KL and DPG. These three designed the study. DK undertook the data collection. DK, KL, and GL analysed the data. DK drafted the paper, which was edited by GL. DK is the guarantor.

Funding: DPG was funded by the NHS Executive to undertake research on depression.

Competing interests: None declared.

REFERENCES

1. **Blackburn, I. M., Bishop, S., Glen, A. T. M.** The efficacy of cognitive therapy in depression: a treatment combination. *British Journal of Psychiatry*, 1981;**139**:181–9.

2. **Hollyman, J. A., Freeling, D., Paykel, E. S.** Double-blind placebo-controlled trail of amitriptyline among depressed patients in general practice. *Journal of the Royal College of General Practitioners*, 1988;**38**:393–7.

3. **Johnstone, A., Goldberg, D.** Psychiatric screening in general practice. *Lancet*, 1976;**i**:605–8

4. **Zung, W. W. K., Magill, M., Moore, J., George, D. T.** Recognition and treatment of depression in a family medicine practice. *Journal of Clinical Psychiatry*, 1983;**44**:3–6

5. **Dowrick, C., Buchan I.** Twelve month outcome of depression in general practice: does detection or disclosure make a difference? *British Medical Journal*, 1995;**311**:1274–6

6. **Shepherd, M., Cooper, B., Brown, A.** *Psychiatric Illness in General Practice.* Oxford: Oxford University Press, 1966.

7. **Goldberg, D., Huxley, P.** *Common Mental Disorders.* London: Routledge, 1992.

8. **Gask, L., Goldberg, D., Porter, R., Creed, F.** The treatment of somatisation: evaluation of a teaching package with general practice trainees. *Journal of Psychosomatic Research*, 1989;**33**:697–703.

9. **Weich, S., Lewis, G., Donmall, R., Mann, A.** Somatic presentation of psychiatric morbidity in general practice. *British Journal of General Practice*, 1995;**45**:143–7.

10. **Bridges, K., Goldberg, D., Evans, B.** Determinations of somatisation in primary care. *Psychological Medicine*, 1991;**21**:473–89.

11. **Kirmayer, L. J., Robbins, J. M., Dwurkind, M., Yaffe, M. J.** Somatisation and the recognition of depression and anxiety in primary care. *American Journal of Psychiatry*, 1993;**150**:734–41.

12. **American Psychiatric Association.** *Diagnostic and Statistical Manual of Mental Disorders.* 4th ed. Washington DC: American Psychiatric Association, 1994.

13. **Bridges, K. W., Goldberg, D.** Somatic presentation of DSM–III disorders in primary care. *Journal of Psychosomatic Research*, 1985;**29**:563–9

14. **King, J.** Attribution theory and the health belief model. In: Hewrone, M., ed. *Attribution Theory: Social and Functional Extensions.* Oxford: Blackwell, 1983.

15. **Robbins, M. J., Kirmayer, L. J.** Attributions of common somatic symptoms. *Psychological Medicine*, 1991;**21**:1029–45.

16. **Goldberg, D., Williams, P.** *A User's Guide in the General Health Questionnaire.* Windsor: Nelson, 1991.

17. **Bashir, K., Blizard, R., Jenkins, R., Mann, A.** A Validation of the 12-item general health questionnaire in British general practice. *Primary Care Psychiatry*, 1996;**2**:4–7.

18. **Statacorp.** *Stata Statistical Software, Version 5.* Texas: College Station, 1997.

19. **Kelley, H. H.** Attribution in social interaction. In *Attribution: Perceiving the Causes of Behaviour* (eds E. E. Jones, D. E. Kanouse, H. H. Kelley, R. E. Nisbett, S. Valins & B. Weiner). Morristown: General Learning, 1971.

(Accepted 16 November 1998)

Early life family disadvantages and major depression in adulthood

H. SADOWSKI, B. UGARTE, I. KOLVIN, C. KAPLAN and J. BARNES

Background   There is evidence that exposure to social and family disadvantages in childhood are a risk factor for adult depression.

Aims   To explore the effects of multiple adversity in early childhood on adult depression, and the relative effects of the different adversities.

Method   This study utilises data from the Newcastle Thousand Family Study. Information on childhood disadvantages was collected when the participants were 5 years old, and information on mental health was gathered when they were 33 years old. Mental health data were scrutinised blind to the evidence of early disadvantage, and best-estimate diagnoses of major depressive disorder were made according to DSM–III–R criteria.

Results   Multiple family disadvantages in childhood substantially increase the risk of suffering a major depressive disorder in adulthood. Such disadvantages include family or marital relationship instability, a combination of poor mothering and poor physical care, and a combination of dependence on social welfare and overcrowding. For females major depression was linked in particular to the quality of parenting in early life.

Conclusions   Social and family (especially multiple family) disadvantages during childhood predispose individuals to an increased risk of major depression in adulthood.

Declaration of interest   I.K. supported by a Leverhulme Emeritus Fellowship.

There is now considerable evidence from population studies (Rodgers, 1990b; Kessler & Magee, 1993) and other cohort studies (Brown & Harris, 1993; Brown & Moran, 1994) that adults who have been exposed to adverse life events in middle or later childhood are at increased risk for adult depression.

Over the past decades there has been an impressive accumulation of evidence that poor maternal care in childhood (Parker, 1979; Perris et al, 1986; Birtchnell, 1988), unsatisfactory child/parent relationships (Abrahams & Whitlock, 1969), parental 'affectionless control' (Mackinnon et al, 1993), and parental marital problems or marital separation (Rodgers, 1994) are associated with an increased risk of suffering from depression in later life.

However, most studies have been retrospective and relied on subjective reports, often from clinical samples. Few studies have utilised evidence gathered prospectively in community studies from an objective external source concerning early life experiences and then related these to depression in adulthood using systematic assessment techniques. Further, Kessler & Magee (1993) have pointed out that very little research has explored "the joint effects of multiple adversities . . . or the comparative effects of different adversities" on adult depression.

THE NEWCASTLE THOUSAND FAMILY STUDY (1947–1980)

The Newcastle Thousand Family Study was originally designed to investigate illness in the first year of life of all children born in the city of Newcastle upon Tyne between 1 May and 30 June 1947. Altogether, 1142 children in 1132 different families were enrolled in the study (Spence et al, 1954). The study was first continued up to age 5 (Miller et al, 1960) and then up to age 15 (Miller et al, 1974). During the first five years of life, deaths, withdrawal from the study, and removals from the area left 847 of the original sample and their families in the survey in 1952.

From 1979 to 1981, Kolvin et al (1988, 1990) followed-up a stratified sample of the 847 index children still in the study in 1952. The reason for focusing on these individuals was that, during the first five years, extensive psychosocial data had been collected, upon which the definitions of early family disadvantages were based (Miller et al, 1960, 1985; Kolvin et al, 1990).

Criteria of disadvantage during the first five years of life

Six categories of long-standing family disadvantages were employed (Kolvin et al, 1990), defined as follows:

(a) Family/marital disruption (divorce, separation or marital instability).

(b) Parental physical illness.

(c) Poor physical care of child and home.

(d) Social dependence (which included serious debt, unemployment, and reliance on National Assistance).

(e) Family overcrowding.

(f) Poor mothering (poor maternal coping skills).

The specific criteria of disadvantage in childhood in this sample population were present with rates ranging from 24% for parental physical illness to 35% for overcrowding (Kolvin et al, 1990).

DESIGN AND METHOD OF THE PRESENT STUDY

The present study is based on the subsequent follow-up study of the subjects of the Newcastle Thousand Family Study (Kolvin et al, 1990) using a 'catch-up longitudinal design' (Robins, 1980). Two hundred and ninety-six index children were selected by random stratification according to the degree of disadvantage of the 847 families that were studied in 1952 (Spence et al, 1954; Miller et al, 1960). The three original selected strata consisted of known proportions of the groups who were not disadvantaged, were disadvantaged in one or two respects, and those who had been exposed to three or more criteria of disadvantage. This stratification allowed the application of an appropriate multiplication factor to estimate one-year prevalence rates of adult depression for the original population.

Efforts were made to trace those families who had moved from the city and eventually 266 (134 females and 132 males) of the 296 individuals and their families were recruited and interviewed between 1979 and 1981 (90% of the selected sample). Extensive psychosocial and mental health data were gathered, which formed the basis for the study of the transmission of deprivation (Kolvin et al, 1990). At the time of the follow-up the participants were 33 years of age.

In the original study (Kolvin et al, 1990) in which the focus was on social and family doctors and offending, the operational decision was to define multiple disadvantage as three or more criteria. While offending is relatively common (Kolvin et al, 1988), major depression is present in only 10% of the population (Kessler et al, 1994). It was therefore decided to focus solely on the dichotomy between multiply disadvantaged and not multiply disadvantaged individuals, and the operational definition of multiple disadvantage in the original study was reviewed and a more stringent definition of multiple disadvantage was adopted. The mean number of disadvantages in the original sample (0.9) plus two standard deviations (2.7) above the mean was used as a cut-off to define multiple disadvantage. The participants were dichotomised as follows: (a) 'no multiple disadvantage' (n=227, 85.3%), those who had experienced up to three coexisting criteria of family disadvantage, and (b) 'multiple disadvantage' (n=39, 14.7%), those who had experienced at least four coexisting family criteria of disadvantages in their first five years of life.

The intercorrelations between specific criteria of disadvantage were either negative or non-significant in both defined groups with the exception of poor maternal care and poor mothering (Spearman correlation coefficient 0.43, $P < 0.001$ in the 'no disadvantage' group and 0.38, $P < 0.05$ in the 'multiple disadvantage' group) and social dependence and parental physical illness in the 'no multiple disadvantage' group (Spearman correlation coefficient 0.32, $P < 0.01$). Thus, the two conceptually and statistically related criteria of poor physical care and poor mothering were combined to form a 'composite index of parenting' (n=24 females and 27 males). In addition, although not significantly

correlated, a conceptually based composite 'social disadvantage index' was created combining both social dependence and overcrowding during childhood (n=21 females and 18 males). The 'index of parenting' is conceptually comparable to Brown & Harris' measure of parental indifference (1993) and the 'social disadvantage index' encompasses disadvantages which Rodgers listed as socio-economic circumstances (1990b). The 'parenting index' was present in 12.5% of subjects in the 'no multiple disadvantage' group and in 80% of the 'multiple disadvantage' group, and the 'social disadvantage index' occurred in 7% of the 'no multiple disadvantage' group and in 60% of those in the 'multiple disadvantage' group.

Diagnoses and classification

The participants were interviewed in their 33rd year of life. They were informed that this was a follow-up study to find out about the general adult functioning of adults who had been studied over the first five years of life. The interviewers were blind to the individuals' experiences of disadvantage and also to other information collected in the first five years of life. All the interviewers had previous training and experience in systematic semi-structured interviewing techniques. Regular quality checks were undertaken to ensure the consistency of the scoring of the information given and any problems were discussed with the senior researcher (I.K.). Satisfactory levels of reliability were achieved (Kolvin et al, 1990, p. 27).

A semi-structured open-ended interview was used enquiring about the experience of a wide range of affective and anxiety symptoms over the year prior to the interview. The definitions of the various abnormal phenomena had been modified from the Standard Psychiatric Interview (Goldberg et al, 1970). The probes included questions comparable to the stem question from the Schedule for Affective Disorders and Schizophrenia (Endicott & Spitzer, 1978): "Over the past year have you had a time when you felt low, miserable and unhappy all the time? Did you find you could not snap out of it? Did it last more than one month?" The responses to these and additional questions about various symptoms of anxiety and depression were rated by the interviewers according to severity on four-point scales (symptom not present,

and symptom present of a mild, moderate, or severe degree).

For the purpose of this study current mental health data on subjects gathered when they were 33 years old were scrutinised blind to the evidence of any childhood disadvantage. First themes relevant to the stem question from the Schedule for Affective Disorders and Schizophrenia (Endicott & Spitzer, 1978) were considered. Fifty-eight subjects (21.6%) – 41 females (30.3%) and 17 males (12.7%) – had experienced dysphoria to a moderate or severe degree lasting for at least one month during the year prior to the interview. Only these individuals were considered to have psychopathology which approximates the mandatory criterion 'depressed mood' of major depressive disorder according to DSM–III–R (American Psychiatric Association, 1987).

In addition all the responses to probes concerning the following symptoms were scrutinised: lack of energy, lack of appetite, sleep disturbance and suicidal ideation. Each was regarded to approximate one of the non-mandatory criteria of major depressive disorder according to DSM–III–R, but only when the symptom had been experienced to a moderate or severe degree. The exception was suicidal ideation which was regarded present if the subject had experienced recurrent suicidal thoughts.

A 'best-estimate' diagnosis of major depressive disorder was made if dysphoria had been present to a moderate or severe degree lasting for one month, and if at least three of the four additional criteria had been judged to approximate the comparable non-mandatory criteria of major depressive disorder according to DSM–III–R. Thus, in order to prevent possible over-inclusion, in this study four of five specified criteria needed to coexist for a diagnosis of an episode of a major depressive disorder over the year prior to the interview. This was considered comparable to the formula of five out of the nine criteria specified in DSM–III–R.

The two research fellows had training and supervision in the use of criteria from the Schedule for Affective Disorders and Schizophrenia and the conversion of the available data into DSM–III–R diagnoses. When a satisfactory level of consensus was achieved, an independent review of the data was conducted on 20 interviews selected randomly. No differences were noted in allocating to groups according to the presence or absence of major depression. Best-estimate diagnoses were then made for the remaining respondents. In most instances the data available were considered sufficient and complete to make a diagnostic rating with reasonable confidence. However, relevant data were unavailable for four women.

Statistical methods

The aim of the analysis was to examine the links between early family disadvantages and depression in adulthood. The stratification procedure allowed population estimates to be calculated to produce a period prevalence of disorder (covering the year prior to the interview at age 33) for the general population of Newcastle upon Tyne.

For the purpose of this paper, univariate analyses of data were undertaken according to the presence and absence of major depressive disorder using χ^2. Intercorrelations between criteria of disadvantage were analysed using the Spearman correlation coefficient.

In order to examine the independent and joint effects of early life disadvantages on the presence of major depressive disorder in adulthood, multivariate analyses were conducted using logistic regression. Backwards stepwise selection was used, with removal based on the probability of the Wald statistic. All procedures were performed using SPSS for Windows software.

RESULTS

Early life adversities and depression in adulthood

It was estimated that at 33 years of age 8.4% of the general population of Newcastle had suffered a major depressive dis-

order over the previous year (Table 1). The rate of depression varied according to the degree of exposure in the first five years of life to social and family disadvantage. In the sample population of those who had experienced no or some disadvantage the one-year prevalence rate was 7.2%; but in those exposed to multiple disadvantages the rate was nearly fourfold (28.2%). In the total sample the rate of major depressive disorder was significantly higher in females than in males ($\chi^2=4.30$, d.f.=1, $P<0.05$, odds ratio 2.7, 95% CI 1.1–6.3).

In males the one-year prevalence rate of major depressive disorder in the 'no multiple disadvantage' group was 3.5%, and those in the 'multiple disadvantage group' were more likely to suffer a major depressive disorder (23.5%) (odds ratio 8.5).

For females the picture is similar albeit against the background of a higher base rate. The rate of depression was 11% for females in the 'no multiple disadvantage' group, but nearly 32% for those from multiply disadvantaged backgrounds (odds ratio 3.7).

In the 'no multiple disadvantage' group females were more likely (odds ratio=3.5) than males to suffer a major depressive disorder at 33 years of age (95% CI 1.1–11.1; $\chi^2=3.79$, d.f.=1, $P<0.06$) but this difference fell just short of statistical significance. In the 'multiple disadvantage' group the female-to-male odds ratio was greatly reduced (odds ratio 1.5, 95% CI 0.4–6.8).

Specific criteria of disadvantage in the pre-school years and subsequent adult depression

Table 2 provides data on the specific criteria of disadvantage in the first five years of

life and their association with depression at 33 years of age.

Most individual criteria of childhood disadvantage were not significantly associated with increased rates of major depression in adulthood, namely social dependence, overcrowding, poor mothering, poor physical care, and parental physical illness during childhood.

In the total sample, the highest rates of major depressive disorder occurred in the presence of the combination of social dependence and overcrowding during early childhood (Table 2). Similarly, there were significant differences in the prevalence of major depressive disorder between the subgroups of individuals who had experienced the 'parenting index' of both poor physical care and poor mothering in childhood and those who had not. Individuals exposed to family or marital instability during their first five years of life were overall three times more likely to receive a best-estimate diagnosis of major depression in adulthood than those who were not.

For females, significantly increased rates of major depression in adulthood were found in the subgroup exposed to the 'parenting index' of both poor physical care and poor mothering. One-third (8/24) of this subgroup experienced recent major depression.

For males, the childhood experience of the composite 'social disadvantage index' and of family or marital instability was significantly associated with increased rates of major depression in adulthood (Table 2).

Logistic regression analyses

Entering multiple disadvantage as a dichotomous variable as present or not, together

Table I One-year prevalence of major depressive disorder at 33 years of age in relation to disadvantage experienced in first five years of life

	n (%)	A 'no multiple disadvantage' group	B 'multiple disadvantage' group	Odds ratio B v. A	95% CI	d.f.	χ^2	P
Sample population								
Total number	27/262 (10.3%)	16/223 (7.2%)	11/39 (28.2%)	5.1	(2.1–12.0)	1	13.69	<0.001
Females	19/130 (14.6%)	12/108 (11.1%)	7/22 (31.8%)	3.7	(1.3–11.0)	1	4.73	<0.05
Males	8/132 (6.1%)	4/115 (3.5%)	4/17 (23.5%)	8.5	(1.9–38.3)	1	7.23	<0.01
Estimated for original sample								
Total number	70/839 (8.4%)	54/781 (6.9%)	16/58 (28.2%)	5.3	(2.8–10.0)	–	–	–
Females	51/423 (12.1%)	41/391 (10.4%)	10/33 (31.8%)	4.0	(1.8–9.0)	–	–	–
Males	19/416 (4.6%)	13/390 (3.4%)	6/25 (23.5%)	8.8	(3.0–25.6)	–	–	–

–, not performed on estimated numbers.

Table 2 Rates of major depressive disorders at 33 years of age in relation to presence and absence of specific criteria of disadvantage in first five years of life

	A Subjects without specific criteria(on)	B Subjects with specific criteria(on)	Odds ratio (B v. A)	95% CI	d.f.	χ^2	P
Sample population							
Both social dependence and overcrowding	16/223 (7.2%)	11/39 (28.2%)	5.1	(2.1–12.0)	1	13.69	<0.001
Both poor physical care and poor mothering	16/211 (7.6%)	11/51 (21.6%)	3.4	(1.4–7.8)	1	7.24	<0.01
Family/marital instability	14/193 (7.3%)	13/69 (18.8%)	3.0	(1.3–6.7)	1	6.18	<0.05
Females							
Both social dependence and overcrowding	13/109 (11.9%)	6/21 (28.6%)	3.0	(1.0–9.0)	1	–	NS
Both poor physical care and poor mothering	11/106 (10.4%)	8/24 (33.3%)	4.3	(1.5–12.4)	1	6.52	<0.01
Family/marital instability	11/93 (11.8%)	8/37 (21.6%)	2.1	(0.8–5.6)	1	–	NS
Males							
Both social dependence and overcrowding	3/114 (2.6%)	5/18 (27.8%)	14.2	(3.0–66.5)	1	13.13	<0.01
Both poor physical care and poor mothering	5/105 (4.8%)	3/27 (11.1%)	2.5	(0.6–11.2)	1	–	NS
Family/marital instability	3/100 (3.0%)	5/32 (15.6%)	6.0	(1.3–26.7)	1	4.75	<0.05

with gender and an interaction variable between gender and disadvantage, into backwards stepwise logistic regression, multiple disadvantage had a highly significant effect (odds ratio 2.22, Table 3). The relative odds ratio of receiving a diagnosis of major depressive disorder was 1.6 times higher for females compared to males. No significant interaction between gender and multiple childhood disadvantage was found.

Another logistic regression was performed to evaluate the cumulative effect of an increasing number of childhood disadvantages on major depression in adulthood. For this purpose six dummy variables were created for those with one, two, three, four, five and six childhood disadvantages. Only three of the variables representing four disadvantages (Wald 5.47, d.f.=1, P<0.05), five disadvantages (Wald 4.17, d.f.=1, P<0.05) and six advantages

Table 3 Results of logistic regression analyses (backwards stepwise) with major depressive disorder as dependent variable for all subjects

Independent variable	n	Odds ratio	95% CI	d.f.	Wald	P
3.1 Degree of disadvantage controlled for gender						
Multiple disadvantage at 5						
Absent	223	1				
Present	39	2.22	(1.43–3.44)	1	12.72	<0.001
Gender						
Male	132	1				
Female	130	1.60	(1.03–2.49)	1	4.29	<0.05
Interaction between gender and multiple disadvantage not selected						
Model predicts 89.7% of outcome (χ^2=16.92, d.f. 2, P<0.001)						
3.2 Specific criteria of disadvantage at five years of age and interaction variables						
Family/marital instability						
Absent	193	1				
Present	69	1.74	(1.11–2.75)	1	5.75	<0.05
Parental illness		–	–	1	–	NS
Social dependence		–	–	1	–	NS
Overcrowding		–	–	1	–	NS
Interaction between social dependence and overcrowding		1.95	(1.17–3.25)	1	6.51	<0.05
Interaction between poor physical care and poor mothering		3.07	(1.04–9.08)	1	4.11	<0.05
Interaction between poor physical care, poor mothering and female gender		1.81	(1.12–2.94)	1	5.83	<0.05
All other variables and interaction variables were not selected						
Model predicts 89.3% of outcome (χ^2=33.44, d.f. 7, P<0.001)						

(Wald 9.76, d.f.=1, $P<0.01$) were selected as significant predictors of major depression in adulthood with odds ratios of 1.95 (95% CI 1.11–3.41), 2.08 (95% CI 1.03–4.19), and 4.40 (95% CI 1.74–11.16). The model accounted for 90% of the overall outcome (χ^2=14.89, d.f.=3, $P<0.01$).

A third logistic regression was performed analysing the independent contribution of each individual criterion of childhood disadvantage to major depressive disorder in adulthood. All individual criteria together with gender, and interaction variables between all criteria, pairs of criteria and gender were entered into logistic regression. Four significant predictors of major depression in adulthood were found, namely: family or marital instability; the interaction between social dependence and overcrowding; the interaction between poor physical care and poor mothering; and a three-way interaction between poor physical care, poor mothering and female gender (Table 3).

DISCUSSION

Multiple family disadvantages during childhood and depression in adulthood

The experience of multiple family disadvantages during early childhood strongly predicted a major depressive disorder at 33 years of age. Although the synergistic effects of multiple risk factors have been examined in studies predicting psychopathology in childhood and adolescence, prospective studies are rare in respect to multiple childhood disadvantages and psychopathology in adulthood. In the National Cohort Study, Rodgers (1990b) showed that those subjects who had experienced multiple adversity during childhood had more affective symptoms during the month prior to the interview than anticipated from the separate effects of each of the independent variables studied.

Using univariate analyses, Cadoret et al (1990) in their study of adult depression in male adoptees showed a significant correlation between two or more adoptive home conditions (including low adoptive home socio-economic status and poor adoptive parent health among others) and affective symptomatology in adulthood. This association did not retain its significance in multivariate (log-linear) analyses. In the current study, when studying all subjects, the experience of multiple childhood disad-

vantages remained significant when the effect of gender was also taken into account.

It should be noted that in both this sample of the Newcastle Thousand Family Study with its revised criteria for multiple disadvantage and in the National Cohort Study only a small proportion of individuals were exposed to 'multiple disadvantage' or a 'high level of childhood adversity' (Rodgers, 1990b). Nevertheless, this small proportion accounted for a relatively high percentage of 'caseness' or 'best-estimate diagnoses' of major depression. This indicates that high risk clusters in a relatively small group of individuals who experienced many childhood disadvantages, and the risk is associated with substantially increased one-year prevalence rates of major depressive disorder in adulthood.

Specific criteria of family disadvantage in childhood and major depression in adulthood

Univariate and multivariate analyses revealed significant differences in the rates of major depressive disorder between those subjects who had and those who had not experienced (a) family or marital instability; (b) both poor physical care and poor mothering; and (c) both social dependence and overcrowding during childhood.

Based on retrospective reports, Kessler & Magee (1993) found a strikingly similar odds ratio for adult major depression where subjects had been exposed to parental divorce, also using logistic regression analyses. After controlling for socio-economic status using MANOVA, Rodgers (1994) demonstrated a significant relationship between parental separation or divorce and an increased affective symptom score for females, but not for males.

Most of the studies supporting the notion that the exposure to poor parental care and other adverse social and family-rearing experiences in childhood is related to depression in adulthood have used retrospective recall measures (Parker, 1979; Perris et al, 1986; Brown & Harris, 1993). Since the other two prospective studies have not employed adequate measures of parenting and care (Cadoret et al, 1990; Rodgers, 1990b), the present study is currently the only one available which used a catch-up longitudinal design to examine the relationship between parenting in childhood and affective disorders in adulthood.

The findings in this study suggest that females are especially vulnerable in view of having a major depression in adulthood, if they experienced both poor mothering and poor physical care in childhood. Thus, it is important to note the convergence between the results in this prospective study and the findings for females where the data were collected retrospectively. The measure of parental indifference used by Brown & Harris (1993) comes nearest to the parenting index employed in the present study. After controlling for adult adversity, they found a comparable odds ratio of 2.6 when comparing groups with and without adverse early parenting experiences.

In the current study, there was a strong association of the experience of both family social dependence and overcrowding in childhood with major depression in adulthood. Rodgers (1990b) did not report an association between an overall index of material home conditions, but there was a link between overcrowding in childhood and affective symptomatology in adult females. However, this link was not confirmed when using multivariate analyses.

Limitations of this study

Post-hoc diagnoses

The 1980 follow-up survey of the Newcastle Thousand Family cohort was intended as a longitudinal study of the transmission of deprivation (Kolvin et al, 1990). The reported findings are based on one-year prevalence rates of major depressive disorders linked to data that were not originally intended for a study of affective disorder in adulthood. The method incorporates a post-hoc diagnostic evaluation of available information about symptoms to ascertain which subjects met DSM–III–R diagnostic criteria based on a one-year recall of symptoms in 1979/80 when the subjects were approximately 33 years of age. Kessler & Magee (1993) employed a similar method, that is making best-estimate diagnoses of major depressive disorder. They derived comparable rates. Face validity of this procedure is also supported by comparing the prevalence rates of major depressive disorder in this study to other epidemiological studies since it was possible to re-estimate the prevalence for the general population in Newcastle upon Tyne based on the known stratification factors.

The estimated one-year prevalence rate of 8.4% for the general population is slightly lower than the 10.3% reported by

Kessler *et al* (1994) from the National Co-morbidity Survey in the United States. Further, the estimated one-year prevalence for females in the general population (12.1%) is very close to the findings for females in the National Comorbidity Survey (12.9%). However, the estimated rate for males (4.6%) is about 3% lower than that recorded in the National Comorbidity Survey (7.7%).

Absence of information about other salient stressors

A crucial limitation is that information was not collected which allowed identification of salient stressors which are known to be important – such as sexual, physical or emotional abuse. Therefore, it was impossible in this study to control for the impact of abuse or the synergistic effect of the forms of abuse and any of the recorded disadvantages during childhood.

Absence of data about relevant childhood psychopathology

Another limitation is that the catch-up longitudinal design of the study precluded collecting information about the onset or prevalence of affective or other disorder in childhood or adolescence. Nor was information available concerning affective disorder in the parental generation, and thus the contribution of parental mental illness could not be explored.

Strengths of this study

Prospective design

The main strength of the current study is that information about disadvantage during the first five years of life had been collected prospectively by professionals visiting the parental home (Kolvin *et al*, 1990). Thus, classification of families according to the degree of disadvantages was not distorted by subjective or retrospective accounts of childhood circumstances (Brewin *et al*, 1993). Further, when the respondents were interviewed at around 33 years of age, the interviewers were blind to the childhood experiences of disadvantage. It is important to note that in this study the results based on prospective research confirm earlier findings from studies employing retrospective designs.

Sampling procedure

The sampling procedure employed in this study allowed an exploration of all degrees of severity of family disadvantages experienced during childhood. The attrition of the baseline cohort of 847 subjects over 25 years by the time of follow-up was estimated to be under 10% (Kolvin *et al*, 1990).

In the original stratification procedure, sub-samples representing strata were selected randomly and thus contained known proportions in relation to the original population. The new and more rigorous definition of multiple disadvantages does not affect the estimations back to the original population as the available data can be calculated either to the new or previous system. Thus, the sub-samples studied were representative of the selected strata.

Avoiding biases of over-sampling

Since all statistical analyses of data were performed on the actual numbers of individuals summating all three original strata, there remained the possibility that over-sampling of multiple disadvantage and the adoption of a more stringent definition of multiple disadvantage could have contributed to distortions. Therefore, the data for the original population were reconstituted employing relevant stratification algorithms. This was followed by repeating the statistical analyses, and all odds ratios were recalculated accordingly and compared with those reported in this study. All odds ratios were slightly higher than those derived by comparing actual numbers, confirming the statistical findings reported in this study.

The elegance of the stratification procedure and over-sampling of individuals who had experienced multiple family disadvantages during childhood was that it had ensured higher actual numbers in the multiply disadvantaged group. Thus, significant differences between groups of the original population were not lost in univariate or multivariate analyses when based on the actual numbers in this study.

Mechanisms

The current findings demonstrate that early life disadvantages predispose to depression in adulthood. Other studies have shown the continuing effect of social and family disadvantages in later childhood and teenage years (Brown & Harris, 1993; Rodgers, 1994). However, there is a need to go beyond the general conclusion that bad

experiences may have bad effects (Rutter, 1981). The future challenge is the search for mechanisms by which disadvantaged children are predisposed to develop specific disorders (Kolvin *et al*, 1990).

First, there is the question of why only a minority of children exposed to such experiences develop a disorder. Environmental experiences may fluctuate over time, some for the better, some for the worse and this may account for substantial discontinuities as well as continuities (Kolvin *et al*, 1990). There may be other operative positive influences.

In brief, when postulating that early life disadvantage is associated with vulnerability to adult depression, there needs to be the appreciation that this can be modified by protective factors. Thus, some of the exposed individuals will be adversely affected, while others may be protected from adverse consequences by their intelligence, strength of character, pre-existing social skills or other positive personal or family qualities. Such qualities may lead the individual to overcome life-term disadvantages – the so-called 'steeling effects'. Other protective factors include the achievement of a positive personal relationship or other continuous or chance experiences between the individual and their life situations.

Second, there are the more precise mechanisms eventually giving rise to depression. Some may consider that the early life adversities have 'sleeper effects' implying that there are hidden operative mechanisms, which only after a long delay give rise to the disorder. A more plausible view is that girls exposed to poor mothering qualities, may be particularly liable to develop insecure attachments giving rise to low self-esteem and poor relational skills; they may have less in the way of academic aspirations and will seek a solution in early cohabitation. In adulthood, exposure to a series of other adverse life events could provoke the emergence of depression (Brown & Harris, 1993). It has been hypothesised by Elder (1973) that adverse economic deprivation often gives rise to marital (spouse) relational strains and in due course, emotional estrangement of the family from the father – with balance of power in the family being changed. Father's role and position may become reduced or undermined. Thus, boys exposed to such family circumstances may tend to identify more strongly with their peer culture. While this culture may serve a function in childhood, it provides only limited skills for solving financial, personal and social problems in adulthood. They do not provide healthy chain reactions, often in social contexts over the course of time. Thus, males are often at greater risk of offending but at lesser risk of emotional problems.

DISADVANTAGES IN EARLY LIFE AND PREDISPOSITION TO DEPRESSION

In conclusion, the current findings demonstrate that early life disadvantages may predispose to depression in adulthood. Individuals exposed to family or marital instability in childhood, to both social dependence and overcrowding, or to both poor mothering and poor physical care were significantly more likely to experience a major depressive disorder at 33 years of age than those who were not. Females were especially sensitive to the quality of early life parenting in respect of vulnerability towards depression in later life.

Strikingly, a cluster of subjects having experienced multiple family disadvantages in childhood are at significant risk of suffering a major depressive disorder in adulthood. It is plausible that the basic mechanism is that as a consequence of these experiences once a threshold has been reached, there is an increased vulnerability to major depression in later life.

Further research is needed to explore the impact of both social disadvantage in the family and the quality of parenting during early childhood on later life psychopathology in males and females. Current concepts about the psychosocial origins of depression need to take into consideration the potential synergistic effects of multiple and diverse disadvantages during early childhood and need to consider how these adversities contribute to greater vulnerability to depression in adult life. Consideration needs to be given to the potential utility of preventive intervention by targeting families at high risk, or in adulthood targeting those individuals previously exposed to high-risk experiences.

ACKNOWLEDGEMENT

We are grateful to Professor G. Brown for helpful advice.

APPENDIX. VALIDATING THE FINDINGS FROM CATEGORICAL ANALYSES USING A DIMENSIONAL APPROACH

Two related crucial issues are the *post hoc* diagnoses and the small number of subjects judged as depressed on a categorical variable – a total of 27 out of 262 subjects. These are the basis of the chi-squared and logistic regression analyses and could give rise to concerns about the validity of the findings. One way of checking the findings is by using a total depression symptom measure or index. Previously Kolvin et al (1990, p. 127) had shown a strong relation between such individual depressive symptoms in adulthood and childhood evidence of family disadvantage. However, these data had not been aggregated into a depression index, nor had they been analysed by gender or according to the individual criteria of disadvantage. In essence, a depression index constitutes a dimension which allows supplementary cross-validity analysis of the data. Further, in previous research total depression symptom scores have proved to be a more robust summary statistic than dichotomous variables in multivariate statistical analysis (Rodgers, 1990a).

Table 4 Univariate analyses of mean depressive symptom score over the year prior to the interview in relation to individual criterion of family disadvantage during first five years of life

	n	Criterion absent (s.d.)	n	Criterion present (s.d.)	t	P
All subjects	262					
Poor mothering	184	6.4 (3.2)	78	7.6 (3.3)	−2.79	<0.01
Poor physical care	197	6.5 (3.2)	65	7.5 (3.3)	−2.26	<0.05
Parental relationship instability	193	6.4 (3.1)	69	7.5 (3.5)	−2.17	<0.05
Parental physical illness	200	6.7 (3.3)	62	6.9 (3.2)	−	NS
Overcrowding	170	6.4 (3.0)	92	7.3 (3.6)	−2.04	<0.05
Social dependence	173	6.3 (2.9)	89	7.5 (3.7)	−2.69	<0.01
Females	130					
Poor mothering	94	6.9 (3.6)	36	8.7 (3.5)	−2.55	<0.05
Poor physical care	99	7.1 (3.5)	31	8.5 (3.8)	(−1.94)	(<0.06)
Parental relationship instability	93	7.3 (3.6)	37	7.7 (3.8)	−	NS
Parental physical illness	100	7.5 (3.6)	30	7.1 (3.6)	−	NS
Overcrowding	84	7.2 (3.5)	46	7.9 (3.9)	−	NS
Social dependence	81	7.2 (3.3)	49	7.9 (4.0)	−	NS
Males	132					
Poor mothering	90	5.7 (2.6)	42	6.6 (2.8)	(−1.79)	(<0.08)
Poor physical care	98	5.8 (2.7)	34	6.6 (2.5)	−	NS
Parental relationship instability	100	5.6 (2.4)	32	7.3 (3.1)	−3.10	<0.01
Parental physical illness	100	5.8 (2.6)	32	6.7 (2.9)	−	NS
Overcrowding	86	5.7 (2.2)	46	6.7 (3.3)	−2.03	<0.05
Social dependence	92	5.6 (2.3)	40	7.0 (3.3)	−2.79	<0.01

Table 5 Multiple regression analysis indicating relative contribution of individual criteria of disadvantage during first five years of life to depressive symptomatology at 33 years of age

Independent variable	Females		Males		All subjects	
	Beta	P	Beta	P	Beta	P
Poor mothering	0.22	<0.05	0.08	NS	0.15	<0.05
Poor physical care	0.05	NS	0.03	NS	0.02	NS
Parental relationship instability	−0.03	NS	0.29	<0.001	0.09	NS
Parental physical illness	−0.09	NS	0.17	<0.05	−0.03	NS
Overcrowding	0.05	NS	0.22	<0.01	0.08	NS
Social dependence	0.03	NS	0.13	NS	0.14	<0.05
Adjusted R^2	0.04	<0.05	0.12	<0.001	0.04	<0.01

Method

The symptom score of all five relevant variables was summated to give a total depressive symptom score. Thus, the range of the total depressive symptom score ranged between 0 and 15. It proved an adequate predictor of a best-estimate diagnosis of major depressive disorder (Spearman correlation coefficient $r=0.53$, $P<0.001$), but the procedure to derive best-estimate diagnoses of major depressive disorder ensured that 'caseness' was not simply a function of any affective symptom cut-off but related rather more to a valid clinical concept.

Statistical analyses

Univariate analyses for the depressive symptom score were conducted using t-tests. In addition, multivariate analyses were conducted using stepwise linear-regression, in order to ascertain which factors had an independent influence on a high total depressive symptom score in adulthood.

Univariate analyses of mean depressive symptom score

When all subjects were included in the analyses then, except for parental illness criteria, the presence of all the other criteria of disadvantage were associated significantly with a higher mean depressive symptom score (Table 4). However, females more commonly reported depressive symptoms than males over the year prior to the interview and had a higher mean depressive symptom score (7.4 v. 6.0; t-value -3.61, $P<0.001$). A contrasting pattern of vulnerability emerged when the data were analysed by gender. In females, only poor mothering in childhood was significantly associated with a higher depressive symptom score in adulthood; whereas in males early life exposure to parental relationship instability, overcrowding and social dependence were associated with depressive symptom score.

Multivariate analyses of mean depressive symptom score

Only two early life disadvantages continued to exert an influence on adult depressive symptoms in the total sample population, namely poor mothering and social dependence (Table 5). They were responsible for about 4% of the variance.

Poor mothering was the only disadvantage experienced in childhood that significantly predicted depressive symptomatology in females, whereas in males parental physical illness assumed significance, with overcrowding and parental relational instability proving the main predictors. These findings corroborate broadly the picture obtained with logistic regression analyses.

REFERENCES

Abrahams, M. J. & Whitlock, F. A. (1969) Childhood experience and depression. *British Journal of Psychiatry*, **115**, 883–888.

American Psychiatric Association (1987) *Diagnostic and Statistical Manual of Mental Disorders* (3rd edn, revised) (DSM–III–R). Washington, DC: APA.

Birtchnell, J. (1988) Depression and family relationships. A study of young married women on a London housing estate. *British Journal of Psychiatry*, **153**, 758–769.

Brewin, C. R., Andrews, B. & Gotlib, I. H. (1993) Psychopathology and early experience: A reappraisal of retrospective reports. *Psychological Bulletin*, **113**, 82–98.

Brown, G. & Harris, T. O. (1993) Aetiology of anxiety and depressive disorders in an inner-city population. I. Early adversity. *Psychological Medicine*, **23**, 143–154.

___, ___, Hepworth, C., et al (1994) Clinical and psychosocial origins of chronic depressive episodes. II: A patient enquiry. *British Journal of Psychiatry*, **165**, 457–465.

___ & Moran, P. (1994) Clinical and psychosocial origins of chronic depressive episodes. I: A community survey. *British Journal of Psychiatry*, **165**, 447–456.

Cadoret, R. J., Troughton, E., Merchant, L. M., et al (1990) Early life psychosocial events and adult affective symptoms. In *Straight and Devious Pathways from Childhood to Adulthood* (eds L. Robins & M. Rutter), pp. 300–313. Cambridge: Cambridge University Press.

Elder, G. H. (1973) *Linking Social Structure and Personality*. Beverly Hills, CA: Sage.

Endicott, J. & Spitzer, R. L. (1978) A diagnostic interview. The Schedule for Affective Disorders and Schizophrenia. *Archives of General Psychiatry*, **35**, 837–844.

Goldberg, D. P., Cooper, B., Eastwood, M. R., et al (1970) A standardised psychiatric interview suitable for use in community surveys. *British Journal of Preventive Social Medicine*, **24**, 18.

Kessler, R. C. & Magee, W. J. (1993) Childhood adversities and adult depression: basic patterns of association in a US national survey. *Psychological Medicine*, **23**, 679–690.

___, McGonagle, K. A., Zhao, S., et al (1994) Lifetime and 12-month prevalence of DSM–III–R psychiatric disorders in the United States. Results from the National Comorbidity Survey. *Archives of General Psychiatry*, **51**, 8–19.

Kolvin, I., Miller, F. J. W., Fleeting, M., et al (1988) Social and parenting factors affecting criminal-offence rates. Findings from the Newcastle Thousand Family Study (1947–1980). *British Journal of Psychiatry*, **152**, 80–90.

___, ___, Scott, D. M., et al (1990) *Continuities of Deprivation? The Newcastle 1000 Family Study*. Avebury: Aldershot.

Mackinnon, A., Henderson, A. S. & Andrews, G. (1993) Parental 'affectionless control' as an antecedent to adult depression: a risk factor refined. *Psychological Medicine*, **23**, 135–141.

Miller, F. J. W., Court, S. D. M., Walton, W. S., et al (1960) *Growing Up in Newcastle upon Tyne*. London: Oxford University Press.

HARTWIN S. SADOWSKI, MRCPsych, BLANCA UGARTE, MRCPsych, ISRAEL KOLVIN, FRCPsych, Tavistock Clinic and Royal Free and University College Medical School, London; CAROLE E. KAPLAN, FRCPsych, Fleming Nuffield Unit, Newcastle upon Tyne; JACQUELINE BARNES, PhD, Tavistock Clinic and Royal Free and University College Medical School, London

Correspondence: Professor I. Kolvin, The Tavistock Clinic, Child and Family Department, 120 Belsize Lane, London NW3 5BA

(First received 9 June 1998, final revision 16 September 1998, accepted 17 September 1998)

___ , ___ , **Knox, E. G., et al (1974)** *The School Years in Newcastle upon Tyne*. London: Oxford University Press.

___ , **Kolvin, I. & Fells, H. (1985)** Becoming deprived: a cross generation study based on the Newcastle upon Tyne 1000 Family Study. In *Longitudinal Studies in Child Psychology and Psychiatry* (ed. A. R. Nicol), pp. 223–240. Chichester: Wiley.

Parker, G. (1979) Parental characteristics in relation to normal depression. *Journal of Psychosomatic Research,* **24**, 67–74.

Perris, C., Arrindell, W. A., Perris, H., et al (1986) Perceived depriving parental rearing and depression. *British Journal of Psychiatry,* **148**, 170–175.

Robins, L. (1980) Longitudinal methods in the study of normal and pathology development. In *Studies of Children* (ed. F. Earls), pp. 34–83. New York: Prodist.

Rodgers, B. (1990a) Behaviour and personality in childhood as predictors of adult psychiatric disorders. *Journal of Child Psychology and Psychiatry,* **31**, 393–414.

___ **(1990b)** Adult affective disorder and early environment. *British Journal of Psychiatry,* **157**, 539–550.

___ **(1994)** Pathways between parental divorce and adult depression. *Journal of Child Psychology and Psychiatry,* **35**, 1289–1308.

Rutter, M. (1981) Stress, coping and development: Some issues and some questions. *Journal of Child Psychology and Psychiatry,* **22**, 323–356.

Spence, J. C., Walton, W. S., Miller, F. J. W., et al (1954) *A Thousand Families in Newcastle upon Tyne.* London: Oxford University Press.